Artificial Intelligence in Otolaryngology

Editors

ANAÏS RAMEAU
MATTHEW G. CROWSON

OTOLARYNGOLOGIC CLINICS OF NORTH AMERICA

www.oto.theclinics.com

Consulting Editor
SUJANA S. CHANDRASEKHAR

October 2024 • Volume 57 • Number 5

ELSEVIER

1600 John F. Kennedy Boulevard • Suite 1800 • Philadelphia, Pennsylvania, 19103-2899

http://www.oto.theclinics.com

OTOLARYNGOLOGIC CLINICS OF NORTH AMERICA Volume 57, Number 5
October 2024 ISSN 0030-6665, ISBN-13: 978-0-443-31352-3

Editor: Stacy Eastman
Developmental Editor: Malvika Shah

Otolaryngologic Clinics of North America (ISSN 0030-6665) is published bimonthly by Elsevier, Inc., 360 Park Avenue South, New York, NY 10010-1710. Months of issue are February, April, June, August, October, and December. Business and Editorial Offices: 1600 John F. Kennedy Blvd., Suite 1800, Philadelphia, PA 19103-2899. Customer Service Office: 6277 Sea Harbor Drive, Orlando, FL 32887-4800. Periodicals postage paid at New York, NY and additional mailing offices. Subscription prices are $478.00 per year (US individuals), $100.00 per year (US & Canadian student/resident), $623.00 per year (Canadian individuals), $679.00 per year (international individuals), $270.00 per year (international student/resident). For institutional access pricing please contact Customer Service via the contact information below. Foreign air speed delivery is included in all *Clinics'* subscription prices. All prices are subject to change without notice. Orders, claims, and journal inquiries: Please visit our Support Hub page https://service.elsevier.com for assistance.

Reprints. For copies of 100 or more of articles in this publication, please contact the Commercial Reprints Department, Elsevier Inc., 360 Park Avenue South, New York, NY 10010-1710. Tel.: 212-633-3874; Fax: 212-633-3820; E-mail: reprints@elsevier.com.

Otolaryngologic Clinics of North America is also published in Spanish by McGraw-Hill Interamericana Editores S.A., P.O. Box 5-237, 06500 Mexico D.F., Mexico.

Otolaryngologic Clinics of North America is covered in *MEDLINE/PubMed (Index Medicus), Current Contents/Clinical Medicine, Excerpta Medica, BIOSIS, Science Citation Index,* and *ISI/BIOMED.*

Contributors

CONSULTING EDITOR

SUJANA S. CHANDRASEKHAR, MD, FACS, FAAO-HNS, FAOS

Consulting Editor, Otolaryngologic Clinics of North America; President, American Otological Society; Past President, American Academy of Otolaryngology-Head and Neck Surgery; Partner, ENT & Allergy Associates, LLP; Clinical Professor, Department of Otolaryngology-Head and Neck Surgery, Zucker School of Medicine at Hofstra-Northwell; Clinical Associate Professor, Department of Otolaryngology-Head and Neck Surgery, Icahn School of Medicine at Mount Sinai, New York, New York, USA

EDITORS

ANAÏS RAMEAU, MDCM, MD, MS, MSc, MPhil, FACS

Assistant Professor, Department of Otolaryngology–Head and Neck Surgery, Sean Parker Institute for the Voice, Weill Cornell Medical College, New York, New York, USA

MATTHEW G. CROWSON, MD, MPA, MASc, MBI, FRCRC

Assistant Professor, Department of Otolaryngology–Head and Neck Surgery, Massachusetts Eye and Ear Hospital, Harvard Medical School, Boston, Massachusetts, USA

AUTHORS

RAHUL ALAPATI, MD

Clinical Research Fellow, Department of Otolaryngology–Head and Neck Surgery, University of Kansas School of Medicine, Kansas City, Kansas, USA

NOEL F. AYOUB, MD, MBA

Fellow, Division of Rhinology and Skull Base Surgery, Department of Otolaryngology–Head and Neck Surgery, Mass Eye and Ear, Harvard Medical School, Boston, Massachusetts, USA

NIKITA BEDI, BS

Student, Division of Head and Neck Surgery, Department of Otolaryngology, Stanford University, Palo Alto, California, USA

YAEL BENSOUSSAN, MD, MSc

Assistant Professor, Department of Otolaryngology–Head and Neck Surgery, University of South Florida, Tampa, Florida, USA

ALEXANDRA T. BOURDILLON, MD

Resident Physician, Department of Otolaryngology–Head and Neck Surgery, University of California-San Francisco, San Francisco, California, USA

ANDRÉS BUR, MD

Associate Professor, Department of Otolaryngology–Head and Neck Surgery, University of Kansas School of Medicine, Kansas City, Kansas, USA

HARVEY CASTRO, MD, MBA
Chief Executive Officer, Medical Intelligence Ops, Dallas, Texas, USA

SI CHEN, MD
Assistant Professor, Department of Otolaryngology–Head and Neck Surgery; Assistant Dean of Continued Medical Education, University of Florida College of Medicine, Gainesville, Florida, USA

FRANCIS X. CREIGHTON Jr, MD
Assistant Professor, Department of Otolaryngology–Head and Neck Surgery, Johns Hopkins Hospital, Baltimore, Maryland, USA

MATTHEW G. CROWSON, MD, MPA, MASc, MBI, FRCRC
Assistant Professor, Department of Otolaryngology–Head and Neck Surgery, Massachusetts Eye and Ear Hospital, Harvard Medical School, Boston, Massachusetts, USA

MOHAMED DIOP, MD
Resident, Department of Otolaryngology–Head and Neck Surgery, Stanford University School of Medicine, Palo Alto, California, USA

EMILY EVANGELISTA, MS
MD Candidate, Morsani College of Medicine, University of South Florida, Yael Bensoussan and Emily Evangelista, Tampa, Florida, USA

DEEPA GALAIYA, MD
Assistant Professor, Department of Otolaryngology–Head and Neck Surgery, Johns Hopkins Hospital, Baltimore, Maryland, USA

JORDAN T. GLICKSMAN, MD, MPH
Attending Surgeon, Department of Otolaryngology–Head and Neck Surgery, Mass Eye and Ear, Harvard Medical School, Boston, Massachusetts, USA

ROSS W. GREEN, MD
Chief Medical Officer, Opollo Technologies, Buffalo, New York, USA

CHRISTOPHER FLOYD HOLSINGER, MD
Professor, Division of Head and Neck Surgery, Department of Otolaryngology, Stanford University, Palo Alto, California, USA

ALICE E. HUANG, MD
Resident Physician, Department of Otolaryngology–Head and Neck Surgery, Stanford University School of Medicine, Stanford, California, USA

ANTHONY LAW, MD, PhD
Assistant Professor, Department of Otolaryngology–Head and Neck Surgery, Emory University, Winship Cancer Institute, Atlanta, Georgia, USA

JÉRÔME R. LECHIEN, MD, PhD, MS, AFACS
Section Chief, Division of Laryngology and Broncho-Esophagology, Professor, Department of Otolaryngology–Head Neck Surgery, EpiCURA Hospital, UMONS Research Institute for Health Sciences and Technology, University of Mons (UMons), Mons, Belgium; Research Committee of Young Otolaryngologists of the International Federation of Otorhinolaryngological Societies (IFOS), Paris, France; Department of Otorhinolaryngology and Head and Neck Surgery, Foch Hospital, Paris Saclay University,

Phonetics and Phonology Laboratory, Paris, France; Department of Otorhinolaryngology and Head and Neck Surgery, CHU Saint-Pierre, Brussels, Belgium

JASON LEE, MD, PhD
Resident Physician, Department of Otolaryngology–Head and Neck Surgery, University of Kansas School of Medicine, Kansas City, Kansas, USA

BRIAN C. LOBO, MD
Assistant Professor, Department of Otolaryngology–Head and Neck Surgery, Associate Chief Medical Informatics Officer, University of Florida College of Medicine, Gainesville, Florida, USA

ANDREW P. MICHELSON, MD
Assistant Professor, Department of Pulmonary Critical Care, Institute for Informatics, Washington University School of Medicine, St Louis, Missouri, USA

MATTHEW R. NAUNHEIM, MD, MBA
Assistant Professor, Department of Otolaryngology–Head and Neck Surgery, Massachusetts Eye and Ear, Assistant Professor, Department of Otolaryngology–Head and Neck Surgery, Harvard Medical School, Boston, Massachusetts, USA

OBINNA I. NWOSU, MD
Resident, Department of Otolaryngology–Head and Neck Surgery, Massachusetts Eye and Ear, Assistant Professor, Department of Otolaryngology–Head and Neck Surgery, Harvard Medical School, Boston, Massachusetts, USA

JAMIE OLIVER, MD
Resident Physician, Department of Otolaryngology–Head and Neck Surgery, University of Kansas School of Medicine, Kansas City, Kansas, USA

ALBERTO PADERNO, MD, PhD
Assistant Professor, Department of Otolaryngology - Head and Neck Surgery, IRCCS Humanitas Research Hospital, Humanitas University, Milan, Italy

KI WAN PARK, MD
Resident, Department of Otolaryngology–Head and Neck Surgery, Stanford University School of Medicine, Palo Alto, California, USA

COLE PAVELCHEK, MD
Otolaryngology Resident, Oregon Health & Science University, Portland, Oregon, USA

JON-PAUL PEPPER, MD
Associate Professor, Department of Otolaryngology–Head and Neck Surgery, Stanford University School of Medicine, Palo Alto, California, USA

ANAÏS RAMEAU, MDCM, MD, MS, MSc, MPhil, FACS
Assistant Professor, Department of Otolaryngology–Head and Neck Surgery, Sean Parker Institute for the Voice, Welll Cornell Medical College, New York, New York, USA

NICHOLAS RAPOPORT, BS
Medical Student, Washington University School of Medicine in St. Louis, St Louis, Missouri, USA

ANITA RAU, PhD
Postdoctoral Scholar, Department of Biomedical Data Science, Stanford University, Palo Alto, California, USA

MATTHEW A. SHEW, MD
Assistant Professor, Department of Otolaryngology–Head and Neck Surgery, Washington University School of Medicine in St. Louis, St Louis, Missouri, USA

SHREYA SRIRAM, BS
Medical Student, Johns Hopkins School of Medicine, Baltimore, Maryland, USA

KATIE TAI, MD
Otolaryngology–Head and Neck Surgery Resident, New York Presbyterian Hospital, New York, New York, USA

TULIO A. VALDEZ, MD, MSc
Professor, Department of Otolaryngology–Head and Neck Surgery, Stanford University School of Medicine, Stanford, California, USA

SIERRA HEWETT WILLENS, BS
Medical Student, Department of Otolaryngology–Head and Neck Surgery, Stanford University School of Medicine, Palo Alto, California, USA

ROBIN ZHAO, BS
Research Assistant, Department of Otolaryngology–Head and Neck Surgery, Sean Parker Institute for the Voice, Weill Cornell Medical College, New York, New York, USA

Contents

This article discusses the role of computer vision in otolaryngology, particularly through endoscopy and surgery. It covers recent applications of artificial intelligence (AI) in nonradiologic imaging within otolaryngology, noting the benefits and challenges, such as improving diagnostic accuracy and optimizing therapeutic outcomes, while also pointing out the necessity for enhanced data curation and standardized research methodologies to advance clinical applications. Technical aspects are also covered, providing a detailed view of the progression from manual feature extraction to more complex AI models, including convolutional neural networks and vision transformers and their potential application in clinical settings.

The role of computer vision in extracting radiographic (radiomics) and histopathologic (pathognomics) features is an extension of molecular biomarkers that have been foundational to our understanding across the spectrum of head and neck disorders. Especially within head and neck cancers, machine learning and deep learning applications have yielded advances in the characterization of tumor features, nodal features, and various outcomes. This review aims to overview the landscape of radiomic and pathognomic applications, informing future work to address gaps. Novel methodologies will be needed to potentially engineer ways of integrating multidimensional data inputs to examine disease features to guide prognosis comprehensively and ultimately clinical management.

The increasing development of artificial intelligence (AI) generative models in otolaryngology—head and neck surgery will progressively change our practice. Practitioners and patients have access to AI resources, improving information, knowledge, and practice of patient care. This article

potential in pattern recognition for early cancer detection, prognostication, and treatment planning, primarily through image analysis using clinical, endoscopic, and histopathologic images. Radiomics is also discussed at length, as well as the many ways that radiologic image analysis can be utilized, including for diagnosis, lymph node metastasis prediction, and evaluation of treatment response. The study highlights AI's promise and limitations, underlining the need for clinician-data scientist collaboration to enhance head and neck cancer care.

Obinna I. Nwosu and Matthew R. Naunheim

Technological advancements in laryngology, broncho-esophagology, and sleep surgery have enabled the collection of increasing amounts of complex data for diagnosis and treatment of voice, swallowing, and sleep disorders. Clinicians face challenges in efficiently synthesizing these data for personalized patient care. Artificial intelligence (AI), specifically machine learning and deep learning, offers innovative solutions for processing and interpreting these data, revolutionizing diagnosis and management in these fields, and making care more efficient and effective. In this study, we review recent AI-based innovations in the fields of laryngology, broncho-esophagology, and sleep surgery.

Noel F. Ayoub and Jordan T. Glicksman

Rhinology, allergy, and skull base surgery are fields primed for the integration and implementation of artificial intelligence (AI). The heterogeneity of the disease processes within these fields highlights the opportunity for AI to augment clinical care and promote personalized medicine. Numerous research studies have been published demonstrating the development and clinical potential of AI models within the field. Most describe in silico evaluation models without direct clinical implementation. The major themes of existing studies include diagnostic or clinical decisions support, clustering patients into specific phenotypes or endotypes, predicting post-treatment outcomes, and surgical planning.

Ki Wan Park, Mohamed Diop, Sierra Hewett Willens, and Jon-Paul Pepper

Artificial intelligence (AI), particularly computer vision and large language models, will impact facial plastic and reconstructive surgery (FPRS) by enhancing diagnostic accuracy, refining surgical planning, and improving post-operative evaluations. These advancements can address subjective limitations of aesthetic surgery by providing objective tools for patient evaluation. Despite these advancements, AI in FPRS has yet to be fully integrated in the clinic setting and faces numerous challenges including algorithmic bias, ethical considerations, and need for validation. This article discusses current and emerging AI technologies in FPRS for the clinic setting, providing a glimpse of its future potential.

GOVERNANCE AND IMPLEMENTATION

OTOLARYNGOLOGIC CLINICS
OF NORTH AMERICA

SERIES OF RELATED INTEREST

Facial Plastic Surgery Clinics
Available at: https://www.facialplastic.theclinics.com/

Foreword

Merging Human and Artificial Intelligence to Improve Otolaryngology Care

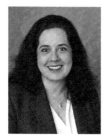

Sujana S. Chandrasekhar, MD, FACS, FAAO-HNS, FAOS
Consulting Editor

I asked ChatGPT4.0 to write me a 600-word foreword for a journal on artificial intelligence and otolaryngology. Here is what I got, with, I am a bit taken aback to say, minimal edits on my end.

In recent years, the intersection of artificial intelligence (AI) and otolaryngology has burgeoned into a fascinating and transformative field. This issue of *Otolaryngologic Clinics of North America*, dedicated to exploring the synergies between AI and the medical subspecialty of otolaryngology, serves as a testament to the innovative strides being made in health care. The mission was to share groundbreaking research, clinical applications, and theoretical advancements that emerge from this interdisciplinary nexus. Guest Editors Drs Anais Rameau and Matthew Crowson, along with all of the authors, have done this admirably.

Otolaryngology has always been a field driven by technological advancement. From the invention of the laryngoscope to the development of cochlear implants, otolaryngologists have leveraged technology to improve diagnostic accuracy and therapeutic outcomes. Today, the integration of AI into otolaryngology promises to elevate this tradition to unprecedented heights.

AI, encompassing machine learning, deep learning, and neural networks, offers powerful tools for data analysis and pattern recognition. In otolaryngology, AI is being employed to enhance various aspects of patient care, from diagnostics to treatment planning and outcome prediction. For instance, machine-learning algorithms can analyze imaging data to detect early signs of head and neck cancers, often with greater accuracy than traditional methods. Similarly, AI-driven tools are aiding in the differentiation of benign and malignant lesions, providing critical information that shapes clinical decision making.

Otolaryngol Clin N Am 57 (2024) xiii–xv
https://doi.org/10.1016/j.otc.2024.06.009
0030-6665/24/© 2024 Published by Elsevier Inc.

One of the most promising applications of AI in otolaryngology is in the realm of personalized medicine. By analyzing vast data sets from diverse patient populations, AI can identify unique patterns and correlations that may not be apparent through human analysis alone. This capability is particularly valuable in understanding complex conditions like chronic rhinosinusitis or hearing loss, where multiple factors interplay. AI-driven insights enable the customization of treatment plans tailored to the individual patient's genetic makeup, lifestyle, and response to previous interventions, thereby optimizing therapeutic outcomes and minimizing adverse effects.

AI is also revolutionizing otolaryngologic surgery. Robotic surgery, augmented by AI, allows for precision that was previously unattainable. Surgeons can now perform minimally invasive procedures with enhanced accuracy, reducing recovery times and improving patient outcomes. AI-driven surgical planning tools can simulate various scenarios, helping surgeons anticipate potential challenges and strategize accordingly. This blend of human expertise and AI is setting new standards in surgical excellence.

AI is already in use to improve patient engagement and education. AI-powered chatbots and virtual assistants are becoming integral to patient care, providing instant responses to queries, facilitating appointment scheduling, and delivering personalized health advice. These tools enhance patient satisfaction and also alleviate some of the administrative burden on health care providers.

However, the integration of AI in otolaryngology is not without challenges. Ethical considerations, data privacy concerns, and the need for robust regulatory frameworks are critical issues that must be addressed. Articles in this issue explore ideas that will foster dialogue on these important topics, ensuring that the deployment of AI technologies aligns with the highest standards of ethical practice, patient safety, and unbiased inclusion.

As we embark on this journey to explore the dynamic interplay between AI and otolaryngology, we are reminded of the words of the renowned computer scientist Alan Kay: "The best way to predict the future is to invent it." Here, Drs Rameau and Crowson have provided a platform for thinkers in the ENT + AI space to share their discoveries, insights, inventions, and visions for the bright future of otolaryngology.

I extend my heartfelt thanks to the Guest Editors and authors, who have cut through the exponentially increasing amount of information on this subject to make it understandable for us, the readers. As we become inspired to collaborate, innovate, and push the boundaries of what is possible, well, then, together, we are not just witnessing the future of otolaryngology, we are actively shaping it.

DECLARATION OF AI AND AI-ASSISTED TECHNOLOGIES IN THE WRITING PROCESS

During the preparation of this work, the author used ChatGPT in order to draft the Foreword. After using this tool/service, the author reviewed and edited the content as needed and takes full responsibility for the content of the publication.

Sujana S. Chandrasekhar, MD, FACS, FAAO-HNS, FAOS
Consulting Editor, Otolaryngologic Clinics of North America
President, American Otological Society
Past President, American Academy of Otolaryngology-Head and Neck Surgery
Partner, ENT & Allergy Associates, LLP
Clinical Professor, Department of Otolaryngology-Head and Neck Surgery, Zucker
School of Medicine at Hofstra-Northwell
Clinical Associate Professor, Department of Otolaryngology–Head and Neck Surgery
Icahn School of Medicine at Mount Sinai
18 East 48th Street, 2nd Floor
New York, NY 10017, USA

E-mail address:
SSC@NYOTOLOGY.COM

Preface

Artificial Intelligence in Otolaryngology - Head and Neck Surgery in the Past Decade

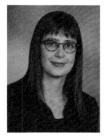
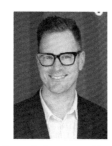

Anaïs Rameau, MDCM, MSc, MPhil, MS, FACS   Matthew G. Crowson, MD, MPA, MASc, MBI, FRCRC
Editors

In 2014, Dr Stanley M. Shapshay, an innovator in laryngology who held numerous leadership positions in our specialty, wrote one of the first pieces on artificial intelligence (AI) and otolaryngology. In "Artificial Intelligence—The Future of Medicine?," Dr Shapshay[1] recounts an interaction with a medical student with engineering training who asserts that "computers will ultimately replace the work of physicians." This leads Dr Shapshay to reflect on the nature of medical reasoning, noting the critical importance of "soft data," such as "complexion, posture, gait, grooming, odor, and status of dentition," information that he does not think a computer system can capture. He concludes, AI "should be an aid and not a substitute for the human encounter. The therapeutic value of the physician-patient encounter [...] is a powerful medicine that is not replaceable by intelligent machines."

Ten years later, more than 500 articles have been published on AI and otolaryngology. The number of manuscripts multiplies every year; the quality of submissions improves, and the performance of algorithms in computer vision, clinical decision support tools, and language production continues to accelerate. And yet, Dr Shapshay's vision could not be truer today. Even with such rapid and exciting developments in machine capability, medicine and its healing potential reside in the physician-patient encounter. AI should only be conceived as an aid to enhance or augment the human element of the encounter and not as a replacement.

With this philosophy in mind, it is with much honor that we have envisioned and edited the first comprehensive review on AI in Otolaryngology. The breadth of topics and

Otolaryngol Clin N Am 57 (2024) xvii–xviii
https://doi.org/10.1016/j.otc.2024.06.001
0030-6665/24/© 2024 Published by Elsevier Inc.

oto.theclinics.com

potentials explored in the following articles is exciting and a testament to the incredible talent of fellow otolaryngologists who have pioneered and relentlessly improved AI applications in all subspecialties, various aspects of clinical workflows, and collaborative research endeavors. Increasing efforts toward AI implementation in otolaryngology beyond research and pilot testing will likely occur in the coming decade. We encourage our colleagues to engage with AI through education, adoption, and inventorship to ensure these digital tools enhance patient care, leveraging our collective expertise and promoting the values of autonomy, beneficence, and justice at the heart of our professional commitment.

DISCLOSURES

A. Rameau was supported by a Paul B. Beeson Emerging Leaders Career Development Award in Aging (K76 AG079040) from the National Institute on Aging and by the Bridge2AI award (OT2 OD032720) from the NIH Common Fund. Such supports do not constitute endorsement by the sponsor of the views expressed in this publication. A. Rameau owns equity of Perceptron Health, Inc. A. Rameau is medical advisor for Sound Health Systems, Inc. M.G. Crowson has no relevant conflicts of interest to disclose.

Anaïs Rameau, MDCM, MSc, MPhil, MS, FACS
Sean Parker Institute for the Voice
Department of Otolaryngology - Head and Neck Surgery
Weill Cornell Medical College
240E 59th Street
New York, NY 10022, USA

Matthew G. Crowson, MD, MPA, MASc, MBI, FRCRC
Department of Otolaryngology–Head & Neck Surgery
Massachusetts Eye and Ear Infirmary
243 Charles Street
Boston, MA 02114, USA

E-mail addresses:
anr2783@med.cornell.edu (A. Rameau)
Matthew_crowson@meei.harvard.edu (M.G. Crowson)

REFERENCE

1. Shapshay SM. Artificial intelligence: the future of medicine? JAMA Otolaryngol Head Neck Surg 2014;140(3):191.

AI MODALITIES IN OTOLARYNGOLOGY - HEAD AND NECK SURGERY

Computer Vision and Videomics in Otolaryngology–Head and Neck Surgery

Bridging the Gap Between Clinical Needs and the Promise of Artificial Intelligence

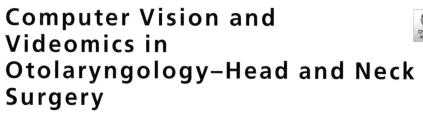

Alberto Paderno, MD, PhD[a,b,]*, Nikita Bedi, BS[c], Anita Rau, PhD[d], Christopher Floyd Holsinger, MD[c]

KEYWORDS

- Artificial intelligence • Computer vision • Otolaryngology • Endoscopy • Surgery
- Videomics

KEY POINTS

- Recent advancements in visual technologies and artificial intelligence (AI) have significantly enhanced the interpretation of medical imaging and introduced new methods for analyzing unstructured medical data.
- There is an ongoing trend toward the development of more complex AI models for analyzing endoscopic and surgical images, focusing on tasks such as lesion detection, segmentation, and lesion characterization.
- The shift toward collaborations across multiple institutions is crucial for developing AI tools that are robust, generalizable, and clinically applicable across diverse patient populations.
- While AI holds substantial potential for enhancing diagnostic accuracy and surgical outcomes in otolaryngology, challenges such as data quality, model validation, and the need for standardization remain.
- Rigorous data curation and comprehensive validation protocols are essential for ensuring the accuracy and reliability of AI models in clinical settings.

[a] IRCCS Humanitas Research Hospital, via Manzoni 56, Rozzano, Milan 20089, Italy; [b] Department of Biomedical Sciences, Humanitas University, Via Rita Levi Montalcini 4, Pieve Emanuele, Milan 20072, Italy; [c] Division of Head and Neck Surgery, Department of Otolaryngology, Stanford University, Palo Alto, CA, USA; [d] Department of Biomedical Data Science, Stanford University, Palo Alto, CA, USA
* Corresponding author. IRCCS Humanitas Research Hospital, via Manzoni 56, Rozzano, Milan 20089, Italy.
E-mail address: albpaderno@gmail.com

Otolaryngol Clin N Am 57 (2024) 703–718
https://doi.org/10.1016/j.otc.2024.05.005
oto.theclinics.com
0030-6665/24/© 2024 Elsevier Inc. All rights reserved, including those for text and data mining, AI training, and similar technologies.

INTRODUCTION

Vision is critical to the practice of otolaryngology and head and neck surgery (OHNS). Endoscopy of the upper aerodigestive tract (UADT) plays a central role in disease diagnosis, tumor staging, and follow-up, encompassing the patient's entire journey from diagnostics through therapeutic. Similarly, surgery hinges on the deep understanding and anticipation of anatomic structures and tissue types, going beyond the mere technical execution of procedural steps. Mastering these visual processing capabilities is central to achieving optimal operative outcomes.

In fact, the evolution of otolaryngology is closely linked to advancements in visual technologies, from the introduction of operative microscopy and endoscopy to more complex equipment such as exoscopes and surgical robots. The last decade has witnessed a surge in the application of software analysis techniques based on computer vision (CV) and artificial intelligence (AI) to medical imaging. These innovations have first enhanced our ability to interpret traditional radiologic examinations and subsequently unlocked new ways to analyze the unstructured data contained in nonradiologic medical images and videos.

This review aims to encapsulate the novel advances in the field of nonradiologic CV applications, or videomics,[1] within Otolaryngology—Head and Neck Surgery. We start by comprehensively examining contemporary research about AI in UADT diseases, focusing on diagnostic endoscopy and surgical video analysis. By integrating insights from adjacent disciplines, we highlight the current research gaps and chart a course toward faster improvement and better clinical transition of these technologies. Through this discourse, we aim to assess the potential of CV and AI in enhancing diagnostic accuracy (Acc), optimizing therapeutic outcomes, and redefining surgical paradigms in Otolaryngology–Head and Neck Surgery.

COMPUTER VISION IN OTOLARYNGOLOGY: DATA SELECTION, ENHANCEMENT, AND CURATION

Recent years have seen significant developments in the deployment of various AI models aimed at analyzing endoscopic and surgical images or videos. Paderno and colleagues[2] proposed an organized structure to frame this effort and distinguish the different studies according to their objective, from quality assurance to classification, detection, segmentation, and in-depth characterization. However, framing objectives and adequately structuring research is only a part of the required process. High-quality data represent the key prerequisite for impactful investigations, extending the field to innovations in data curation, postprocessing, and frame selection (the entire AI development pipeline is summarized in **Fig. 1**). The importance of data curation has been recently highlighted by Yao and colleagues[3] who developed a deep learning pipeline for the classification of vocal fold polyps, emphasizing the need for peer-reviewed frame classification in dataset assembly. Furthermore, to enhance data quality, Gómez and colleagues[4] presented a U-Net-based method for enhancing the brightness of low-light high-speed endoscopic videos and informative frame selection. The selection of informative frames was indeed a recurrent theme also in earlier research, with different authors developing machine learning (ML)- and convolutional neural network (CNN)-based classifiers to accelerate the video review process for clinicians, potentially saving valuable time and resources.[5,6] Relevant studies are summarized in **Table 1**.

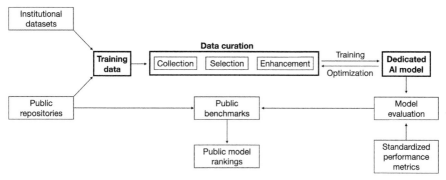

Fig. 1. Proposed pipeline for AI models development and validation.

COMPUTER VISION IN UPPER AERODIGESTIVE TRACT ENDOSCOPY

Research in the field of UADT endoscopy is varied and can be distinguished in applications focusing on structural and functional evaluations. In the structural domain, the ultimate goal is to refine diagnostic Acc in determining mucosal alterations, while in the functional one, the authors have attempted to automate and objectify dynamic aspects of the UADT, such as vocal fold motility and pharyngeal collapse leading to sleep apnea.

Not surprisingly, CV research has extensively explored the neoplastic and preneoplastic tissue detection domains. However, recent studies were also targeted at benign lesions, foreign bodies, and inflammatory/traumatic conditions. In particular, Parker and colleagues[7] employed CNNs to recognize postextubation laryngeal lesions (granulomas and ulcerations), and Tao and colleagues[8] tackled the detection of concealed fish bones by leveraging the YOLO-V5 algorithm, an out-of-the-box solution employed in many CV tasks.

Finally, various authors[1,2,9] provided a comprehensive review of AI-based investigations in the field of UADT endoscopy, detailing their domain of application, objectives, and outcomes. While providing a similar list of studies on the topic is beyond the scope of this narrative review, different compelling concepts can be drawn from the overview of available papers.

Developments in Model Architecture

In the preliminary stages of development of CV, studies were based on a combination of feature extraction from images and ML-based analysis of their numerical features. This approach was burdened by significant biases related to manual feature selection, with potential overfitting to each specific dataset or task. Each problem had to be addressed by a specifically tailored workflow and dedicated features, potentially hampering generalizability, and scalability. The advent of CNNs and advancements in neural network-based algorithms have substantially alleviated these limitations. By automatically learning hierarchical feature representations directly from data, a sort of automatic feature extraction, CNNs have emerged as the preferred architecture in contemporary CV research. This shift enhances model robustness and data adaptability and facilitates the development process, allowing for more scalable and universally applicable solutions across diverse domains. In future studies, exploring the implications of even more recent model architectures, transformers, and hybrid structures (combining transformer and CNN architectures) presents a promising development route. Transformers, having demonstrated their effectiveness in natural language processing

Table 1
Summary of studies focusing on data selection, enhancement, and standardization

Author, Year	Methods or Models Used	Results or Outcomes
Yao et al,[3] 2022	Developed a deep learning classifier using a pretrained ResNet-18 model to automatically select informative frames from flexible laryngoscopic videos	Precision 94.4%, recall 90.2%, and F-1 score of 92.3%. Used Grad-CAM to provide visual explanations for the CNNs decisions.
Gómez et al,[4] 2019	Using CNN (U-Net) architecture, Gómez et al focus on improving the quality of high-speed video endoscopic images under low-light conditions.	The model's performance was assessed using metrics such as peak signal-to-noise ratio and structural similarity index, and when compared with other state-of-the-art models such as SRIE, NPE, LDR, and CVC, this U-Net architecture showed superior results of enhancing image quality more effectively and with fewer artifacts.
Patrini et al,[5] 2020	Study used a transfer learning approach using 6 different pretrained CNNs for feature selection and then used SVM and CNNs for robust classification of NBI laryngoscopy videos as informative, blurry, saliva or specular reflections, or underexposed.	The VGG 16 model combined with SVMs achieved the highest recall for informative (I) frames, showing a recall of 0.97 and 0.98 when using SVMs and CNN-based classification, respectively.
Moccia et al,[6] 2018	Primary model used in the study was SVM with a radial bases function kernel, and features were extracted for classification into 4 categories: informative, blurry, saliva or specular reflections, or underexposed.	Precision, recall, and F1 scores of informative frames was 91%,
Gómez et al,[34] 2020	Introduces the Benchmark for Automatic Glottis Segmentation (BAGLS), a multihospital dataset aimed at improving automatic glottis segmentation techniques using high-speed videoendoscopy (HSV) frames to facilitate the training and validation of deep learning models on a diverse array of data from different institutions, enhancing the generalizability and accuracy of these models in clinical settings	The BAGLS dataset was used to train a state-of-the-art deep learning segmentation network, achieving robust segmentation results. It showed a high median Intersection over Union (IoU) score of 0.772 across different expert validations, indicating strong agreement and effectiveness in segmenting the glottis from HSV frames.

Abbreviations: CVC, contextual and variational context enhancement; HSV, high-speed videolaryngoscopy; LDR, layered difference representation; NBI, narrow band imaging; NPE, naturalness preserved enhancement; SRIE, simultaneous reflectance and illumination estimation; SVM, support vector machine.

(eg, ChatGPT, Llama-2, and Gemini),[10] are now starting to be applied to visual tasks with promising initial results.[11,12] The potential of transformers lies in their ability to model complex dependencies and capture long-range interactions within images, a feature particularly advantageous for handling complex visual information. Recently, You and colleagues[13] included a basic vision transformer in their evaluation of vocal cord leukoplakia; however, outcomes were still inferior to CNN-based algorithms. This may be related to these algorithms' higher training data requirements that often lead to underwhelming results when dealing with small datasets. In contrast, within gastrointestinal (GI) endoscopy, hybrid or transformer-based architectures are the basis for 9 of the top 10 models across the 2 main benchmarks (ie, Kvasir-SEG and CVC-ClinicDB) in the field. These benchmarks, not available in otolaryngology, are designed to evaluate AI models' performance in segmenting and identifying polyps and other abnormalities within the GI tract, allowing for fair comparison between different studies and improving the identification of emerging trends in the field.[14,15]

Finally, from a technical standpoint, the authors recently shifted from simple general-purpose "pre-made" models to more complex dedicated architectures tailored to UADT endoscopy frames.[16] This concept can be further observed in the constant technical progression both in clinical and engineering studies.

Downstream Tasks and Algorithm Validation: Objectives and Clinical Validity

In terms of scope, a clear advancement toward complex tasks can also be seen, with earlier studies mainly focusing on classification and recent research venturing into more advanced technical solutions, such as lesion detection or segmentation, up to complex workflows including multiple sequential analytical steps.[17] Yet, most studies are still presented as "proof-of-concept" projects analyzing a single disease site and a cohort of patients originating from a single institution. An attempt at multisite segmentation has been made by Paderno and colleagues,[18] underlining the marked difference in performance when addressing different anatomic areas, with a significant reduction in segmentation performance in the oral cavity. Furthermore, a shift to multi-institutional collaborative studies represents the next step to obtain more generalizable and clinically relevant applications. Azam and colleagues[16] and Xiong and colleagues[19] focusing on laryngeal cancer endoscopic detection, evaluated their outcomes with an external validation cohort, demonstrating the impact of independent data on performance.

Following this recent trend of increasing algorithm tailoring and validation, Tran and colleagues[20] and Mohamed and colleagues[21] not only developed models for classifying vocal fold images and automated laryngeal cancer detection but also highlighted areas for improvement, such as the need for better noise filtering techniques and the enhancement of hyperparameter tuning. These technical improvements also extended to processing speed, with the introduction by Sampieri and colleagues[22] of the SegMENT-Plus algorithm, allowing its application on videolaryngoscopies simulating real-time use.

Furthermore, the research landscape exhibits a trend toward multimodal data utilization, as demonstrated by Li and colleagues,[23] who developed an AI-assisted system incorporating multimodal data (both white light and narrow band imaging frames) for the real-time detection of laryngopharyngeal cancer. This effort underscores AIs versatility in integrating diverse data types for enhanced diagnostic precision.

Finally, when considering innovative tasks outside conventional endoscopy, Esmaeili and colleagues[24,25] introduced automated approaches for vascular pattern characterization during contact endoscopy. These contributions aimed to reduce subjectivity in an area where the increased amount of information provided by high magnification may enhance diagnostic potential but also require specialized training to achieve consistent results.

Functional Endoscopic Evaluation

From a functional standpoint (**Table 2**), research has been mainly focused on providing a new way to reliably determine objective measures from unstructured data (ie, endoscopic images and videos). Starting from this concept, Lin and colleagues[26] developed a CNN-based algorithm aimed at quantifying upper airway obstruction by automating the delineation of vocal folds, glottic opening, and supraglottic structures.

Interesting applications have also been developed in the field of sleep medicine, such as an AI model for automatic scoring of drug-induced sleep endoscopy (DISE) videos for obstructive sleep apnea and a CV system that calculates the epiglottis obstruction ratio using a deep learning-based method.[27,28]

However, vocal fold motility remains the central topic for functional evaluation of the UADT. A series of studies demonstrated the possibility of identifying vocal fold paralysis during conventional endoscopy by automatically tracking the free border of the vocal folds and estimating the anterior glottic angle.[29–31] Furthermore, in cases where neoplastic lesions subverted the vocal folds, Villani and colleagues[32] demonstrated the value of a 3 dimensional key point-based reconstruction of the glottic and supraglottic larynx to achieve the same outcome. In adjunction, Wang and colleagues[33] proposed a novel deep learning system for automated detection of laryngeal adductor reflex events in laryngeal endoscopy videos, achieving promising performance for objective and quantitative analysis.

However, the bulk of research in the field of endoscopic functional evaluation is aimed at improving and automating the evaluation of high-speed videoendoscopy (ie, precisely segmenting the vocal folds free border and glottic opening), starting with specific datasets and benchmarks,[34] to software tools and open-source platforms,[35,36] with the final aim of improving automated glottal segmentation.[37–39] These coordinated research efforts have facilitated a swift transition of proposed solutions from proof-of-concept to clinical application, highlighting the profound impact of open-source resources and collaborative efforts across multiple institutions.

SURGERY

The increasing potential of CV algorithms led to extending the research effort to the surgical domain (**Table 3**). Different authors have preliminarily explored various fields, from laryngology to head and neck surgery, skull base, and otologic surgery. Early approaches by Laves and colleagues[40] and Aubreville and colleagues[41] introduced automatic segmentation and classification systems for tissues in endomicroscopy images of the larynx and oral cavity using deep learning. These systems showed promising preliminary results, outperformed previous methods, and set the stage for subsequent studies.

In the field of traditional "open" surgery, Gong and colleagues[42] presented a deep learning algorithm aimed at soft tissue discrimination during thyroidectomy, specifically to segment and measure nerves, focusing on the recurrent laryngeal nerve. The authors identified the significant impact of optimal image capture conditions, with the algorithm showing strong segmentation performance in the medium-lighting and close-up combination.

In otologic surgery, Gao and colleagues[43] proposed a method to track the malleus bone during endoscopic ventilation grommet insertion surgery using the optical flow

Table 2
Artificial intelligence in functional endoscopic evaluation

Author, Year	Methods or Models Used	Results or Outcomes
Lin et al,[26] 2019	Developed a computer vision algorithm for quantifying laryngeal closure from endoscopic videos, utilizing a 2 stage CNN for region detection and FCN for structure segmentation	The method achieved segmentation speeds of 16 FPS with Intersection over Union (IoU) scores ranging from 0.65 to 0.85
Su et al,[27] 2023	Developed a deep learning-based epiglottis obstruction ratio calculation system using the YOLOv4 model for precise localization and analysis of epiglottis cartilage in endoscopic images	The system demonstrated high precision, capable of calculating obstruction ratios with a granularity of 0.1%, across a spectrum from 0% to 100%
Hanif et al,[28] 2023	Aims to automate the scoring of drug-induced sleep endoscopy (DISE) for obstructive sleep apnea diagnosis using deep learning	The model achieved a mean F1 score of 70% across all DISE examinations, with site-specific scores of 85% for velum, 72% for oropharynx, 57% for tongue, and 65% for epiglottis
Adamian et al,[29] 2021	Introduces an open-source computer vision tool named AGATI (Automated Glottic Action Tracking by Artificial Intelligence), designed for automated quantitative tracking of vocal fold (VF) motion from videolaryngoscopy using a deep learning algorithm to estimation of glottic opening angles.	AGATI achieved a correlation of 0.97 with manual expert markings and predicted unilateral VF paralysis with 85% sensitivity and specificity, demonstrating an AUC of 0.888
Wang et al,[30] 2021	Validate AGATI for automated tracking of true VF paralysis by analyzing videolaryngoscopy recordings to calculate AGAs in patients with UVFP.	AGATI accurately differentiated between UVFP and control groups, predicting UVFP with 77% sensitivity and 92% specificity, particularly using the 97th percentile AGA cutoff of 48.12°
DeVore et al,[31] 2023	Utilized a deep learning-based computer vision tool to quantitatively assess the anterior glottic angle (AGA) from videolaryngoscopy in patients with bilateral and unilateral vocal fold immobility, correlating AGA with patient-reported outcomes and predicting the necessity for airway interventions	Demonstrated high accuracy with an area under the curve (AUC) of 0.92 for diagnosing bilateral VF immobility, and an AUC of 0.77 for predicting surgical intervention needs, effectively correlating reduced AGA with increased dyspnea severity

(*continued on next page*)

Table 2 (continued)		
Author, Year	**Methods or Models Used**	**Results or Outcomes**
Villani et al,[32] 2023	Classifies VFs motility from endoscopic videos, aiming to improve the objectivity and reliability of clinical assessments for functional deficits and staging of neoplastic diseases of the glottis by using several machine learning classifiers, including XGBoost.	The study reported precision, recall, F1 score, accuracy, average precision, AUC as metrics for the classifiers used in classifying VFs motility from endoscopic videos:
Wang et al,[33] 2022	Uses a deep learning-based system for detecting laryngeal closure events in endoscopy videos without the need for prior region segmentation by incorporating a novel spatiotemporal orthogonal region selection network that integrates both local and global image features, along with temporal context, to enhance the detection and classification of VF states directly from video frames.	LARNet-STC achieved high detection accuracy for laryngeal adductor reflex (LAR) events with over 90% F1 score for LAR frames and 99% for non-LAR frames
Kist et al,[35] 2021	Introduces OpenHSV, an open-source, modular platform for laryngeal high-speed videoendoscopy that combines state-of-the-art hardware with an advanced, fully automated data analysis pipeline using deep neural networks for segmentation of the glottal area, aiming to standardize data acquisition and analysis for voice physiology research and clinical assessments	In a preliminary clinical validation involving 28 healthy individuals, OpenHSV demonstrated robust performance with its deep learning-based segmentation methods achieving high image and audio quality using the natural image quality evaluator (NIQE) and traditional voice quality metrics such as jitter and shimmer.
Kist et al,[36] 2021	Introduces Glottis Analysis Tools (GAT), a software developed to automate segmentation and analysis of laryngeal dynamics from high-speed videoendoscopy data by incorporating deep learning techniques and utilizing CNNs and region of interest (ROI)-based segmentation to facilitate the evaluation of VF vibrations in order to improve diagnostic accuracy and research productivity in voice pathology.	GAT demonstrated robust performance with mean IoU scores of 0.830 using custom U-Net, 0.812 with EfficientNetB0, and 0.842 with ResNet-50

(continued on next page)

Table 2
(continued)

Author, Year	Methods or Models Used	Results or Outcomes
Fehling et al,[37] 2020	Automate segmentation of the glottis and VFs in endoscopic laryngeal high-speed videos using a deep convolutional LSTM network	The deep learning model exhibited robust performance, achieving a mean Dice coefficient of 0.85 for the glottis, 0.91 for the right VF, and 0.90 for the left VF.
Kist et al,[38] 2022	Demonstrates that a single latent channel in an encoder–decoder architecture is sufficient for glottis segmentation by employing a U-Net architecture.	Findings reveal that a single latent channel can effectively encode glottal area segmentation, achieving high IoU scores with both enabled and disabled skip connections.
Kruse et al,[39] 2023	Introduces GlottisNetV2, a deep learning model that enhances glottal midline detection through temporal and spatial analysis, utilizing a dual-decoder architecture to perform segmentation and midline detection simultaneously on a dataset of laryngeal images.	Results demonstrate that GlottisNetV2 significantly outperforms previous models with a mean IoU of 84.7%, and the model's temporal analysis improves median prediction accuracy

Abbreviations: LSTM, long short term memory; UVFP, unilateral vocal fold palsy.

technique and gradient vector flow active contours algorithm. Adjunctively, Miwa and colleagues[44] assessed the potential of AI in combination with image enhancement techniques for identifying cholesteatoma matrix, debris, and normal middle ear mucosa during endoscopic ear surgery in a preliminary study involving 14 consecutive patients. The CNN-based model could detect cholesteatoma matrix lesions with a sensitivity of 34.6% and 42.3% and with a specificity of 81.3% and 87.5%, respectively, using SPECTRA A and SPECTRA B image enhancement modalities. To add to these two previous studies, Nwosu and colleagues[45] developed a proof-of-concept CV model for detecting instruments and anatomy during transcanal endoscopic ear surgery.

Finally, shifting to transnasal surgery, King and colleagues[46] created a multistage video summarization procedure using a CNN with a Hidden Markov Model to output a representative summary of endoscopic endonasal skull base surgical videos, reducing video length by 98.2% while preserving 84% of key medical scenes.

CURRENT RESEARCH GAPS

Overviewing the recent literature can be valuable in understanding the current state of development of AI and CV in otolaryngology. However, this evaluation can also help identify research needs and gaps in the field, guiding further progression in an organized manner.

Standardization

Despite the growing number of studies on AI and CV, reporting remains inconsistent, leading to significant challenges when analyzing and interpreting research. Standardized evaluation metrics are required to allow quick evaluations and fair comparison of

Table 3
Artificial intelligence in surgery, summary

Author, Year	Methods or Models Used	Results or Outcomes
Laves et al,[40] 2019	Evaluates the effectiveness of deep learning-based segmentation methods (SegNet, UNet, ENet, and ErfNet) on a novel dataset of transoral endoscopic images of the human larynx.	The ensemble of UNet and ErfNet models achieved the best performance with a mean Intersection over Union (IoU) of 84.7%, while ENet demonstrated the highest efficiency with an average inference time of 9.22 ms per image.
Auberville et al,[41] 2017	Automatically classify cancerous tissue in laser endomicroscopy images of the oral cavity using CNN and textural feature-based ML models in order to improve accuracy of early detection of OSCC	The deep learning model had an AUC of 0.96 and mean accuracy of 88.3%, sensitivity 86.6%, and specificity at 90%.
Gong et al,[42] 2021	Utilizes a deep learning algorithm designed for identifying the recurrent laryngeal nerve during thyroidectomy	The deep learning model achieved a Dice similarity coefficient (DSC) of 0.707 under optimal conditions for close-up images and medium lighting, demonstrating effective nerve segmentation capabilities.
Gao et al,[43] 2016	Using optical flow techniques and gradient vector flow, this study explores the use of an intelligent vision guide for automatic ventilation grommet insertion into the tympanic membrane, focusing on real-time tracking of the malleus under the endoscope to avoid insertion failure and damage during surgery.	Demonstrates superior stability and accuracy in tracking the malleus compared to traditional methods in preclinical tests.
Miwa et al,[44] 2022	Using a CNN trained on endoscopically enhanced images to identify cholesteatoma matrix, debris, and normal mucosa during ear surgeries, they employed image enhancement systems and assessed the CNNs diagnostic accuracy using an independent dataset from surgeries.	Sensitivity of 34.6% for SPECTRA A and 42.3% for SPECTRA B, with specificities of 81.3% and 87.5%, respectively. The positive prediction values were 60.0% for SPECTRA A and 73.3% for SPECTRA B, indicating moderate diagnostic performance in identifying cholesteatoma matrix during endoscopic ear surgery

(continued on next page)

Table 3 *(continued)*		
Author, Year	**Methods or Models Used**	**Results or Outcomes**
Nwosu et al,[45] 2023	Proof-of-concept computer vision model developed to accurately estimate the size of tympanic membrane perforations using deep learning techniques, demonstrating the model's superior accuracy compared to traditional clinical estimates by otolaryngologists	Model performance: Achieved a mean average precision (mAP) of 83% across IoU thresholds from 0.5 to 0.95, indicating robust model performance. Confidence levels: The model's predictions were associated with a high average confidence level of 96.4%.
King et al,[46] 2023	Automatically summarize endoscopic skull base surgical videos using deep learning techniques (CNN) model for feature extraction and classification and using Markov modeling for surgical stage estimation.	The model achieved 98.2% reduction in video length while preserving 84% of key surgical stages significantly outperforming other available tools.

Abbreviation: OSCC, oral squamous cell carcinoma.

results, this being especially true when considering detection and segmentation tasks. For example, a commonly used parameter is Acc, which measures the percentage of pixels that are correctly classified. However, endoscopic frames are commonly highly class-imbalanced, containing a single region of interest involving only a small portion of pixels, whereas the remaining image is labeled as background (ie, true negatives). Consequently, because of the positive impact of true negatives, Acc tends to result in high scores even in case of poor diagnostic performance. This issue can be mitigated by the use of overlap metrics such as the Dice similarity coefficient and Intersection over Union. Addressing this field, Sampieri and colleagues[9] and Paderno and colleagues[47] have recently highlighted and addressed the need for adequate technical knowledge and carefully selected outcome metrics in studies applying AI to endoscopy.

However, widely accepted guidelines specifically focused on reporting of AI techniques in endoscopic and surgical images are still lacking. In the overall medical AI literature, several reports have been published to encourage authors to provide information to allow their work to be evaluated appropriately. The MINimum Information for Medical AI Reporting proposal describes the minimum information necessary to understand intended predictions and the ability to generalize AI models.[48] The authors positioned the study as a starting point for a broader discussion, aiming to provide transparency and help disseminate AI algorithms across health care systems. Similarly, the minimum information about clinical AI modeling checklist covered comparable aspects such as the description of the data used, the specifics of the AI model, the evaluation methods, and the reproducibility of the results.[49] Each item in the checklist is aimed at providing precise information about different stages of AI model development and deployment in a clinical setting. Finally, the Checklist for Artificial Intelligence in Medical Imaging has been developed for AI applications in radiology and includes points related to study design, data description, ground truth establishment, data partitioning, model details, training procedures, evaluation metrics, and results reporting.[50] For image analysis specifically, it covers items such as data preprocessing, definitions of data elements, de-identification methods, annotation tools, model input and output descriptions, validation on external data, and performance metrics for optimal models. These are useful frameworks that can be translated and adapted to the field of nonradiologic medical image analysis with the aim of guiding future research and enhancing comparability. Adapting these useful guidelines for CV analysis in endoscopy and surgery, especially those involving multimodal data, will serve as a roadmap for future investigations and foster standardized reporting practices vital for advancement in OHNS.

Repositories and Benchmarks

Since its inception, CV research has been driven by shared data repositories and standardized benchmarks. ImageNet is a notable example when considering natural image detection and classification, with its expansive image repository meticulously categorized into numerous categories.[51] This dataset has served as a foundational benchmark in the field, enabling the development and evaluation of innovative image recognition algorithms. Ultimately, by providing a diverse range of annotated images it allowed recognition of the CNN architecture as an ideal technical solution for complex vision tasks.[52]

However, the available repositories in the medical field are far from the depth and breadth of ImageNet, a significant issue that represents the bottleneck in current research. As previously stated, the Benchmark for Automatic Glottis Segmentation (BAGLS) dataset provides an interesting case study in Otolaryngology—Head and Neck Surgery.[34] Capturing the vocal fold's mucosal wave with high-speed video endoscopy requires expert segmentation, a tedious process ideal for deep learning-based automation. Nevertheless, the absence of comprehensive datasets had previously hindered advancements in the field. Addressing this, the BAGLS dataset emerged as an essential resource with over 59,000 high-speed videoendoscopy frames, each with detailed segmentation masks. This dataset, developed thanks to a multi-institutional effort, exemplifies a new research model based on collaboration and data sharing, with the common objective of advancing AI research toward practical clinical applications.

However, public repositories and benchmarks are still not available for the broader UADT endoscopy and surgery domains, significantly hampering the pace of development of these fields. In this context, the GI endoscopy literature offers exemplary practices that could be usefully adopted in our field. Among these, "KVASIR: A Multi-Class Image Dataset for Computer Aided Gastrointestinal Disease Detection" is a notable example, a dataset containing endoscopic images of the GI tract, providing a varied collection of classified images that can be used for training models and conducting experiments in image and video analysis.[53] By offering a standardized dataset, Kvasir facilitates easier comparison and ranking of experimental results, which is crucial for advancing the field of medical image analysis. Similarly, the datasets CVC-ClinicDB, ETIS-Larib, and ASU-Mayo Clinic Colonoscopy Video Database, focused on colonoscopy, offer valuable source data to track and compare model diagnostic Acc and organize Grand Challenges to allow competition on the development of the best performing algorithms (see **Fig. 1**).[54–56] The success of these repositories in promoting research and development emphasizes the need for similar resources in UADT endoscopy and surgery.

SUMMARY

AI and CV are enhancing the precision of endoscopic evaluations, improving surgical planning, and offering new insights into patient care. Despite the progress, challenges such as the need for standardized reporting, data sharing, and validation of AI models remain. Addressing these will be crucial for fully integrating AI and CV into clinical practice. Ultimately, the integration of these technologies holds the promise of refining current practice through more accurate diagnoses and personalized treatments.

CLINICS CARE POINTS

- Recent advancements in visual technologies and AI can significantly enhance the interpretation of medical imaging and introduce new methods for analyzing unstructured medical data.

- There is an ongoing trend toward developing more complex AI models for analyzing endoscopic and surgical images, focusing on tasks like lesion detection, segmentation, and characterization.

- Automating dynamic evaluations, such as vocal fold motility and airway obstructions, provides reliable, objective measures from these unstructured data.

- Enhanced tissue segmentation capabilities can assist surgeons in identifying critical structures, potentially reducing operative risks.

- Advanced noise filtering and hyperparameter tuning techniques enhance image quality and processing speed, facilitating smoother clinical workflows.

- Collaborative efforts across institutions ensure AI tools are robust, generalizable, and applicable across diverse patient populations.

- Creating comprehensive datasets, like the BAGLS dataset, enhances the development and validation of AI models.

- Adopting standardized metrics and reporting guidelines, like MINIMAR and MI-CLAIM, ensures consistent and transparent AI model evaluations.

DISCLOSURE

The authors have nothing to disclose.

ACKNOWLEDGMENTS

The authors acknowledge support from the Isackson Family Foundation and the Stanford Head and Neck Surgery Research Fund.

REFERENCES

1. Paderno A, Holsinger FC, Piazza C. Videomics: bringing deep learning to diagnostic endoscopy. Curr Opin Otolaryngol Head Neck Surg 2021;29(2):143–8.
2. Paderno A, Gennarini F, Sordi A, et al. Artificial intelligence in clinical endoscopy: Insights in the field of videomics. Frontiers in Surgery 2022;9. Available at: https://www.frontiersin.org/articles/10.3389/fsurg.2022.933297. [Accessed 7 February 2024].
3. Yao P, Witte D, Gimonet H, et al. Automatic classification of informative laryngoscopic images using deep learning. Laryngoscope Investig Otolaryngol 2022; 7(2):460–6.
4. Gómez P, Semmler M, Schützenberger A, et al. Low-light image enhancement of high-speed endoscopic videos using a convolutional neural network. Med Biol Eng Comput 2019;57(7):1451–63.

5. Patrini I, Ruperti M, Moccia S, et al. Transfer learning for informative-frame selection in laryngoscopic videos through learned features. Med Biol Eng Comput 2020;58(6):1225–38.

6. Moccia S, Vanone GO, Momi ED, et al. Learning-based classification of informative laryngoscopic frames. Comput Methods Programs Biomed 2018;158:21–30.

7. Parker F, Brodsky MB, Akst LM, et al. Machine Learning in Laryngoscopy Analysis: A Proof of Concept Observational Study for the Identification of Post-Extubation Ulcerations and Granulomas. Ann Otol Rhinol Laryngol 2021;130(3):286–91.

8. Tao X, Zhao X, Liu H, et al. Automatic Recognition of Concealed Fish Bones under Laryngoscopy: A Practical AI Model Based on YOLO-V5. Laryngoscope 2023. https://doi.org/10.1002/lary.31175.

9. Sampieri C, Baldini C, Azam MA, et al. Artificial Intelligence for Upper Aerodigestive Tract Endoscopy and Laryngoscopy: A Guide for Physicians and State-of-the-Art Review. Otolaryngol Head Neck Surg 2023. https://doi.org/10.1002/ohn.343.

10. Vaswani A, Shazeer N, Parmar N, et al. Attention Is All You Need. Published online August 1, 2023. https://doi.org/10.48550/arXiv.1706.03762.

11. Dosovitskiy A, Beyer L, Kolesnikov A, et al. An Image is Worth 16x16 Words: Transformers for Image Recognition at Scale. 2021. Available at: http://arxiv.org/abs/2010.11929. [Accessed 16 September 2023].

12. Oquab M, Darcet T, Moutakanni T, et al. DINOv2: Learning Robust Visual Features without Supervision. arvix 2023. https://doi.org/10.48550/arXiv.2304.07193.

13. You Z, Han B, Shi Z, et al. Vocal cord leukoplakia classification using deep learning models in white light and narrow band imaging endoscopy images. Head Neck 2023;45(12):3129–45.

14. Papers with Code - Kvasir-SEG Benchmark (Medical Image Segmentation). Available at: https://paperswithcode.com/sota/medical-image-segmentation-on-kvasir-seg. [Accessed 7 February 2024].

15. Papers with Code - CVC-ClinicDB Benchmark (Medical Image Segmentation). Available at: https://paperswithcode.com/sota/medical-image-segmentation-on-cvc-clinicdb. [Accessed 7 February 2024].

16. Azam MA, Sampieri C, Ioppi A, et al. Videomics of the Upper Aero-Digestive Tract Cancer: Deep Learning Applied to White Light and Narrow Band Imaging for Automatic Segmentation of Endoscopic Images. Front Oncol 2022;12:900451.

17. Yao P, Witte D, German A, et al. A deep learning pipeline for automated classification of vocal fold polyps in flexible laryngoscopy. Eur Arch Otorhinolaryngol 2023. https://doi.org/10.1007/s00405-023-08190-8.

18. Paderno A, Villani FP, Fior M, et al. Instance segmentation of upper aerodigestive tract cancer: site-specific outcomes. Acta Otorhinolaryngol Ital 2023;43(4):283–90.

19. Xiong H, Lin P, Yu JG, et al. Computer-aided diagnosis of laryngeal cancer via deep learning based on laryngoscopic images. eBioMedicine 2019;48:92–9.

20. Tran BA, Dao TTP, Dung HDQ, et al. Support of deep learning to classify vocal fold images in flexible laryngoscopy. Am J Otolaryngol 2023;44(3):103800.

21. Mohamed N, Almutairi RL, Abdelrahim S, et al. Automated Laryngeal Cancer Detection and Classification Using Dwarf Mongoose Optimization Algorithm with Deep Learning. Cancers (Basel) 2023;16(1). https://doi.org/10.3390/cancers16010181.

22. Sampieri C, Azam MA, Ioppi A, et al. Real-Time Laryngeal Cancer Boundaries Delineation on White Light and Narrow-Band Imaging Laryngoscopy with Deep Learning. Laryngoscope 2024. https://doi.org/10.1002/lary.31255.

23. Li Y, Gu W, Yue H, et al. Real-time detection of laryngopharyngeal cancer using an artificial intelligence-assisted system with multimodal data. J Transl Med 2023; 21(1):698.
24. Esmaeili N, Sharaf E, Gomes Ataide EJ, et al. Deep Convolution Neural Network for Laryngeal Cancer Classification on Contact Endoscopy-Narrow Band Imaging. Sensors (Basel) 2021;21(23). https://doi.org/10.3390/s21238157.
25. Esmaeili N, Illanes A, Boese A, et al. Novel automated vessel pattern characterization of larynx contact endoscopic video images. Int J Comput Assist Radiol Surg 2019;14(10):1751–61.
26. Lin J, Walsted ES, Backer V, et al. Quantification and Analysis of Laryngeal Closure From Endoscopic Videos. IEEE Trans Biomed Eng 2019;66(4):1127–36.
27. Su HH, Lu CP. Development of a Deep Learning-Based Epiglottis Obstruction Ratio Calculation System. Sensors (Basel) 2023;23(18). https://doi.org/10.3390/s23187669.
28. Hanif U, Kiaer EK, Capasso R, et al. Automatic scoring of drug-induced sleep endoscopy for obstructive sleep apnea using deep learning. Sleep Med 2023; 102:19–29.
29. Adamian N, Naunheim MR, Jowett N. An Open-Source Computer Vision Tool for Automated Vocal Fold Tracking From Videoendoscopy. Laryngoscope 2021; 131(1):E219–25.
30. Wang TV, Adamian N, Song PC, et al. Application of a Computer Vision Tool for Automated Glottic Tracking to Vocal Fold Paralysis Patients. Otolaryngol Head Neck Surg 2021;165(4):556–62.
31. DeVore EK, Adamian N, Jowett N, et al. Predictive Outcomes of Deep Learning Measurement of the Anterior Glottic Angle in Bilateral Vocal Fold Immobility. Laryngoscope 2023;133(9):2285–91.
32. Villani FP, Paderno A, Fiorentino MC, et al. Classifying Vocal Folds Fixation from Endoscopic Videos with Machine Learning. Annu Int Conf IEEE Eng Med Biol Soc 2023;2023:1–4.
33. Wang YY, Hamad AS, Palaniappan K, et al. LARNet-STC: Spatio-temporal orthogonal region selection network for laryngeal closure detection in endoscopy videos. Computers in Biology and Medicine 2022;144:105339.
34. Gómez P, Kist AM, Schlegel P, et al. BAGLS, a multihospital Benchmark for Automatic Glottis Segmentation. Sci Data 2020;7(1):186.
35. Kist AM, Dürr S, Schützenberger A, et al. OpenHSV: an open platform for laryngeal high-speed videoendoscopy. Sci Rep 2021;11(1):13760.
36. Kist AM, Gómez P, Dubrovskiy D, et al. A Deep Learning Enhanced Novel Software Tool for Laryngeal Dynamics Analysis. J Speech Lang Hear Res 2021; 64(6):1889–903.
37. Fehling MK, Grosch F, Schuster ME, et al. Fully automatic segmentation of glottis and vocal folds in endoscopic laryngeal high-speed videos using a deep Convolutional LSTM Network. PLoS One 2020;15(2):e0227791.
38. Kist AM, Breininger K, Dörrich M, et al. A single latent channel is sufficient for biomedical glottis segmentation. Sci Rep 2022;12(1):14292.
39. Kruse E, Dollinger M, Schutzenberger A, et al. GlottisNetV2: Temporal Glottal Midline Detection Using Deep Convolutional Neural Networks. IEEE J Transl Eng Health Med 2023;11:137–44.
40. Laves MH, Bicker J, Kahrs LA, et al. A dataset of laryngeal endoscopic images with comparative study on convolution neural network-based semantic segmentation. Int J Comput Assist Radiol Surg 2019;14:483–92.

41. Aubreville M, Knipfer C, Oetter N, et al. Automatic Classification of Cancerous Tissue in Laserendomicroscopy Images of the Oral Cavity using Deep Learning. Sci Rep 2017;7(1):11979.
42. Gong J, Holsinger FC, Noel JE, et al. Using deep learning to identify the recurrent laryngeal nerve during thyroidectomy. Sci Rep 2021;11(1):14306.
43. Gao W, Tan KK, Liang W, et al. Intelligent vision guide for automatic ventilation grommet insertion into the tympanic membrane. Int J Med Robot 2016;12(1): 18–31.
44. Miwa T, Minoda R, Yamaguchi T, et al. Application of artificial intelligence using a convolutional neural network for detecting cholesteatoma in endoscopic enhanced images. Auris Nasus Larynx 2022;49(1):11–7.
45. Nwosu O, Suresh K, Lee DJ, et al. Proof-of-Concept Computer Vision Model for Instrument and Anatomy Detection During Transcanal Endoscopic Ear Surgery. Otolaryngol Head Neck Surg 2023;17. https://doi.org/10.1002/ohn.613. Published online December.
46. King D, Adidharma L, Peng H, et al. Automatic summarization of endoscopic skull base surgical videos through object detection and hidden Markov modeling. Comput Med Imaging Graph 2023;108:102248.
47. Paderno A, Villani FP, Sordi A, et al. Deep learning in endoscopy: the importance of standardisation. Acta Otorhinolaryngol Ital 2023;43(6):430–2.
48. Hernandez-Boussard T, Bozkurt S, Ioannidis JPA, et al. MINIMAR (MINimum Information for Medical AI Reporting): Developing reporting standards for artificial intelligence in health care. J Am Med Inform Assoc 2020;27(12):2011–5.
49. Norgeot B, Quer G, Beaulieu-Jones BK, et al. Minimum information about clinical artificial intelligence modeling: the MI-CLAIM checklist. Nat Med 2020;26(9): 1320–4.
50. Mongan J, Moy L, Kahn CE. Checklist for Artificial Intelligence in Medical Imaging (CLAIM): A Guide for Authors and Reviewers. Radiol Artif Intell 2020;2(2): e200029.
51. Deng J, Dong W, Socher R, et al. ImageNet: A large-scale hierarchical image database. In: 2009 IEEE conference on computer vision and pattern recognition. 2009. p. 248–55.
52. Krizhevsky A, Sutskever I, Hinton GE. ImageNet Classification with Deep Convolutional Neural Networks. In: Advances in neural information processing systems. Curran Associates, Inc.; 2012. Available at: https://papers.nips.cc/paper_files/paper/2012/hash/c399862d3b9d6b76c8436e924a68c45b-Abstract.html. [Accessed 7 February 2024].
53. Pogorelov K, Randel KR, Griwodz C, et al. KVASIR: A Multi-Class Image Dataset for Computer Aided Gastrointestinal Disease Detection. In: Proceedings of the 8th ACM on multimedia systems conference. MMSys'17. Association for Computing Machinery; 2017. p. 164–9.
54. Bernal J, Sánchez FJ, Fernández-Esparrach G, et al. WM-DOVA maps for accurate polyp highlighting in colonoscopy: Validation vs. saliency maps from physicians. Computerized Medical Imaging and Graphics 2015;43:99–111.
55. Tajbakhsh N, Gurudu SR, Liang J. Automated Polyp Detection in Colonoscopy Videos Using Shape and Context Information. IEEE Transactions on Medical Imaging 2016;35(2):630–44.
56. Silva J, Histace A, Romain O, et al. Toward embedded detection of polyps in WCE images for early diagnosis of colorectal cancer. Int J CARS 2014;9(2): 283–93.

Computer Vision— Radiomics & Pathognomics

Alexandra T. Bourdillon, MD

KEYWORDS

- Radiomics • Pathognomics • Computer vision • Radiology • Histopathology
- Machine learning • Deep learning

KEY POINTS

- Computer vision or the extraction of salient imaging features has ushered the fields of radiomics and pathognomics for identifying imaging biomarkers of radiographic and histopathologic data.
- Radiomic classifiers have yielded impressive results for detecting distinct tumor pathologic features, such as extranodal extension, and prognostication of various outcomes with the potential to help guide oncologic management.
- Breakthrough pathognomic methods have demonstrated feasible tools for enhancing intraoperative evaluation of tumor margins.
- The majority of studies examine squamous cell carcinomas, although applications exist broadly for other head and neck neoplasms.

INTRODUCTION
An Overview of Artificial Intelligence

Artificial intelligence (AI) is an umbrella term that broadly encompasses a wide array of computational methodologies from traditional statistical inferences such as linear regression to multidimensional non-linear machine learning (ML) methods. A subset of ML, deep learning (DL), is marked by artificial neural networks (ANNs) which consist of an assembly of perceptrons or *nodes* whose relationships are parameterized through learned *weights* determined through a gradient-based back-propagation fitting algorithm on a training dataset.[1] To process images, multilayer ANNs were expanded and named convolutional neural networks (CNNs) for their convoluting windows that sequentially evaluate subregions of an image to extract sub-features from which "high-level" 2-dimensional (2D) and 3-dimensional (3D) relationships are inferred.[2,3] This type of modeling has ultimately given way to the field of computer vision, which has enabled the evolution of self-driving cars, facial recognition, and impressive image classifiers. In medicine, such classifiers yield tremendous

Department of Otolaryngology–Head & Neck Surgery, University of California-San Francisco, San Francisco, CA 94115, USA
E-mail address: alexandra.bourdillon@ucsf.edu

Otolaryngol Clin N Am 57 (2024) 719–751
https://doi.org/10.1016/j.otc.2024.05.003
0030-6665/24/© 2024 Elsevier Inc. All rights reserved, including those for text and data mining, AI training, and similar technologies.

oto.theclinics.com

opportunities for characterizing, detecting, and evaluating pathologies across many disciplines, including radiology, pathology, dermatology, and surgery.

Artificial Intelligence and Otolaryngology

The role of computer vision in otolaryngology spans the breadth of the discipline.[4] Breakthrough discoveries about tumor biology's genomic and transcriptomic drivers have been foundational to our understanding of many head and neck neoplasms. The evolution of extracting radiographic and histopathologic features extends those molecular biomarkers, ushering the fields of *radiomics* and *pathognomics*, both hinging on computer vision techniques.[5] The potential in head and neck pathophysiology is vast, with numerous challenges and opportunities to interpret one of the most anatomically complex and cellularly diverse regions of the body. Already, many studies have spanned diagnosis, prognosis, and prediction of treatment response across critical clinical decisions: surgical, radiation, and systemic therapies.

Most computer vision methods rely on supervised learning in which the desired outcome is explicitly labeled and used to train a model and iteratively perceive the salient features between the data inputs and the outcome(s). The model can be fine-tuned with a validation set before assessing performance on a testing set composed of fresh, unseen inputs. Model performance is frequently evaluated using various biologic and computational metrics such as accuracy (or precision), sensitivity (or recall), specificity, positive predictive value (or precision), and area under the curve (AUC). In some instances, a dataset from another institution or cohort is used independently for *external* validation to evaluate the model's generalizability.

Radiomics & Pathognomics

Altogether, radiomic and pathognomic methods offered promising advancement for integrating complex clinical and pathologic features to aid in diagnosis, patient risk stratification, and potentially guide treatment decisions. However, AI methods are not without their criticisms including vulnerability to noise and limited generalizability to dissimilar datasets. Furthermore, deep learning is especially susceptible to what is referred to as a *black box phenomenon*, which underscores difficulties in interpreting what features the model relies on and, therefore, the inability to leverage human domain expertise for verification. This often introduces a large degree of ambiguity that is generally unacceptable in medicine. Although such limitations are beyond the scope of this article, it is worth mentioning. The remainder of the article will explore cohort studies in head and neck pathologies employing computer vision techniques across radiomic and pathognomic biomarkers, separately. Studies will be listed by type of neoplasm and then further examined in sequence: diagnostic classifiers, other clinicopathologic classifiers, prognostic biomarkers, and predictors of treatment response and adverse events.

RADIOMICS AND OTOLARYNGOLOGY

In head and neck oncology, machine-learning applications of clinicopathologic data have frequently been used to characterize and enhance the prognostication of various tumors. Radiomics methods typically consist of either 1 of 2 methodologies: feature extraction packages that infer tissue properties (ranging from size to texture to computed third-order attributes), or, deep learning algorithms that internalize relevant 2D or 3D features captured by a CNN model (**Fig. 1**).[6] Because of the large number of features that can be extracted, a feature selection process is often used to generate a subset or signature of relevant features. Radiomic methods have the advantage of

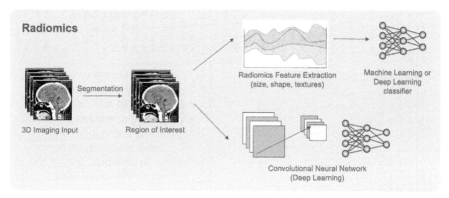

Radiomics

3D Imaging Input → Segmentation → Region of Interest → Radiomics Feature Extraction (size, shape, textures) → Machine Learning or Deep Learning classifier

Convolutional Neural Network (Deep Learning)

Fig. 1. Depiction of radiomic pathways. (Figure created using select icons rendered from Bioicons.com.)

corresponding to inherent tissue properties such as heterogeneity, which in some studies is associated with unfavorable treatment response.[7,8] Furthermore, another methodology has incorporated radiologic analyses across an interval of scans, so called *delta-radiomics*, to detect tumor alterations and responses to treatment. Numerous radiomic studies have determined that models with combination clinical and radiomic inputs outperformed algorithms based on either clinical factors or radiomic features alone.[9–14]

Head & Neck Squamous Cell Carcinoma

Diagnostic and pathologic classifiers

Among radionics-based diagnostic classifiers (**Table 1**) in head & neck squamous cell carcinomas (HNSCCs), MRI-based inputs have been used to distinguish oropharyngeal squamous cell carcinoma (SCC) from lymphoma (AUC of 0.750 in a cohort with 68 oropharyngeal squamous cell carcinomas [OPSCC] tumors and 19 lymphoma),[15] while arterial-phase and venous-phase computed tomography (CT) studies were able to differentiate HNSCC from hyperplasia in a small cohort of 60 SCC and 40 hyperplastic (AUC 0.96).[16] Many studies have examined tumor and lymph node (LN) pathologic features, for example, characterizing histologic grade in HNSCCs (AUC >0.90).[10,17,18] A hybrid radiomic and deep learning method trained on a 124-patient cohort, however, only achieved an AUC of 0.822.[19] Another area of focus has been detecting human papilloma virus (HPV) status. Work by Haider and colleagues devised 360 candidate classification models (6 feature selection methods × 5 machine-learning classification algorithms × 4 volume of interest (VOI) sources of radiomics input × 3 imaging modalities). It ultimately achieved an AUC of 0.83 using tumor and metastatic LN volumes from a PET scans using an XGBoost ML classifier.[20]

Detection of lymph node metastasis has also been widely studied to guide elective neck dissections or irradiation. Kubo and colleagues examined 161 patients with oral tongue SCC who received local treatment and sought to detect level-specific nodal involvement using ML-based classifiers on radiomic features, ultimately achieving an accuracy, precision, recall, and AUC greater than 0.95 each.[21] A fusion method by Chen and colleagues employing radiomics and DL achieved an AUC of 0.95 in detecting LN metastases in oral cavity SCCs (OCSCCs), although with lower specificity and higher sensitivity compared to clinician determinations.[22] Other nodal classifiers ranged in performance.[23,24]

Table 1
Radiomic classifiers for head and neck squamous cell carcinomas tumor and nodal pathologic features

	Tumor Type	Author, Year	Outcome	Imaging Modality	Data Input	Feature Selection	Machine Learning	Deep Learning	Model Type	Cohort Size	Performance
Diagnosis	Oropharyngeal squamous cell carcinoma (OPSCC)	Bae et al,[15] 2020	Classify oropharyngeal lymphoma	MRI	Radiomics features: 19 out of 202 =	Selected twice using 5-fold cross-validation	✓		Elastic-net regularized generalized model (GLM)	n = 87 patients with oropharyngeal SCC (n = 68) and lymphoma (n = 19)	The mean area under the ROC curve (AUC) of the radiomics classifier was 0.750 (95% confidence interval [CI]: 0.613–0.887), with a sensitivity of 84.2%, specificity of 60.3%, and an accuracy of 65.5%. Two human readers yielded AUCs of 0.613 (95% CI, 0.467–0.759) and 0.663 (95% CI, 0.531–0.795), respectively.
Diagnosis	Head and neck squamous cell carcinoma (HNSCC)	Khodrog et al,[16] 2021	Classify squamous cell carcinoma from hyperplasia	CTA, computed tomography venogram (CTV), CECT	Radiomic features	MRMR and LASSO	✓		Multivariate LR	n = 100 (n = 60 with squamous cell carcinoma (SCC) and n = 40 with squamous cell hyperplasia (SCH) split into training group (70%) and test group (30%).	The diagnostic accuracy, specificity, positive predictive value (PPV), negative predictive value (NPV), and AUC values obtained for the training cohort were 0.91, 0.9, 0.93, 0.9, and 0.96 CTA 0.93, 0.93, 0.95, 0.90, and 0.96 computed tomography normal (CTN), and 0.92, 0.87, 0.91, 0.96, and 0.96 CT venogram (CTV).

Tumor Pathologic Feature	OPSCC	HPV status	MRI	Radiomics: 1618 features	LASSO	✓	3 machine learning (ML) classifiers: LR, RF, and XGBoost	n = 60 patients (48 HPV-positive and 12 HPV-negative)	LR And RF classifiers yielded higher accuracy compared with that of the XGboost classifier (AUC: 0.77, 0.76, and 0.71, respectively).
Tumor Pathologic Feature	OPSCC	HPV status	MRI	Radiomics: 77 features from T1-weighted postcontrast images	Mann-Whitney U testing and interclass correlation coefficient	✓	LR; nomogram	n = 153 patients, subdivided into training (91) and test (62)	Model performance showed AUCs of 0.794, 0.764, and 0.871 for the clinical, radiomic, and combined models, respectively.
Tumor Pathologic Feature	OPSCC	HPV status	MRI	Radiomics: 170 features from semi-automatically segmented tumors	LASSO	✓	LR	n = 62 subjects divided into training (n = 43) and test sets (n = 19)	Ultimately using 6 radiomic features, the model achieved an AUC of 0.744 [95% CI, 0.496–0.991] on the testing set.
Tumor Pathologic Feature	OPSCC	HPV Status	MRI	Radiomics: tumor volumes	Mann-Whitney U testing and Pearson correlation	✓	Logistic regression	n = 153, divided into a training (60%, n = 91) and test (40%, n = 62) subset	Models constructed and tested using single-slice delineations (AUC/Sensitivity/Specificity: 0.84/0.75/0.84) perform better compared to 3D experienced observer delineations, 4 mm sphere delineation and largest diameter delineations (AUC 0.76–0.77)

Row author/year labels (first column): Suh et al,[164] 2020 · Bos et al,[11] 2021 · Sohn et al,[165] 2021 · Eos et al,[166] 2022

(continued on next page)

Table 1
(continued)

Tumor Type	Author, Year	Outcome	Imaging Modality	Data Input	Feature Selection	Machine Learning	Deep Learning	Model Type	Cohort Size	Performance
Tumor Pathologic Feature OPSCC	Bagher-Ebadian et al,[167] 2022	HPV Status	CT	Radiomics	LASSO	✓		GLM	n = 128 total patients with known HPV-status (60-HPV+ and 68-HPV-)	Performances for prediction of HPV for the 3 classifiers were Radiomics-Lasso-GLM: AUC/PPV/NPV = 0.789/0.755/0.805; Clinical-Lasso-GLM: 0.676/0.747/0.672, and Integrated/Ensemble-Lasso-GLM: 0.895/0.874/0.844.
Tumor Pathologic Feature OPSCC	Bagher-Ebadian et al,[168] 2020	HPV status	CT	Radiomic: 172 features from pretreatment tumor volumes	Kolmogorov-Smirnov's testing yielding 12 significant features (from 3 categories)	✓		8 different classifiers, including a GLM	187 patients; Group A: 95 patients (19 HPV- and 76 HPV+); Group B: 92 patients (52 HPV- and 40 HPV+) from author institution	The GLM high prediction power was AUC/PPV/NPV = 0.849/0.731/0.788 and AUC/PPV/NPV = 0.869/0.807/0.870 for unseen test datasets for groups A and B, respectively. Radiomic analysis implies that gross tumor volumes for HPV+ patients exhibit higher intensities, smaller lesion size, greater sphericity/roundness, and higher spatial intensity-variation/heterogeneity.

Tumor Pathologic Feature	OPSCC	Haider et al,[20] 2020	HPV status	PET/(CT)	Radiomics	Hierarchical clustering, MRMR, PCA, LR with Ridge regularization and no feature selection	✓ ✓	LR with elastic net regularization, Naive Bayes classifier, RF, SVM, and XGBoost	435 primary tumors (326 for training, 109 for validation) and 741 metastatic cervical lymph nodes (518 for training, 223 for validation)	Among 360 combinations of classifiers, the best model was achieved from the volume model derived from primary tumor and metastatic LNs, validated on an external PET-only MAASTRO cohort, with the XGBoost classifier (AUC of 0.83, 95% CI = 0.68–0.98).
Tumor Path. Feature	OCC: tongue and FOM	Ren et al,[173] 2021	Histologic differentiation Grade	MRI	Radiomics from apparent diffusion coefficient (ADC) maps	LASSO	✓	GLM	n = 88 patients (training cohort: n = 59; testing cohort: n = 29)	The radiomics signature achieved accuracies of 0.78 and 0.79, sensitivities of 0.65 and 0.71, and specificities of 0.85 and 0.82 in the training and testing cohorts, respectively.

(continued on next page)

Table 1
(continued)

Tumor Type	Author, Year	Outcome	Imaging Modality	Data Input	Feature Selection	Machine Learning	Deep Learning	Model Type	Cohort Size	Performance
Tumor Pathologic Feature										
HNSCC	Wu et al,[10] 2019	Histologic differentiation Grade	CT	Radiomics: 670 features	Kernel principal component analysis	✓		RF	n = 206 consecutive HNSCC patients (training cohort: n = 137; testing cohort: n = 69)	A combined radiomic/clinical model (specificity 0.83, accuracy 0.93, sensitivity 0.97, PPV 0.90, NPV 0.92, and AUC 0.97) and a radiomics-only model (specificity 0.83, accuracy 0.92, sensitivity 0.96, PPV 0.94, NPV 0.91, and AUC 0.96) both performed significantly better than a clinical model (specificity 0.38, accuracy 0.68, sensitivity 0.87, PPV 0.69, NPV 0.68, and AUC 0.63).

		Author	Pathologic Feature	Imaging Modality	Feature	Feature Selection		Model	n	Results
Tumor Pathologic Feature	HNSCC	Li et al,[17] 2022	Histologic differentiation Grade	CT: virtual monoenergetic images (VMI) and iodine-based material decomposition images (IMDI)	Radiomics signatures	LASSO selection method with cross-validation and Spearman's rank correlation testing	✓	LR	n = 178 patients (112 in the training and 66 in the validation cohorts)	The tumor location, VMI-signature, and IMDI-signature were associated with the degree of HNSCC differentiation, and AUCs were 0.729, 0.890, and 0.833 in the training cohort and 0.627, 0.859, and 0.843 in the validation cohort, respectively. The nomogram incorporating tumor location and 2 radiomics-signature models yielded the best performance in training (AUC = 0.987) and validation (AUC = 0.968) cohorts.
Tumor Pathologic Feature	HNSCC	Zheng et al,[19] 2023	Histologic differentiation grade	CT	CECT-based manually-extracted radiomics (MER) features and deep learning (DL) features	LASSO and cross-validation	✓	Multivariate LR	n = 204 total (training set with 1 hospital cohort of n = 124, and testing set from external hospital cohort with n = 80)	Ultimately a combination model with 3 MER features and 7 DL features achieved the best performance in distinguishing poorly and moderately-well differentiated lesions: training (AUC, 0.878) and test (AUC, 0.822) sets

(continued on next page)

Table 1
(continued)

Tumor Type	Author, Year	Outcome	Imaging Modality	Data Input	Feature Selection	Machine Learning	Deep Learning	Model Type	Cohort Size	Performance
Tumor & Nodal Pathologic Features HNSCC	Mukherjee et al,[169] 2020	Tumor Grade and Nodal features: LVI, PNI, ENE	CT	Radiomics: 2131 features	PCA	✓		Regularized regression	The Cancer Genome Atlas (n = 113) and an institutional test cohort (n = 71)	In the test cohort, the model achieved a mean AUC of 0.66 for tumor grade, 0.70 for PNI, 0.65 for LVI; 0.67 for ENE, and 0.80 for HPV status.
Nodal Pathologic Features HPV + OPSCC	Kann et al,[26] 2023	ENE	CT	CT volumes of LNs	-		✓	DL: 3D convolutional neural networks (CNN) based on DualNet	178 collected scans obtained from E3311, 313 nodes were annotated: 71 (23%) with ENE in general, 39 (13%) with ENE larger than 1 mm.	DL modeling for ENE identification was superior to each of the 4 specialized head and neck radiologist readers (algorithm AUC 0.857, 95% CI 0.82–0.90; vs 0.63–0.71; $P<.001$).
Nodal Pathologic Features OCSCC	Ariji et al,[28] 2020	ENE	CT	CT Voxels consisting of individual nodes	-		✓	CNN based on AlexNet	n = 51 patients with 703 nodes (178 with ENE and 525 without ENE)	The DL accuracy of ENE was 84.0%. The radiologists' accuracies based on minor axis ≥ 11 mm, central necrosis, and irregular borders were 55.7%, 51.1%, and 62.6%, respectively.

Nodal Pathologic Features	OCSCC	Chen et al,[22] 2023	LN metastasis	CT	Radiomics (1454 features) and DL (3D DenseNet architecture)	LASSO	✓	ML classifiers: SVM, LR, XGBoost, and artificial neural networks	n = 100 patients with OSCC (76 patients for training; 24 patients for test set)	A hybrid model combining deep learning with radiomics showed the best performance (Acc: 89.2%; sensitivity, 92.0%; specificity, 88.9%; and AUC, 0.950 [95% CI: 0.908–0.993, $P<.001$] in the test set. In comparison with the clinicians, the fusion model showed higher sensitivity (92.0 vs 72.0% and 60.0%) but lower specificity (88.9 vs 97.5% and 98.8%).
Nodal Pathologic Features	OCSCC tongue	K Jbo et al,[21] 2022	Occult nodal metastasis	CT	Radiomics: ipsilateral neck levels	LASSO	✓	5 ML classifiers: KNN, SVM, classification and regression tree (CART), (RF), and AdaBoost; each with and without SMOTE	n = 161, including 46 with OCLNM	After applying SMOTE pre-processing, SVM was the best model, with accuracy of 0.96. The precision, recall, and AUC scores were 0.96, 0.95, and 0.98, respectively.

(continued on next page)

Table 1
(continued)

	Tumor Type	Author, Year	Outcome	Imaging Modality	Data Input	Feature Selection	Machine Learning	Deep Learning	Model Type	Cohort Size	Performance
Nodal Pathologic Features	OCSCC: tongue	Konishi & Kakimoto,[170] 2023	LN metastasis	Ultrasound (intraoral)	Radiomics	LASSO	✓		3 ML classifiers: Bootstrap forest (BF), SVM, and neural tanh boost (NTB)	n = 120 patients with tongue cancer who underwent intraoral ultrasonography (30 with cervical lymph node metastasis)	The sensitivity, specificity, accuracy, and AUC in the validation group were, respectively, 0.600, 0.967, 0.875, and 0.923 for the BF model; 0.700, 0.967, 0.900, and 0.950 for the SVM model; and 0.900, 0.967, 0.950, and 0.967 for NTB model.
Nodal Pathologic Features	Laryngeal SCC	Jia et al,[171] 2020	LN metastasis	MRI	Radiomics: from enhanced T1- and T2-weighted sequences	ANOVA and LASSO	✓		Multivariate regression, nomogram	n = 117, subdivided into a training cohort (n = 89) and test cohort (n = 28)	The model yielded an AUC, specificity, and sensitivity of 0.930, 0.930 and 0.875 in the training cohort, and 0.883, 0.889 and 0.800 in the testing cohort.
Nodal Pathologic Features	Laryngeal SCC	Zhao et al,[172] 2023	LN metastasis	CT	Radiomics: 9 features	LASSO	✓		Multivariate LR, nomogram	n = 464; split into primary and validation cohorts at a ratio of 7:3 (325 vs 139).	A radiomics model incorporating independent predictors of LNM (the radiomics signature, tumor subsite, and CT report) detected nodal status significantly better than either the clinical model or the CT report in the primary cohort (AUC 0.91 vs 0.84 vs 0.68) and validation cohort (AUC 0.89 vs 0.83 vs 0.70).

Nodal Pathologic Features	HNSCC or salivary gland carcinoma	Kann et al,[25] 2018	ENE	CT	CT volumes of LNs	-	↘	DL: 3D CNNs based on BoxNet, SmallNet, and DualNet	n = 270 with preoperative scans and in total 653 lymph nodes were segmented in total (range: 1–5 per patient): 380 negative nodes, 153 NM without ENE, and 120 NM with ENE	For ENE prediction (n = 98 LNs), the DLNN demonstrated AUC: 0.91 (95% CI: 0.85–0.97), (accuracy: 85.7%, sensitivity: 0.88, FNR rate: 0.12, specificity: 0.85, FPR: 0.15, PPV: 0.66, and NPV: 0.95), outperforming the random forest model (AUC: 0.88, 95% CI: 0.81–0.95), and the benchmark model (AUC: 0.81, 95% CI: 0.76–0.86). For NM prediction (n = 131), the DLNN (AUC: 0.91, 95% CI: 0.86–0.96); the random forest model (AUC: 0.91, 95% CI: 0.86–0.97), and benchmark model (AUC: 0.86, 95% CI: 0.83–0.89) performed similarly.
Nodal Pathologic Features	HNSCC	Wang et al,[24] 2022	LN metastasis	MRI	Radiomic features: 48 examined features from nodes, ADC, and node size	Nonparametric testing	↘	Linear combination of inputs	120 lymph node volumes	The AUC value of 0.797 for radiomics was better than that of lymph node size (AUC 0.71) and ADC (AUC: 0.638). The AUC of the predicted value from the combined model was 0.81

(continued on next page)

Table 1
(continued)

Tumor Type	Author, Year	Outcome	Imaging Modality	Data Input	Feature Selection	Machine Learning	Deep Learning	Model Type	Cohort Size	Performance
Nodal Pathologic Features	Bardosi et al,[23] 2022	LN metastasis, ENE	CT	Radiomics	Eliminative feature selection: sparse discriminant analysis and genetic optimization	✓		Linear discriminant analysis	Total of 252 LNs; including n-182 pathologic, and 52 additionally with ENE	The combination of sparse discriminant analysis and genetic optimization retained up to 90% of the classification accuracy with only 10% of the original numbers of features.
Nodal Pathologic Features	Kann et al,[27] 2020	ENE	CT	CT volumes of LNs	NA		✓	DL: 3D CNN based on DualNet	n = 270 patients (653 LNs) and tested on 2 external datasets: Mt Sinai cohort (n = 82, 130 LNs) and TCIA-TCGA cohort (n = 62, 70 LNs)	AUC of the DL algorithm was superior to that of 2 specialized head and neck radiologist observers (P=.01 [DL v R1]; P=.02 [DL v R2]) for the external institution data set. For the TCIA-TCGA data set, AUC of DL algorithm was superior to R1 (P<.0001), and similar to R2 (P = .16).

| Nodal Pathologic Features | HNSCC | Chen et al,[68] 2019 | LN metastasis | PET/CT | Radiomics: 257 features and nodal voxels for CNN input | Many-objective optimization algorithm | ✓ | ✓ | 3D-CNN, conventional radiomics, hybrid model, XmasNet, and MaO-radiomics model | n = 59 patients with HNC; subdivided into training (n = 41 patients, including 85 involved nodes, 55 suspicious nodes, and 30 normal nodes) and validation set (n = 18 patients, with 22 involved nodes, 27 suspicious nodes, and 17 normal nodes) | The hybrid method achieved an accuracy of 0.88 withXmasNet compared to 0.81 and 0.75 with 2 radiomics methods. |

Abbreviations: Acc, accuracy; ANOVA, analysis of variance; CECT, contrast enhanced computed tomography; CTA, computed tomography angiogram; DLNN, deep learning neural network; ENE, extranodal extension; FNR, false negative rate; FOM, floor of mouth; FPR, false positive rate; HPV, human papilloma virus; KNN, k-nearest neighbors; LASSO, least absolute shrinkage and selection operator; LN, lymph node; LR, logistic regression; LVI, lymphvascular invasion; MRMR, minimum redundancy maximum relevance; NM, nodal metastases; OCLNM, occult lymph node metastases; PCA, principle component analysis; PNI, perineural invasion; RF, random forest; SMOTE, synthetic minority oversampling technique; SVMs, support vector machine; TCIA, the cancer imaging archive; TCGA, the canger genome atlas; XGBoost, extreme gradient boosting.

Extranodal extension (ENE) classification is another potentially treatment-altering diagnosis, and radiographic evaluation has been challenging even for expert eyes. Kann and colleagues trained DL models in a cohort of 270 subjects and 653 LNs using CT volumes of lymph nodes and 3D CNNs, which outperformed specialized head and neck radiologists (AUC: 0.91, 95% confidence interval [CI]: 0.85–0.97, vs AUC: 0.81, 95% CI: 0.76–0.86).[25] The same group externally validated their results. It demonstrated significantly better detection of ENE by the DL algorithm compared to human experts in separate studies: on a subset of from the E3311 trial (311 nodes from 178 subjects) with an AUC of 0.857[26] and additional datasets from Mt. Sinai (n = 82, 130 LNs) and also the Cancer Genome Atlas, or TCGA, (n = 62, 70 LNs).[27] Ariji and colleagues similarly developed a CNN algorithm that was superior to radiologist predictions (accuracy of 84% compared to 55%–63%).[28]

Prognostic and predictive classifiers

Dozens of studies have examined radiographic markers for various oncologic outcomes: locoregional recurrence, overall survival (OS), progression-free survival (PFS), nodal failure, which are captured in detail in Supplementary Table 1. Additionally, many studies investigate sensitivity or response to specific treatments, such as radiotherapy (RT), induction chemotherapy (IC), concurrent treatments, or some combination of chemoradiotherapy (CRT), which are captured in Supplementary Table 2.

Oropharyngeal squamous cell carcinomas. By tumor subtype, OPSCCs are among the most examined head & neck tumors using computer vision techniques. Park and colleagues developed an ML classifier using MRI radiomic features that reliably prognosticated disease recurrence (AUC 0.86) and OS (AUC: 0.82), and was superior to predictions regarding HPV status, and other pathologic features.[29] Cheng and colleagues integrated a DL-based methodology on tumor volumes from fluorodeoxyglucose (FDG)-PET/CT with clinical risk factors that was able to reliably prognosticate 5-year OS (AUC at 5 years: 0.801 [95% CI: 0.727–0.874]).[30] Multivariate regression radiomic textures of both primary tumors and metastatic lymph nodes have been shown to successfully stratify OPSCC patients.[31]

Varied results have been reported by ML radiomic classifiers for prognosis of HNCs across MRI,[32–34] CT[31,35–38] or PET-CT[39] data inputs. A preliminary study (n = 124) by Giraud and colleagues investigated the benefit tumor shape and tissue uniformity in predicting locoregional recurrence at 18 months after RT (accuracy: 0.64, PPV 0.92).[40] A delta-radiomic study by Lafata and colleagues showed that intra-treatment radiomics features of the tumor volume from interval FDG-PET/CT scans (2 weeks into a 7-week RT treatment) were more prognostic than baseline scans in predicting recurrence-free survival.[41]

Hypopharyngeal squamous cell carcinomas. In prognosticating SCCs of the hypopharynx, integration of radiomic features enhanced clinical models of.[42] Among the most reliable PFS classifiers is a radiomic logistic regression (AUC: 0.80, accuracy: 0.70), outperforming other ML algorithms.[43,44] Lin and colleagues demonstrated that mid-treatment CT features of peritumoral and intratumoral volumes outperformed pre-treatment features in predicting PFS and OS after definitive RT.[45]

Laryngeal squamous cell carcinomas. A k-nearest neighbor algorithm highly discriminated early recurrence in a cohort of 140 laryngeal SCCs (AUC 0.936) compared to other ML algorithms (AUC 0.79–0.86) using 4 CT-feature signature.[46] In a cohort of 136 patients (testing n = 40), Chen and colleagues developed a CT-radiomics model that relied on 3 texture features and was able to outperform cancer staging in prognosticating overall survival (c-index, 0.913 vs 0.699; *P* =.019).[47] Preliminary studies have suggested that other imaging features may be predictive.[48]

Oral cavity squamous cell carcinomas. A model by Liu and colleagues demonstrated that MRI-based radiomics outperformed clinical modeling in prognosticating PFS in oral tongue SCCs (AUC: 0.870, 95% CI [0.761–0.942] vs AUC: 0.730, 95% CI [0.602–0.835], *P* = .033).[12] Certain gray-distributions and texture features are also strongly associated with survival outcomes.[36]

Head & neck squamous cell carcinomas. Many additional studies have examined HNSCCs generally or across other subsites, spanning a variety of image processing, feature extraction, and machine learning techniques. Some have yielded great promise, demonstrating that an MRI-based radiomic signature outperformed TNM staging in prognosticating OS[49] or that pre-treatment FDG-PET/CT features better predicted local failure after CRT compared to clinical variables alone (c-index 0.76 vs 0.65).[50] Wang and colleagues developed a multi-class model for prognosticating locoregional recurrence after CRT from pre-treatment and post-treatment PET/CT scans, achieving an AUC of 0.75 to 0.77 on 2 distinct datasets.[51] Some studies have further sought to extrapolate guidance on clinical therapy: Ou and colleagues showed that combination of HPV status and 24-feature CT radiomic signature significantly improved risk stratification of locally advanced HNSCC warranting benefit from CRT over bioradiotherapy (BRT).[52]

Novel strategies in image segmentation volumes that are generated from radiotherapy targets have given way to generation of *dosiomic* features. Using this strategy, Pan and colleagues demonstrated in a cohort of 228 patients that dosiomics outperformed traditional radiomic features from gross tumor volumes, especially when combined with clinical factors (c-index 0.766 vs 0.624, *P*<.0001 via Wilcoxon test).[53] Wu and colleagues showed that integration of dosiomic and tumor radiomic features from PET/CT scans enhanced multivariate modeling of locoregional recurrence after intensity-modulated radiotherapy, yielding a c-index 0.66 versus 0.59 for radiomics alone (*P*<.001).[54]

Fluoromisonidazole positron emission tomography (FMISO-PET) has risen as another promising imaging modality, due to its ability to capture hypoxic features. Sorensen and colleagues showed that tumor hypoxic features detected from significantly predicted overall survival outcome after CRT, especially when comparing the decrease in non-uniformity features from pre-treatment scans to the second week of treatment (*P*=.04, hazard ratio [HR] = 9.4).[55] Larger cohort studies using FMISO-PET/CT predicted 2-year locoregional control after radiotherapy alone with an AUC of 0.59 on a 47-subject validation cohort.[56] Carles and colleagues examined radiomic features from FMISO-PET/CT scans at intervals of week 0, 2, and 5 during definitive CRT and determined that specifically low gray zone emphasis texture at weeks 2 and 5 reliably predicted PFS with an AUC of 0.79 to 0.80, although they did not validate their data on untrained inputs.[57] Similarly, Beichel and colleagues examined interval scans and demonstrated that peritumoral signals from pre-RT FDG-PET/CT and post-RT FDG-PET/CT scans in a cohort of 58 subjects and showed significant prediction of PFS (HR: 1.95, 95% CI: 1.27–2.99).[58]

Still many studies have reported that ML classifiers are less reliable than traditional methods. For example, Keek and colleagues reported that a clinical model outperformed a random survival forest model trained on peritumoral radiomic features in predicting distant metastasis in stage III-IV HNSCC after CRT.[59] Gangil and colleagues also showed that a clinical-radiomic classifier for post-radiotherapy outcomes performed similarly to a clinical model, both of which outperformed the CT-radiomic model alone.[60] Zhai and colleagues showed that clinical models faired similarly to CT-based image biomarkers from tumor and nodal volumes in HNSCC patients treated with CRT, across multiple outcomes: local control (c-index: 0.62 for both), regional control (c-index: 0.76 for clinical, 0.80 for radiomic), distant metastasis-free survival (c-index: 0.70 for clinical, 0.68 for radiomic) and also disease-free survival (c-index: 0.66 for clinical, 0.65 for radiomic).[61] However, the same group showed that radiomic and combined imaging and clinical model outperformed the clinical model on an external validation cohort (c-index 0.71 vs c-index 0.57, $P=.0005$).[62]

Additionally, models combining radiomic features from both tumor and lymph node volumes have yielded mixed results. Bogowicz and colleagues reported marginal benefit when compared to primary tumor volumes alone (c-index 0.67 vs 0.63).[63] The same group also examined radiosensitivity in a small cohort (n = 40) using tumor sub-volumes from CT scans.[8] Studies examining nodal failure in isolation[64,65] remain limited.

Interestingly, some models exhibited divergent performance on distinct subsites. For example, Mes and colleagues demonstrated that a selection of 50 MRI radiomic features was more prognostic for oropharyngeal cancer for both overall survival (AUC 0.81) and recurrence-free survival (AUC: 0.78) compared to oral cavity cancer (AUC 0.72 and 0.74, respectively).[66]

Deep learning methods have been sparsely employed and with variable performance. Starke and colleagues trained a 3D-CNN ensemble method on 206 subjects for predicting locoregional tumor control after definitive CRT, and achieved a c-index of 0.31 on a validation cohort of 85 subjects.[67] A hybrid radiomic-CNN methodology was able to detect PET/CT features consistent with lymph node involvement with an accuracy of 0.88.[68]

Predicting treatment complications
Other studies have yet examined the risk of adverse events such as post-treatment xerostomia[69–72] and ototoxicity.[73,74] Such insights can inform semi-automated registration of image-guided radiation therapy[75] to mitigate such risks.

Other Neoplasms

Sinonasal malignancies
Among other radiomic studies of head and neck neoplasms, sinonasal tumors have been among the most commonly studied.[76] Reliable classifiers based on MRI radiomic features have achieved AUC 0.80 to 0.96 for discriminating benign and malignant sinonasal tumors,[77,78] distinguishing high-grade and low-grade tumors,[79] classifying T stage,[80] and prognosticating PFS,[81,82] OS,[83,84] and response to induction chemotherapy.[85,86] Lin and colleagues used a deep learning algorithm to generate automated segmentations from preoperative MRIs to extract radiomic features that would predict recurrence-free survival of advanced sinonasal SCCs with an AUC of 0.854 (95% CI: 0.749–0.927).[87] A radiogenomic study by Gao and colleagues showed that a 24-feature radiomic signature for PFS was significantly correlated with expression of certain genes: CDKL2, PLIN5, and SPAG1.[88] Furthermore, Zhang and colleagues investigated imaging biomarkers from pretreatment MRI scans and digital histopathologic slides, and predicted treatment failure in patients with nasopharynageal carcinoma with a c-index of 0.834 on an external validation dataset. Their analysis also showed a correlation between tumor texture features and chromatin remodeling pathways.[89] Finally, similar radiologic techniques have been employed for nasopharyngeal lymphoma.[90]

Thyroid & salivary tumors

ML classifiers use CT radiomic features of papillary thyroid cancers (PTCs) for enhanced diagnosis,[91] and detection of thyroid capsule invasion[92,93] and lymph node metastasis.[94–97] CNN-based algorithms for detecting PTC have been promising with both ultrasound (accuracy of 93.5%) [98] and CT-inputs (AUC 0.81–0.84).[99] Zhu and colleagues developed an ANN model on Doppler ultrasound features to classify malignant thyroid nodules with an AUC of 0.898. A radiogenomic study by Tong and colleagues showed that ultrasound-based radiomic features reliably predicted lymph node involvement (AUC 0.831 on validation cohort) and correlated with telomere maintenance and cell-cell adhesion gene expression.[100] Similarly, Liu and colleagues used preoperative ultrasound studies in 450 PTC patients and predicted lymph node involvement with an AUC of 0.727 on a validation dataset.[101] A CNN-based risk prediction of thyroid cancer using ultrasonography independently predicted BRAFV600 E mutation, in addition to older age and smaller size.[102]

Parotid tumors have been frequently studied using various ML[103] and DL[104] methods. In a study of 57 patients with various parotid gland tumors (including pleomorphic adenomas, Warthin tumors, and malignancies), Vernuccio and colleagues showed that MRI-based texture analysis outperformed general radiologists but not subspecialized radiologists in detecting malignancies. The authors reported similar accuracies when distinguishing pleomorphic adenomas from Warthin tumors.[105] Radiomic signatures from T1-weighted and T2-weighted MRIs of 38 patients with parotid malignancies yielded an accuracy of 97.5% when using 4-fold cross-validation testing.[106] While another ML classifier trained on and tested on 298 patient MRIs achieved an accuracy of 80.8% compared to 49.2% by a radiologist.[107] In a study on FDG-PET/CT features from a cohort of 75 patients with minor salivary gland carcinomas, a prognostic model based on maximum standardized uptake value (SUV_{max}) and certain imaging features in combination with N-classification, outperformed traditional American Joint Committee on Cancer (AJCC) staging when prognosticating overall survival (c-index 0.83 vs vs 0.65, $P=.005$).[108]

Other disorders

Initial studies characterizing vestibular schwannomas have demonstrated some potential in detecting tumor histology[109] and predicting tumor enlargement[110] and radiosensitivity.[111] Still other radiomic applications exist across vestibular aqueduct syndromes,[112] Meniere's disease,[113] middle ear disorders,[114] inverted papilloma,[115] and sialadenitis.[116] An ML classifier was also able to detect occult nodes with an AUC of 0.734 using a cohort of 8466 individuals from the national cancer database.[117]

PATHOGNOMICS AND OTOLARYNGOLOGY

Advances in digital pathology including whole sliding imaging (WSI) and multiomic assays have given way to computer vision and the development of histopathologic biomarkers.[118–120] CNNs have been used to diagnose and prognosticate head and neck cancers using Hematoxylin and Eosin (H&E) staining or other immunohistochemistry (IHC) biomarkers, so-called *optical biopsy*. Hyperspectral imaging (HSI) is another quantitative technique that enhances a 2D spatial image with spectral information related to absorption, reflect or fluorescence across multiple wavelengths, constructing a 3D data cube. HSI among other modalities has been used to elucidate tumor microenvironment (TME) and the profile of immune cells such as Tumor-Infiltrating Lymphocytes (TILs).[118,119,121] Furthermore, CNNs and other DL methods have been applied to diagnosing oral carcinoma from benign or precancerous lesions.[122,123] Intra-operative tissue evaluation for surgical margin status has also unleashed new opportunities for ensuring tumor clearance that may have profound implications.

Head & Neck Squamous Cell Carcinoma

Tumor classification

DL methods complement the imaging data that are generated in histopathology. Halicek and colleagues developed a CNN pathognomic classifier with HSI inputs to detect SCCs (AUC: 0.82–0.92, Accuracy: 0.74–0.81) and thyroid cancers (AUC 0.95, Accuracy: 0.88–0.92).[124–126] Hybrid CNN models using RGB (red, green, blue) images and HSI have yielded similar results.[127] Similarly, polarized HSI data inputs reliably detect SCC using ML[128] and DL methods[129] with accuracies ranging 79% to 96%. Multispectral narrow-band imaging has also been shown to detect OPSCC better than white light endoscopy (AUC>0.80 vs AUC<0.55, P<.0001).[130]

Pathognomic methods have also been applied to stratify risk of malignant transformation in precancerous lesions. In a multicenter cohort of 759 H&E slides of oral leukoplakia, Cai and colleagues showed that a hybrid DL/ML pathognomic model predicted malignant transformation better than traditional dysplasia grading (AUC 0.899 vs 0.743 on the validation subset of 196 subjects).[131] A separate study by Zhang and colleagues showed that a CNN-based model of H&E slides was able to significantly stratify 5-year malignant transformation of oral leukoplakia even after controlling for age, site, and dysplasia grading (HR = 4.52, 1.5–13.7).[132] Yuan and colleagues developed a CNN method using optical coherence tomography, classifying OCSCC with an AUC of 0.92.[133]

The implications of HPV-driven disease, especially within OPSCCs, have led to the development of automated HPV classifiers. Digital HPV-classifiers have shown to achieve AUCs ranging from 0.79 to 0.92 across multiple studies.[134] CNN algorithms based on ISH (in situ hybridization) assays have also yielded comparable performance (accuracy > 90% when compared to pathologists).[135] Weyers and colleagues trialed an ML classifier for detecting p16+ OPSCC intraoperatively using extracted image features from da Vinci integrated fluorescence imaging during transoral robotic surgery (TORS).[136] Other pathologic factors such as perineural invasion (PNI) have also been modeled with DL algorithms with an accuracy of 89.0%.[137] (**Fig. 2**).

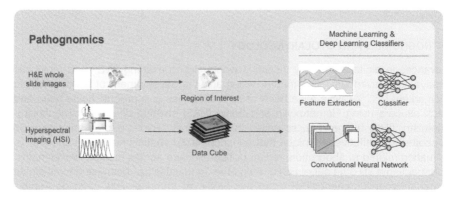

Fig. 2. Depiction of pathognomic pathways. (Figure created using select icons rendered from Bioicons.com.)

Tumor microenvironment characteristics

The tumor microenvironment (TME) interface as a critical prognosticator and predictor of treatment response yields distinct opportunities for guiding management and therapeutic de-escalation. Sharma and colleagues studied a cohort of 462 patients from TCGA-HNSC and used compressed spatially represented patches of H&E WSIs to train a CNN model to predict RNA-seq gene expression of 10 distinct genes that span various immunologic and gene regulatory functions.[138]

Prognostication

A computerized tumor multinucleation index (MuNI) derived from automated segmentations of H&E WSI was validated to prognosticate survival outcomes and anti-tumor immune suppression in *P*16+ OPSCC.[139,140] Among HNSCCs, Chen and colleagues determined that ML models trained on extracted histopathological imaging features significantly correlate with transcriptional subtypes and can enhance prognostication of 5-year OS.[141] CNN modeling of Cyclin-D1 expression patterns has been shown to prognosticate OS and PFS in HPV- OCSCC and OPSCCs.[142] Hue and colleagues examined digital pathology texture features associated with 5-year disease-free survival in HPV + OPSCCs.[143] Klein and colleagues demonstrated that CNN-based stratification of HPV status was not only reliable but also clinically prognostic of 5-year survival, outperforming molecular HPV testing.[144] The same group reported similar prognostication benefit across 3 distinct validation cohorts.[145]

To date only 1 study has studied treatment response by way of scoring immune marker (such as PD-L1) expression in an automated fashion. Puladi and colleagues integrated 3 distinct DL methods combining tumor classification, cell classification, and ultimately inference of the tumor proportion score (percentage of tumor cells expressing PD-L1), achieving a concordance with human experts of 0.84.[146]

Surgical margin status

Computer vision techniques in fresh pathologic slides hold incredible promise for intraoperative margin assessments. A preliminary study by Lu and colleagues demonstrated that ML classifiers using HSI from 450 to 900 nm wavelengths of fresh surgical specimens from a cohort of 36 HNC patients were significantly more reliable in distinguishing cancer from benign tissue compared to imaging modalities such as autofluorescence, and other dyes.[147] Halicek and colleagues also examined HSI on fresh surgical specimens, and developed CNN models that achieved an AUC of 0.80 to 0.95 in detecting carcinoma.[148,149] Others have shown that HIS is reliable in tongue tumor detection using HSI.

In in-vivo specimens, Dittberner and colleagues published a proof of trial using confocal laser endomicroscopy to distinguish neoplastic and non-neoplastic tissue intraoperatively with an AUC of 0.50 to 0.94.[150] Another technique for intraoperative imaging is Raman scattering microscopy.[151]

Other neoplasms

Pathognomic techniques have been sparsely studied across other neoplasms, although with impressive performance among sinonasal tumors. CNN approaches have been used to classify nasopharyngeal cancers (NPCs) using H&E WSIs (AUC 0.905–0.972)[152] and anti-Epstein-Barr virus (EBV) immunofluorescence assays (AUC 0.926 for the model vs 0.821 for human performance).[153] Additionally, H&E features have enhanced prognostication of 5-year PFS (c-index: 0.723), superseding both EBV DNA (c-index: 0.612) and N staging (c-index: 0.593).[154] Additional studies have also examined nasal polyps.[155,156]

Among thyroid pathology, ML models have proven to perform comparably to humans in classifying malignancy from fine-needle aspiration (FNA) biopsies with high concordance (AUC 0.932 and k-score of 0.924).[157,158] A general model for diagnosing goiters, adenomas, and medullary and follicular thyroid carcinomas in addition to PTCs was able to achieve AUCs 0.822 to 0.994 across all subclasses.[159] DL models on liquid-based FNA predictions of low-risk papillary thyroid microcarcinoma performed slightly worse (AUC: 0.850), but still superior to humans.[160] HSI was shown to identify aggressive histopathologic features using fresh surgical specimens in PTCs.[161] CNNs have also been trained to classify rates of mutations such as telomerase reverse transcriptase promoter mutations (sensitivity 99.9% and specificity 60%) in thyroid cancers[162] and BRAF (V600 E) mutations in papillary thyroid carcinoma (accuracy 87%, sensitivity 91% and specificity 71%).[163]

SUMMARY

Applications of computer vision in radiologic and histopathologic inputs are varied in data inputs, pre-processing, feature selection, model architecture, and ultimately also performance. The sea of studies and reporting of results can be difficult to interpret, but a few principles stand out. Robust cohort curation including data protocolization, normalization, and pre-processing techniques in conjuction with a sizable, balanced dataset are requisite for ensuring wider generalizability. Study designs with very precise outcomes or tumor subtypes are advantageous and multi-class classifiers may risk performance without augmentation of suspected correlates. Head-to-head comparisons are needed to evaluate which distinct imaging modalities (MRI vs ultrasound vs PET/CT, etc.) or model architectures are superior, because no one methodology appears distinctly more reliable based on standard criteria. While ML radiomic classifiers are more commonly developed than DL methodologies for characterizing HNCs, many studies evaluating NPCs, thyroid, and salivary gland lesions employ DL algorithms. Comparatively, pathognomic studies benefit from the possibility of generating up to dozens or even hundreds of highly enriched imaging inputs for training DL models, which are frequently employed. However, the nature of using replicate samples can compromise the model's overall generalizability. Altogether, the most promising revelations include the benefit of merging multiple data inputs such as clinical and radiomic or pathognomic. Ultimately, we must engineer sophisticated ways of integrating multidimensional data from various inputs across multiple timepoints (ie, pre- and post-treatment) for the most comprehensive characterization of disease features and prognosis.

CLINICS CARE POINTS

- ML and DL methods can be applied widely but generally succeed when tasked with classifying specific traits.
- Hybrid methods using imaging and clinicopathologic features generally outperform models using clinical data alone.
- Multi-institutional studies are needed to assess the generalizability of such methods in new contexts.

DISCLOSURES

The author has nothing to disclose.

SUPPLEMENTARY DATA

Supplementary data related to this article can be found online at https://doi.org/10.1016/j.otc.2024.05.003.

REFERENCES

1. Zhang Z, Beck MW, Winkler DA, et al. Opening the black box of neural networks: methods for interpreting neural network models in clinical applications. Ann Transl Med 2018;6(11):216.
2. Albawi S, Mohammed TA, Al-Zawi S. Understanding of a convolutional neural network. In: 2017 International Conference on engineering and technology (ICET). 2017. p. 1–6.
3. Yamashita R, Nishio M, Do RKG, et al. Convolutional neural networks: an overview and application in radiology. Insights Imaging 2018;9(4):611–29.
4. Crowson MG, Ranisau J, Eskander A, et al. A contemporary review of machine learning in otolaryngology-head and neck surgery. Laryngoscope 2020;130(1):45–51.
5. Peng Z, Wang Y, Wang Y, et al. Application of radiomics and machine learning in head and neck cancers. Int J Biol Sci 2021;17(2):475–86.
6. Bibault JE, Xing L, Giraud P, et al. Radiomics: A primer for the radiation oncologist. Cancer Radiother 2020;24(5):403–10.
7. Ulrich EJ, Menda Y, Boles Ponto LL, et al. FLT PET Radiomics for Response Prediction to Chemoradiation Therapy in Head and Neck Squamous Cell Cancer. Tomography 2019;5(1):161–9.
8. Bogowicz M, Pavic M, Riesterer O, et al. Targeting Treatment Resistance in Head and Neck Squamous Cell Carcinoma - Proof of Concept for CT Radiomics-Based Identification of Resistant Sub-Volumes. Front Oncol 2021;11:664304.
9. Wang K, Zhou Z, Wang R, et al. A multi-objective radiomics model for the prediction of locoregional recurrence in head and neck squamous cell cancer. Med Phys 2020;47(10):5392–400.
10. Wu W, Ye J, Wang Q, et al. CT-Based Radiomics Signature for the Preoperative Discrimination Between Head and Neck Squamous Cell Carcinoma Grades. Front Oncol 2019;9:821.
11. Bos P, van den Brekel MWM, Gouw ZAR, et al. Clinical variables and magnetic resonance imaging-based radiomics predict human papillomavirus status of oropharyngeal cancer. Head Neck 2021;43(2):485–95.
12. Liu J, Song L, Zhou J, et al. Prediction of Prognosis of Tongue Squamous Cell Carcinoma Based on Clinical MR Imaging Data Modeling. Technol Cancer Res Treat 2023;22:15330338231207006.
13. Franzese C, Lillo S, Cozzi L, et al. Predictive value of clinical and radiomic features for radiation therapy response in patients with lymph node-positive head and neck cancer. Head Neck 2023;45(5):1184–93.
14. Mo X, Wu X, Dong D, et al. Prognostic value of the radiomics-based model in progression-free survival of hypopharyngeal cancer treated with chemoradiation. Eur Radiol 2020;30(2):833–43.
15. Bae S, Choi YS, Sohn B, et al. Squamous Cell Carcinoma and Lymphoma of the Oropharynx: Differentiation Using a Radiomics Approach. Yonsei Med J 2020;61(10):895–900.

16. Khodrog OA, Cui F, Xu N, et al. Prediction of squamous cell carcinoma cases from squamous cell hyperplasia in throat lesions using CT radiomics model. Saudi Med J 2021;42(3):284–92.

17. Li Z, Liu Z, Guo Y, et al. Dual-energy CT-based radiomics nomogram in predicting histological differentiation of head and neck squamous carcinoma: a multi-center study. Neuroradiology 2022;64(2):361–9.

18. Ren J, Qi M, Yuan Y, et al. Radiomics of apparent diffusion coefficient maps to predict histologic grade in squamous cell carcinoma of the oral tongue and floor of mouth: a preliminary study. Acta Radiol 2021;62(4):453–61.

19. Zheng YM, Che JY, Yuan MG, et al. A CT-Based Deep Learning Radiomics Nomogram to Predict Histological Grades of Head and Neck Squamous Cell Carcinoma. Acad Radiol 2023;30(8):1591–9.

20. Haider SP, Mahajan A, Zeevi T, et al. PET/CT radiomics signature of human papilloma virus association in oropharyngeal squamous cell carcinoma. Eur J Nucl Med Mol Imag 2020;47(13):2978–91.

21. Kubo K, Kawahara D, Murakami Y, et al. Development of a radiomics and machine learning model for predicting occult cervical lymph node metastasis in patients with tongue cancer. Oral Surg Oral Med Oral Pathol Oral Radiol 2022; 134(1):93–101.

22. Chen Z, Yu Y, Liu S, et al. A deep learning and radiomics fusion model based on contrast-enhanced computer tomography improves preoperative identification of cervical lymph node metastasis of oral squamous cell carcinoma. Clin Oral Invest 2023;28(1):39.

23. Bardosi ZR, Dejaco D, Santer M, et al. Benchmarking Eliminative Radiomic Feature Selection for Head and Neck Lymph Node Classification. Cancer 2022;14(3):477.

24. Wang Y, Yu T, Yang Z, et al. Radiomics based on magnetic resonance imaging for preoperative prediction of lymph node metastasis in head and neck cancer: Machine learning study. Head Neck 2022;44(12):2786–95.

25. Kann BH, Aneja S, Loganadane GV, et al. Pretreatment Identification of Head and Neck Cancer Nodal Metastasis and Extranodal Extension Using Deep Learning Neural Networks. Sci Rep 2018;8(1):14036.

26. Kann BH, Likitlersuang J, Bontempi D, et al. Screening for extranodal extension in HPV-associated oropharyngeal carcinoma: evaluation of a CT-based deep learning algorithm in patient data from a multicentre, randomised de-escalation trial. Lancet Digit Health 2023;5(6):e360–9.

27. Kann BH, Hicks DF, Payabvash S, et al. Multi-Institutional Validation of Deep Learning for Pretreatment Identification of Extranodal Extension in Head and Neck Squamous Cell Carcinoma. J Clin Oncol 2020;38(12):1304–11.

28. Ariji Y, Sugita Y, Nagao T, et al. CT evaluation of extranodal extension of cervical lymph node metastases in patients with oral squamous cell carcinoma using deep learning classification. Oral Radiol 2020;36(2):148–55.

29. Park YM, Lim JY, Koh YW, et al. Machine learning and magnetic resonance imaging radiomics for predicting human papilloma virus status and prognostic factors in oropharyngeal squamous cell carcinoma. Head Neck 2022;44(4): 897–903.

30. Cheng NM, Yao J, Cai J, et al. Deep Learning for Fully Automated Prediction of Overall Survival in Patients with Oropharyngeal Cancer Using FDG-PET Imaging. Clin Cancer Res 2021;27(14):3948–59.

31. Chang YS, Nair JR, McDougall CC, et al. Risk Stratification for Oropharyngeal Squamous Cell Carcinoma Using Texture Analysis on CT - A Step Beyond HPV Status. Can Assoc Radiol J 2023;74(4):657–66.

32. Bos P, van den Brekel MWM, Taghavi M, et al. Simple delineations cannot substitute full 3d tumor delineations for MR-based radiomics prediction of locoregional control in oropharyngeal cancer. Eur J Radiol 2022;148:110167.

33. Bos P, Martens RM, de Graaf P, et al. External validation of an MR-based radiomic model predictive of locoregional control in oropharyngeal cancer. Eur Radiol 2023;33(4):2850–60.

34. Boot PA, Mes SW, de Bloeme CM, et al. Magnetic resonance imaging based radiomics prediction of Human Papillomavirus infection status and overall survival in oropharyngeal squamous cell carcinoma. Oral Oncol 2023;137:106307.

35. Kwan JYY, Su J, Huang SH, et al. Radiomic Biomarkers to Refine Risk Models for Distant Metastasis in HPV-related Oropharyngeal Carcinoma. Int J Radiat Oncol Biol Phys 2018;102(4):1107–16.

36. Ling X, Alexander GS, Molitoris J, et al. Identification of CT-based non-invasive radiomic biomarkers for overall survival prediction in oral cavity squamous cell carcinoma. Sci Rep 2023;13(1):21774.

37. Choi Y, Nam Y, Jang J, et al. Prediction of Human Papillomavirus Status and Overall Survival in Patients with Untreated Oropharyngeal Squamous Cell Carcinoma: Development and Validation of CT-Based Radiomics. AJNR Am J Neuroradiol 2020;41(10):1897–904.

38. Song B, Yang K, Garneau J, et al. Radiomic Features Associated With HPV Status on Pretreatment Computed Tomography in Oropharyngeal Squamous Cell Carcinoma Inform Clinical Prognosis. Front Oncol 2021;11:744250.

39. Xu H, Abdallah N, Marion JM, et al. Radiomics prognostic analysis of PET/CT images in a multicenter head and neck cancer cohort: investigating ComBat strategies, sub-volume characterization, and automatic segmentation. Eur J Nucl Med Mol Imag 2023;50(6):1720–34.

40. Giraud P, Giraud P, Nicolas E, et al. Interpretable Machine Learning Model for Locoregional Relapse Prediction in Oropharyngeal Cancers. Cancers 2020; 13(1):57.

41. Lafata KJ, Chang Y, Wang C, et al. Intrinsic radiomic expression patterns after 20 Gy demonstrate early metabolic response of oropharyngeal cancers. Med Phys 2021;48(7):3767–77.

42. Liu X, Sun C, Long M, et al. Computed tomography-based radiomics signature as a pretreatment predictor of progression-free survival in locally advanced hypopharyngeal carcinoma with a different response to induction chemotherapy. Eur Arch Oto-Rhino-Laryngol 2022;279(7):3551–62.

43. Nakajo M, Kawaji K, Nagano H, et al. The Usefulness of Machine Learning-Based Evaluation of Clinical and Pretreatment [18F]-FDG-PET/CT Radiomic Features for Predicting Prognosis in Hypopharyngeal Cancer. Mol Imag Biol 2023;25(2):303–13.

44. Siow TY, Yeh CH, Lin G, et al. MRI Radiomics for Predicting Survival in Patients with Locally Advanced Hypopharyngeal Cancer Treated with Concurrent Chemoradiotherapy. Cancers 2022;14(24):6119.

45. Lin CH, Yan JL, Yap WK, et al. Prognostic value of interim CT-based peritumoral and intratumoral radiomics in laryngeal and hypopharyngeal cancer patients undergoing definitive radiotherapy. Radiother Oncol 2023;189:109938.

46. Yao Y, Jia C, Zhang H, et al. Applying a nomogram based on preoperative CT to predict early recurrence of laryngeal squamous cell carcinoma after surgery. J X Ray Sci Technol 2023;31(3):435–52.

47. Chen L, Wang H, Zeng H, et al. Evaluation of CT-based radiomics signature and nomogram as prognostic markers in patients with laryngeal squamous cell carcinoma. Cancer Imag 2020;20(1):28.

48. Nakajo M, Nagano H, Jinguji M, et al. The usefulness of machine-learning-based evaluation of clinical and pretreatment 18F-FDG-PET/CT radiomic features for predicting prognosis in patients with laryngeal cancer. Br J Radiol 2023;96(1149):20220772.

49. Yuan Y, Ren J, Shi Y, et al. MRI-based radiomic signature as predictive marker for patients with head and neck squamous cell carcinoma. Eur J Radiol 2019; 117:193–8.

50. Feliciani G, Fioroni F, Grassi E, et al. Radiomic Profiling of Head and Neck Cancer: 18F-FDG PET Texture Analysis as Predictor of Patient Survival. Contrast Media Mol Imaging 2018;2018:3574310.

51. Wang K, Dohopolski M, Zhang Q, et al. Towards reliable head and neck cancers locoregional recurrence prediction using delta-radiomics and learning with rejection option. Med Phys 2023;50(4):2212–23.

52. Ou D, Blanchard P, Rosellini S, et al. Predictive and prognostic value of CT based radiomics signature in locally advanced head and neck cancers patients treated with concurrent chemoradiotherapy or bioradiotherapy and its added value to Human Papillomavirus status. Oral Oncol 2017;71:150–5.

53. Pan Z, Men K, Liang B, et al. A subregion-based prediction model for local-regional recurrence risk in head and neck squamous cell carcinoma. Radiother Oncol 2023;184:109684.

54. Wu A, Li Y, Qi M, et al. Dosiomics improves prediction of locoregional recurrence for intensity modulated radiotherapy treated head and neck cancer cases. Oral Oncol 2020;104:104625.

55. Sörensen A, Carles M, Bunea H, et al. Textural features of hypoxia PET predict survival in head and neck cancer during chemoradiotherapy. Eur J Nucl Med Mol Imag 2020;47(5):1056–64.

56. Socarrás Fernández JA, Mönnich D, Leibfarth S, et al. Comparison of patient stratification by computed tomography radiomics and hypoxia positron emission tomography in head-and-neck cancer radiotherapy. Phys Imaging Radiat Oncol 2020;15:52–9.

57. Carles M, Fechter T, Grosu AL, et al. 18F-FMISO-PET Hypoxia Monitoring for Head-and-Neck Cancer Patients: Radiomics Analyses Predict the Outcome of Chemo-Radiotherapy. Cancers 2021;13(14):3449.

58. Beichel RR, Ulrich EJ, Smith BJ, et al. FDG PET based prediction of response in head and neck cancer treatment: Assessment of new quantitative imaging features. PLoS One 2019;14(4):e0215465.

59. Keek S, Sanduleanu S, Wesseling F, et al. Computed tomography-derived radiomic signature of head and neck squamous cell carcinoma (peri)tumoral tissue for the prediction of locoregional recurrence and distant metastasis after concurrent chemo-radiotherapy. PLoS One 2020;15(5):e0232639.

60. Gangil T, Sharan K, Rao BD, et al. Utility of adding Radiomics to clinical features in predicting the outcomes of radiotherapy for head and neck cancer using machine learning. PLoS One 2022;17(12):e0277168.

61. Zhai TT, Langendijk JA, van Dijk LV, et al. The prognostic value of CT-based image-biomarkers for head and neck cancer patients treated with definitive (chemo-)radiation. Oral Oncol 2019;95:178–86.

62. Zhai TT, Wesseling F, Langendijk JA, et al. External validation of nodal failure prediction models including radiomics in head and neck cancer. Oral Oncol 2021;112:105083.

63. Bogowicz M, Tanadini-Lang S, Guckenberger M, et al. Combined CT radiomics of primary tumor and metastatic lymph nodes improves prediction of loco-regional control in head and neck cancer. Sci Rep 2019;9(1):15198.

64. Zhai TT, Langendijk JA, van Dijk LV, et al. Pre-treatment radiomic features predict individual lymph node failure for head and neck cancer patients. Radiother Oncol 2020;146:58–65.

65. Zhang MH, Cao D, Ginat DT. Radiomic Model Predicts Lymph Node Response to Induction Chemotherapy in Locally Advanced Head and Neck Cancer. Diagnostics 2021;11(4):588.

66. Mes SW, van Velden FHP, Peltenburg B, et al. Outcome prediction of head and neck squamous cell carcinoma by MRI radiomic signatures. Eur Radiol 2020;30(11):6311–21.

67. Starke S, Leger S, Zwanenburg A, et al. 2D and 3D convolutional neural networks for outcome modelling of locally advanced head and neck squamous cell carcinoma. Sci Rep 2020;10(1):15625.

68. Chen L, Zhou Z, Sher D, et al. Combining many-objective radiomics and 3D convolutional neural network through evidential reasoning to predict lymph node metastasis in head and neck cancer. Phys Med Biol 2019;64(7):075011.

69. van Dijk LV, Thor M, Steenbakkers RJHM, et al. Parotid gland fat related Magnetic Resonance image biomarkers improve prediction of late radiation-induced xerostomia. Radiother Oncol 2018;128(3):459–66.

70. Berger T, Noble DJ, Yang Z, et al. Assessing the generalisability of radiomics features previously identified as predictive of radiation-induced sticky saliva and xerostomia. Phys Imaging Radiat Oncol 2023;25:100404.

71. Li Y, Sijtsema NM, de Vette SPM, et al. Validation of the 18F-FDG PET image biomarker model predicting late xerostomia after head and neck cancer radiotherapy. Radiother Oncol 2023;180:109458.

72. Gabryś HS, Buettner F, Sterzing F, et al. Design and Selection of Machine Learning Methods Using Radiomics and Dosiomics for Normal Tissue Complication Probability Modeling of Xerostomia. Front Oncol 2018;8:35.

73. Abdollahi H, Mostafaei S, Cheraghi S, et al. Cochlea CT radiomics predicts chemoradiotherapy induced sensorineural hearing loss in head and neck cancer patients: A machine learning and multi-variable modelling study. Phys Med 2018;45:192–7.

74. Amiri S, Abdolali F, Neshastehriz A, et al. A machine learning approach for prediction of auditory brain stem response in patients after head-and-neck radiation therapy. J Cancer Res Therapeut 2023;19(5):1219–25.

75. Stoiber EM, Bougatf N, Teske H, et al. Analyzing human decisions in IGRT of head-and-neck cancer patients to teach image registration algorithms what experts know. Radiat Oncol 2017;12(1):104.

76. Spadarella G, Calareso G, Garanzini E, et al. MRI based radiomics in nasopharyngeal cancer: Systematic review and perspectives using radiomic quality score (RQS) assessment. Eur J Radiol 2021;140:109744.

77. Zhang H, Wang H, Hao D, et al. An MRI-Based Radiomic Nomogram for Discrimination Between Malignant and Benign Sinonasal Tumors. J Magn Reson Imag 2021;53(1):141–51.

78. Deng Y, Huang Y, Jing B, et al. Deep learning-based recurrence detector on magnetic resonance scans in nasopharyngeal carcinoma: A multicenter study. Eur J Radiol 2023;168:111084.

79. Lin N, Yu S, Xia Z, et al. Apparent Diffusion Coefficient-Based Radiomic Nomogram in Sinonasal Squamous Cell Carcinoma: A Preliminary Study on Histological Grade Evaluation. J Comput Assist Tomogr 2022;46(5):823–9.

80. Yang Q, Guo Y, Ou X, et al. Automatic T Staging Using Weakly Supervised Deep Learning for Nasopharyngeal Carcinoma on MR Images. J Magn Reson Imag 2020;52(4):1074–82.

81. Kim MJ, Choi Y, Sung YE, et al. Early risk-assessment of patients with nasopharyngeal carcinoma: the added prognostic value of MR-based radiomics. Transl Oncol 2021;14(10):101180.

82. Zhang Q, Wu G, Yang Q, et al. Survival rate prediction of nasopharyngeal carcinoma patients based on MRI and gene expression using a deep neural network. Cancer Sci 2023;114(4):1596–605.

83. Bologna M, Corino V, Tenconi C, et al. Methodology and technology for the development of a prognostic MRI-based radiomic model for the outcome of head and neck cancer patients. In: 2020 42nd Annual International Conference of the IEEE engineering in medicine & biology society (EMBC), July 20-24, 2020; held virtually. 2020. p. 1152–1155.

84. Meng M, Gu B, Bi L, et al. DeepMTS: Deep Multi-Task Learning for Survival Prediction in Patients With Advanced Nasopharyngeal Carcinoma Using Pretreatment PET/CT. IEEE J Biomed Health Inform 2022;26(9):4497–507.

85. Bologna M, Calareso G, Resteghini C, et al. Relevance of apparent diffusion coefficient features for a radiomics-based prediction of response to induction chemotherapy in sinonasal cancer. NMR Biomed 2022;35(4):e4265.

86. Yang Y, Wang M, Qiu K, et al. Computed tomography-based deep-learning prediction of induction chemotherapy treatment response in locally advanced nasopharyngeal carcinoma. Strahlenther Onkol 2022;198(2):183–93.

87. Lin M, Lin N, Yu S, et al. Automated Prediction of Early Recurrence in Advanced Sinonasal Squamous Cell Carcinoma With Deep Learning and Multi-parametric MRI-based Radiomics Nomogram. Acad Radiol 2023;30(10):2201–11.

88. Gao Y, Mao Y, Lu S, et al. Magnetic resonance imaging-based radiogenomics analysis for predicting prognosis and gene expression profile in advanced nasopharyngeal carcinoma. Head Neck 2021;43(12):3730–42.

89. Zhang F, Zhong LZ, Zhao X, et al. A deep-learning-based prognostic nomogram integrating microscopic digital pathology and macroscopic magnetic resonance images in nasopharyngeal carcinoma: a multi-cohort study. Ther Adv Med Oncol 2020;12:1758835920971416.

90. Tomita H, Yamashiro T, Iida G, et al. Unenhanced CT texture analysis with machine learning for differentiating between nasopharyngeal cancer and nasopharyngeal malignant lymphoma. Nagoya J Med Sci 2021;83(1):135–49.

91. Zhou H, Jin Y, Dai L, et al. Differential Diagnosis of Benign and Malignant Thyroid Nodules Using Deep Learning Radiomics of Thyroid Ultrasound Images. Eur J Radiol 2020;127:108992.

92. Wu X, Yu P, Jia C, et al. Radiomics Analysis of Computed Tomography for Prediction of Thyroid Capsule Invasion in Papillary Thyroid Carcinoma: A Multi-Classifier and Two-Center Study. Front Endocrinol 2022;13:849065.

93. Qi Q, Huang X, Zhang Y, et al. Ultrasound image-based deep learning to assist in diagnosing gross extrathyroidal extension thyroid cancer: a retrospective multicenter study. EClinicalMedicine 2023;58:101905.
94. Li J, Wu X, Mao N, et al. Computed Tomography-Based Radiomics Model to Predict Central Cervical Lymph Node Metastases in Papillary Thyroid Carcinoma: A Multicenter Study. Front Endocrinol 2021;12:741698.
95. Yu J, Deng Y, Liu T, et al. Lymph node metastasis prediction of papillary thyroid carcinoma based on transfer learning radiomics. Nat Commun 2020;11(1):4807.
96. Wang J, Dong C, Zhang YZ, et al. A novel approach to quantify calcifications of thyroid nodules in US images based on deep learning: predicting the risk of cervical lymph node metastasis in papillary thyroid cancer patients. Eur Radiol 2023;33(12):9347–56.
97. Zheng G, Zhang H, Lin F, et al. Performance of CT-based deep learning in diagnostic assessment of suspicious lateral lymph nodes in papillary thyroid cancer: a prospective diagnostic study. Int J Surg 2023;109(11):3337–45.
98. Li H, Weng J, Shi Y, et al. An improved deep learning approach for detection of thyroid papillary cancer in ultrasound images. Sci Rep 2018;8(1):6600.
99. Wang C, Yu P, Zhang H, et al. Artificial intelligence-based prediction of cervical lymph node metastasis in papillary thyroid cancer with CT. Eur Radiol 2023;33(10):6828–40.
100. Tong Y, Sun P, Yong J, et al. Radiogenomic Analysis of Papillary Thyroid Carcinoma for Prediction of Cervical Lymph Node Metastasis: A Preliminary Study. Front Oncol 2021;11:682998.
101. Liu T, Zhou S, Yu J, et al. Prediction of Lymph Node Metastasis in Patients With Papillary Thyroid Carcinoma: A Radiomics Method Based on Preoperative Ultrasound Images. Technol Cancer Res Treat 2019;18:1533033819831713.
102. Yoon J, Lee E, Koo JS, et al. Artificial intelligence to predict the BRAFV600E mutation in patients with thyroid cancer. PLoS One 2020;15(11):e0242806.
103. Chang YJ, Huang TY, Liu YJ, et al. Classification of parotid gland tumors by using multimodal MRI and deep learning. NMR Biomed 2021;34(1):e4408.
104. Liu X, Pan Y, Zhang X, et al. A Deep Learning Model for Classification of Parotid Neoplasms Based on Multimodal Magnetic Resonance Image Sequences. Laryngoscope 2023;133(2):327–35.
105. Vernuccio F, Arnone F, Cannella R, et al. Diagnostic performance of qualitative and radiomics approach to parotid gland tumors: which is the added benefit of texture analysis? Br J Radiol 2021;94(1128):20210340.
106. Ikushima K, Arimura H, Yasumatsu R, et al. Topology-based radiomic features for prediction of parotid gland cancer malignancy grade in magnetic resonance images. Magma 2023;36(5):767–77.
107. He Z, Mao Y, Lu S, et al. Machine learning–based radiomics for histological classification of parotid tumors using morphological MRI: a comparative study. Eur Radiol 2022;32(12):8099–110.
108. Cheng NM, Hsieh CF, Fang YHD, et al. Development and validation of a prognostic model incorporating [18F]FDG PET/CT radiomics for patients with minor salivary gland carcinoma. EJNMMI Res 2020;10:74.
109. George-Jones NA, Chkheidze R, Moore S, et al. MRI Texture Features are Associated with Vestibular Schwannoma Histology. Laryngoscope 2021;131(6):E2000–6.
110. Wang K, George-Jones NA, Chen L, et al. Joint Vestibular Schwannoma Enlargement Prediction and Segmentation Using a Deep Multi-task Model. Laryngoscope 2023;133(10):2754–60.

111. Langenhuizen PPJH, Zinger S, Leenstra S, et al. Radiomics-Based Prediction of Long-Term Treatment Response of Vestibular Schwannomas Following Stereotactic Radiosurgery. Otol Neurotol 2020;41(10):e1321–7.

112. Duan B, Xu Z, Pan L, et al. Prediction of Hearing Prognosis of Large Vestibular Aqueduct Syndrome Based on the PyTorch Deep Learning Model. J Healthc Eng 2022;2022:4814577.

113. van der Lubbe MFJA, Vaidyanathan A, de Wit M, et al. A non-invasive, automated diagnosis of Menière's disease using radiomics and machine learning on conventional magnetic resonance imaging: A multicentric, case-controlled feasibility study. Radiol Med 2022;127(1):72–82.

114. Arendt CT, Leithner D, Mayerhoefer ME, et al. Radiomics of high-resolution computed tomography for the differentiation between cholesteatoma and middle ear inflammation: effects of post-reconstruction methods in a dual-center study. Eur Radiol 2021;31(6):4071–8.

115. Liu GS, Yang A, Kim D, et al. Deep learning classification of inverted papilloma malignant transformation using 3D convolutional neural networks and magnetic resonance imaging. Int Forum Allergy Rhinol 2022;12(8):1025–33.

116. Ito K, Muraoka H, Hirahara N, et al. Quantitative assessment of normal submandibular glands and submandibular sialadenitis using CT texture analysis: A retrospective study. Oral Surg Oral Med Oral Pathol Oral Radiol 2021;132(1):112–7.

117. Oliver JR, Karadaghy OA, Fassas SN, et al. Machine learning directed sentinel lymph node biopsy in cutaneous head and neck melanoma. Head Neck 2022;44(4):975–88.

118. Classe M, Lerousseau M, Scoazec JY, et al. Perspectives in pathomics in head and neck cancer. Curr Opin Oncol 2021;33(3):175.

119. Lee K, Lockhart JH, Xie M, et al. Deep Learning of Histopathology Images at the Single Cell Level. Front Artif Intell 2021;4:754641.

120. Alabi RO, Almangush A, Elmusrati M, et al. Deep Machine Learning for Oral Cancer: From Precise Diagnosis to Precision Medicine. Front Oral Health 2021;2:794248.

121. Sarode GS, Kumari N, Sarode SC. Oral cancer histopathology images and artificial intelligence: A pathologist's perspective. Oral Oncol 2022;132:105999.

122. Araújo ALD, da Silva VM, Kudo MS, et al. Machine learning concepts applied to oral pathology and oral medicine: A convolutional neural networks' approach. J Oral Pathol Med 2023;52(2):109–18.

123. Mahmood H, Shaban M, Indave BI, et al. Use of artificial intelligence in diagnosis of head and neck precancerous and cancerous lesions: A systematic review. Oral Oncol 2020;110:104885.

124. Halicek M, Lu G, Little JV, et al. Deep convolutional neural networks for classifying head and neck cancer using hyperspectral imaging. J Biomed Opt 2017;22(6):060503.

125. Halicek M, Little JV, Wang X, et al. Optical Biopsy of Head and Neck Cancer Using Hyperspectral Imaging and Convolutional Neural Networks. Proc SPIE-Int Soc Opt Eng 2018;10469:104690X.

126. Halicek M, Shahedi M, Little JV, et al. Detection of Squamous Cell Carcinoma in Digitized Histological Images from the Head and Neck Using Convolutional Neural Networks. Proc SPIE-Int Soc Opt Eng 2019;10956:109560K.

127. Ma L, Little JV, Chen AY, et al. Automatic detection of head and neck squamous cell carcinoma on histologic slides using hyperspectral microscopic imaging. J Biomed Opt 2022;27(4):046501.

128. Zhou X, Ma L, Brown W, et al. Automatic detection of head and neck squamous cell carcinoma on pathologic slides using polarized hyperspectral imaging and machine learning. Proc SPIE-Int Soc Opt Eng 2021;11603:116030Q.

129. Ma L, Zhou X, Little JV, et al. Hyperspectral Microscopic Imaging for the Detection of Head and Neck Squamous Cell Carcinoma on Histologic Slides. Proc SPIE-Int Soc Opt Eng 2021;11603:116030P.

130. Mascharak S, Baird BJ, Holsinger FC. Detecting oropharyngeal carcinoma using multispectral, narrow-band imaging and machine learning. Laryngoscope 2018;128(11):2514–20.

131. Cai X, Li L, Yu F, et al. Development of a Pathomics-Based Model for the Prediction of Malignant Transformation in Oral Leukoplakia. Lab Invest 2023;103(8): 100173.

132. Zhang X, Gleber-Netto FO, Wang S, et al. Deep learning-based pathology image analysis predicts cancer progression risk in patients with oral leukoplakia. Cancer Med 2023;12(6):7508–18.

133. Yuan W, Yang J, Yin B, et al. Noninvasive diagnosis of oral squamous cell carcinoma by multi-level deep residual learning on optical coherence tomography images. Oral Dis 2023;29(8):3223–31.

134. Wang R, Khurram SA, Walsh H, et al. A Novel Deep Learning Algorithm for Human Papillomavirus Infection Prediction in Head and Neck Cancers Using Routine Histology Images. Mod Pathol 2023;36(12):100320.

135. Fouad S, Landini G, Robinson M, et al. Human papilloma virus detection in oropharyngeal carcinomas with in situ hybridisation using hand crafted morphological features and deep central attention residual networks. Comput Med Imag Graph 2021;88:101853.

136. Weyers BW, Birkeland AC, Marsden MA, et al. Intraoperative delineation of p16+ oropharyngeal carcinoma of unknown primary origin with fluorescence lifetime imaging: Preliminary report. Head Neck 2022;44(8):1765–76.

137. Lee LY, Yang CH, Lin YC, et al. A domain knowledge enhanced yield based deep learning classifier identifies perineural invasion in oral cavity squamous cell carcinoma. Front Oncol 2022;12:951560.

138. Sharma S, Ragothaman S, Vahadane A, et al. Spatial-context-aware RNA-sequence prediction from head and neck cancer histopathology images. In: 2021 43rd Annual International Conference of the IEEE engineering in medicine & biology Society (EMBC). 2021. p. 1711–4.

139. Koyuncu CF, Lu C, Bera K, et al. Computerized tumor multinucleation index (MuNI) is prognostic in p16+ oropharyngeal carcinoma. J Clin Invest 2021; 131(8):e145488.

140. Koyuncu CF, Frederick MJ, Thompson LDR, et al. Machine learning driven index of tumor multinucleation correlates with survival and suppressed anti-tumor immunity in head and neck squamous cell carcinoma patients. Oral Oncol 2023; 143:106459.

141. Chen L, Zeng H, Zhang M, et al. Histopathological image and gene expression pattern analysis for predicting molecular features and prognosis of head and neck squamous cell carcinoma. Cancer Med 2021;10(13):4615–28.

142. Yang K, Zhu G, Sun Y, et al. Prognostic significance of cyclin D1 expression pattern in HPV-negative oral and oropharyngeal carcinoma: A deep-learning approach. J Oral Pathol Med 2023;52(10):919–29.

143. Hue J, Valinciute Z, Thavaraj S, et al. Multifactorial estimation of clinical outcome in HPV-associated oropharyngeal squamous cell carcinoma via automated

image analysis of routine diagnostic H&E slides and neural network modelling. Oral Oncol 2023;141:106399.

144. Klein S, Wuerdemann N, Demers I, et al. Predicting HPV association using deep learning and regular H&E stains allows granular stratification of oropharyngeal cancer patients. NPJ Digit Med 2023;6(1):152.

145. Klein S, Quaas A, Quantius J, et al. Deep Learning Predicts HPV Association in Oropharyngeal Squamous Cell Carcinomas and Identifies Patients with a Favorable Prognosis Using Regular H&E Stains. Clin Cancer Res 2021;27(4):1131–8.

146. Puladi B, Ooms M, Kintsler S, et al. Automated PD-L1 Scoring Using Artificial Intelligence in Head and Neck Squamous Cell Carcinoma. Cancers 2021; 13(17):4409.

147. Lu G, Little JV, Wang X, et al. Detection of Head and Neck Cancer in Surgical Specimens Using Quantitative Hyperspectral Imaging. Clin Cancer Res 2017; 23(18):5426–36.

148. Halicek M, Dormer JD, Little JV, et al. Hyperspectral Imaging of Head and Neck Squamous Cell Carcinoma for Cancer Margin Detection in Surgical Specimens from 102 Patients Using Deep Learning. Cancers 2019;11(9):1367.

149. Halicek M, Fabelo H, Ortega S, et al. Hyperspectral imaging for head and neck cancer detection: specular glare and variance of the tumor margin in surgical specimens. J Med Imaging 2019;6(3):035004.

150. Dittberner A, Rodner E, Ortmann W, et al. Automated analysis of confocal laser endomicroscopy images to detect head and neck cancer. Head Neck 2016; 38(S1):E1419–26.

151. Zhang L, Wu Y, Zheng B, et al. Rapid histology of laryngeal squamous cell carcinoma with deep-learning based stimulated Raman scattering microscopy. Theranostics 2019;9(9):2541–54.

152. Diao S, Hou J, Yu H, et al. Computer-Aided Pathologic Diagnosis of Nasopharyngeal Carcinoma Based on Deep Learning. Am J Pathol 2020;190(8): 1691–700.

153. Samanta S, Swaminathan M, Hu J, et al. Deep Learning Fuzzy Inference: An Interpretable Model for Detecting Indirect Immunofluorescence Patterns Associated with Nasopharyngeal Cancer. Am J Pathol 2022;192(9):1295–304.

154. Liu K, Xia W, Qiang M, et al. Deep learning pathological microscopic features in endemic nasopharyngeal cancer: Prognostic value and protentional role for individual induction chemotherapy. Cancer Med 2020;9(4):1298–306.

155. Ding J, Yue C, Wang C, et al. Machine learning method for the cellular phenotyping of nasal polyps from multicentre tissue scans. Expet Rev Clin Immunol 2023;19(8):1023–8.

156. Wang K, Ren Y, Ma L, et al. Deep learning-based prediction of treatment prognosis from nasal polyp histology slides. Int Forum Allergy Rhinol 2023;13(5): 886–98.

157. Elliott Range DD, Dov D, Kovalsky SZ, et al. Application of a machine learning algorithm to predict malignancy in thyroid cytopathology. Cancer Cytopathol 2020;128(4):287–95.

158. Dov D, Kovalsky SZ, Feng Q, et al. Use of Machine Learning-Based Software for the Screening of Thyroid Cytopathology Whole Slide Images. Arch Pathol Lab Med 2022;146(7):872–8.

159. Deng C, Li D, Feng M, et al. The value of deep neural networks in the pathological classification of thyroid tumors. Diagn Pathol 2023;18(1):95.

160. Ren W, Zhu Y, Wang Q, et al. Deep learning prediction model for central lymph node metastasis in papillary thyroid microcarcinoma based on cytology. Cancer Sci 2023;114(10):4114–24.
161. Edwards K, Halicek M, Little JV, et al. Multiparametric Radiomics for Predicting the Aggressiveness of Papillary Thyroid Carcinoma Using Hyperspectral Images. Proc SPIE-Int Soc Opt Eng 2021;11597:1159728.
162. Kim J, Ko S, Kim M, et al. Deep Learning Prediction of TERT Promoter Mutation Status in Thyroid Cancer Using Histologic Images. Medicina 2023;59(3):536.
163. Wang CW, Muzakky H, Lee YC, et al. Annotation-Free Deep Learning-Based Prediction of Thyroid Molecular Cancer Biomarker BRAF (V600E) from Cytological Slides. Int J Mol Sci 2023;24(3):2521.
164. Suh CH, Lee KH, Choi YJ, et al. Oropharyngeal squamous cell carcinoma: radiomic machine-learning classifiers from multiparametric MR images for determination of HPV infection status. Sci Rep 2020;10(1):17525.
165. Sohn B, Choi YS, Ahn SS, et al. Machine Learning Based Radiomic HPV Phenotyping of Oropharyngeal SCC: A Feasibility Study Using MRI. Laryngoscope 2021;131(3):E851–6.
166. Bos P, van den Brekel MWM, Taghavi M, et al. Largest diameter delineations can substitute 3D tumor volume delineations for radiomics prediction of human papillomavirus status on MRI's of oropharyngeal cancer. Phys Med 2022;101: 36–43.
167.. Bagher-Ebadian H, Siddiqui F, Ghanem AI, et al. Radiomics outperforms clinical factors in characterizing human papilloma virus (HPV) for patients with oropharyngeal squamous cell carcinomas. Biomed Phys Eng Express 2022; 8(4):045010.
168. Bagher-Ebadian H, Lu M, Siddiqui F, et al. Application of radiomics for the prediction of HPV status for patients with head and neck cancers. Med Phys 2020; 47(2):563–75.
169. Mukherjee P, Cintra M, Huang C, et al. CT-based Radiomic Signatures for Predicting Histopathologic Features in Head and Neck Squamous Cell Carcinoma. Radiol Imaging Cancer 2020;2(3):e190039.
170. Konishi M, Kakimoto N. Radiomics analysis of intraoral ultrasound images for prediction of late cervical lymph node metastasis in patients with tongue cancer. Head Neck 2023;45(10):2619–26.
171. Jia CL, Cao Y, Song Q, et al. [Radiomics nomogram of MR: a prediction of cervical lymph node metastasis in laryngeal cancer]. Zhonghua er bi yan hou tou jing wai ke za zhi 2020;55(12):1154–61.
172. Zhao X, Li W, Zhang J, et al. Radiomics analysis of CT imaging improves preoperative prediction of cervical lymph node metastasis in laryngeal squamous cell carcinoma. Eur Radiol 2023;33(2):1121–31.
173.. Ren J, Qi M, Yuan Y, Tao X. Radiomics of apparent diffusion coefficient maps to predict histologic grade in squamous cell carcinoma of the oral tongue and floor of mouth: a preliminary study. Acta Radiol 2021;62(4):453–61.

Generative AI and Otolaryngology—Head & Neck Surgery

Jérôme R. Lechien, MD, PhD, MS, AFACS[a,b,c,d]

KEYWORDS

- Otorhinolaryngology • Otolaryngology • Head neck • Surgery • Artificial intelligence
- ChatGPT • GPT • Generative

KEY POINTS

- The current literature on generative artificial intelligence (AI) has been booming since the launch of AI-powered language models, such as Chatbot Generative Pre-trained Transformer (ChatGPT).
- Most studies investigated the accuracy of ChatGPT in providing general information on disease basic science and clinical research, clinical vignette management, scientific paper referencing, and improvement.
- ChatGPT may provide accurate theoretic information on otolaryngologic disorders commonly found in general otolaryngology, head and neck surgery, oncology, and sleep practices.
- The performance of ChatGPT as an adjunctive clinical tool for managing clinical vignettes or true clinical cases may be limited, especially in providing the most adequate additional examinations.
- The AI may revolutionize the otolaryngology—head and neck surgery field, which should lead to the improvement of patient care. The next few years will be decisive for applying the new AI technologies in the office-based practice.

INTRODUCTION

Artificial intelligence (AI) can revolutionize many fields in medicine and surgery. The mediatization related to the launch of Chatbot Generative Pre-trained Transformer

[a] Research Committee of Young Otolaryngologists of the International Federation of Otorhinolaryngological Societies (IFOS), Paris, France; [b] Division of Laryngology and Bronchoesophagology, Department of Otolaryngology-Head Neck Surgery, EpiCURA Hospital, UMONS Research Institute for Health Sciences and Technology, University of Mons (UMons), Mons, Belgium; [c] Department of Otorhinolaryngology and Head and Neck Surgery, Foch Hospital, Paris Saclay University, Phonetics and Phonology Laboratory (UMR 7018 CNRS, Université Sorbonne Nouvelle/Paris 3), Paris, France; [d] Department of Otorhinolaryngology and Head and Neck Surgery, CHU Saint-Pierre, Brussels, Belgium
E-mail address: Jerome.Lechien@umons.ac.be

Otolaryngol Clin N Am 57 (2024) 753–765
https://doi.org/10.1016/j.otc.2024.04.006
0030-6665/24/© 2024 Elsevier Inc. All rights reserved.

(ChatGPT) in November 2022 has led to a significant increase in public and practitioner interest in generative AI, and, particularly, artificial intelligence-powered language models (AILM).[1] Indeed, 2023 was the year associated with the highest number of publications dedicated to AI in otolaryngology—head and neck surgery and available on PubMED central (**Fig. 1**). Many AILM are available online for patients or practitioners, including ChatGPT (OpenAI, San Francisco, USA), Large Language Model Meta AI (Lamaa; MetaAI Palo Alto, CA, USA), Google Bidirectional Encoder Representations from Transformer (BERT; Mountain View, CA, USA), or Google DeepMind's Gopher.[2,3] AILM have been found to respond to simple-to-complicated questions related to clinical and basic science research,[4] referencing,[5,6] medical examinations,[7] clinical vignettes,[8] and they may improve scientific reports through spelling correction.[9,10] The mediatization, accessibility, and popularity of AILM may encourage patients to use them for medical and surgical education, while some young practitioners may consider AILM as adjunctive clinical tools to improve their knowledge and practice.[11] This article summarizes the application of AILM in Otolaryngology—Head and Neck Surgery.

HISTORY

The intelligent machine concept was born in Greek mythology where Hephaestus crafted golden robot-like statues to serve him.[12] In the Renaissance, Leonardo da Vinci imagined automatons capable of mimicking human actions. At the same time, in the eighteenth century, Gottfried Wilhelm Leibniz discussed a "universal language" and a machine that could reason, like human logical reasoning.[13] The technological revolution of the twentieth century made possible the development of AI-based processes in economic, law, or medical fields. Yet, in 1943, McCulloch and Pitts developed a computer model able to learn through a process that was comparable to human neurons.[14] A few years after this publication (1950), Alan Turing developed a test for model intelligence, which consisted of a blinded human interrogator questioning human and machine respondents (Turing test).[15,16] In 1956, AI was officially recognized at a Dartmouth College (Hanover, USA) conference in which researchers proposed the following statement "every aspect of learning or any other feature of intelligence can be so precisely described that a machine can be made to simulate it.[15,17]" Since then, more studies have been conducted in medicine and surgery to simulate, supplement, or efficiently augment human intelligence and skills in improving patient care.[15] The AI field currently involves machine learning and natural language processing subfields.[12] Machine learning consists of algorithms that learn from simple-to-complicated tasks for developing predictive models.[15]

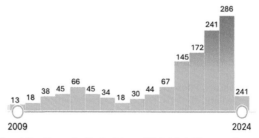

Fig. 1. Evolution of publications dedicated to artificial intelligence in otolaryngology in the past 15 years. (*Source:* figure was generated through PubMED (January 19, 2024) with the following key words: Artificial Intelligence Otolaryngology.)

Deep learning, which can be considered a subfield of machine learning, is based on artificial neural networks that can perform computations like the human brain. Recent developments in deep learning have led to many machine learning applications in medicine or surgery, which may analyze numerical data, clinical images, or videos through various databases.[12,15] AILM may consist of an association between machine learning and natural language processing and, consequently, may support practitioners in clinical decision-making, the proposition of additional examinations, or treatments.

BRIEF FUNCTIONING OF GENERATIVE ARTIFICIAL INTELLIGENCE

Generative artificial intelligence (AI) models are based on language processing, machine learning, and deep learning.[12,18–20] They include neural networks (mathematical models mimicking human brain functioning) and variational autoencoders, which rely on machine learning algorithms training on large databases, allowing them to recognize some specific patterns, understand complex relationships, and generate new outputs. In summary, the neural network is composed of many units (like neurons) connected by connections (weights). They communicate through inputs from the other units or the outside world, and may generate outputs for the others.[18,19] According to the received and potentially repeated inputs, units may learn from each other and adjust the related weights. AILM, such as GPT, are trained through a large corpus of text data used as input to a neural network composed of up to 175 billion parameters.[18,20] The weights between units may be improved with human use and related corrections. In practice, the input text is tokenized into individual words embedded into a vector space using the same embedding matrix used during training.[18] The embedded input text is subsequently passed via the encoder and decoder components. Then, AILM can generate creative, coherent, and contextually relevant sentences, making it a valuable tool for patient engagement, medical education, and clinical decision support.[20] It is important to note that the functioning of AILM is influenced by hyperparameters, which consist of settings controlling how the model learns from data, such as the learning rate, the batch size, the number of layers, and the activation function.[18,19] They are important because they influence the AILM performance, speed, and accuracy. In practice, they influence the content of the responses, leading to more coherent responses and better management of different inputs and outputs. For example, hyperparameters of ChatGPT-3.5 differ from hyperparameters of ChatGPT-4, which is the most recent model release. Importantly, all AILM have limitations, such as hallucination of facts (false positive), lack of common-sense knowledge, restricted context window, and potential privacy concerns.[18,20] All of them may be corrected by human feedback.

APPLICATIONS OF ARTIFICIAL INTELLIGENCE-POWERED LANGUAGE MODELS IN OTOLARYNGOLOGY

Patients have access to AILM to get information about symptoms of ear, nose, and throat conditions, surgery risks, and alternatives. In that way, several otolaryngologists have investigated the accuracy, precision, and performance of AILM, especially ChatGPT, in providing patient information.[11,18] Moreover, the accuracy of ChatGPT was similarly investigated in the management of theoretic or true clinical cases in the different subspecialties of otolaryngology head and neck surgery.[5–9] The current applications of ChatGPT in otolaryngology—head and neck surgery are summarized in **Fig. 2**.

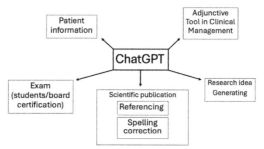

Fig. 2. Current applications of Chatbot Generative Pre-trained Transformer in otolaryngology—head and neck surgery.

Applications in General Otolaryngology

Student and resident board certification examinations

The ChatGPT accuracy in medical, surgical, and otolaryngologic questions was investigated from students or resident in-service examinations.[21–23] The first study was conducted by Hoch and colleagues to evaluate the accuracy of ChatGPT-3 on 2576 practice quiz questions designed for German otolaryngology board certification.[21] The authors reported an overall accuracy rate of 57% and observed that ChatGPT-3 responded better to single-choice questions than multiple-choice questions (34% vs 63%), while the performance of ChatGPT-3 was particularly high in allergology (72%), and low in the legal field (30%), respectively.[21] In the same vein, Mahajan and colleagues investigated the performance of ChatGPT-3.5 in responding to practice examination questions in otolaryngology head and neck surgery. The comparison of outputs from ChatGPT-3.5 with the benchmark of answers and explanations reported that ChatGPT-3.5 correctly answered 53% of the questions and provided correct explanations in 54% of the cases, respectively.[22] Long and colleagues submitted to ChatGPT-4.0 21 common questions of the licensing examination in otolaryngology, which were analyzed by 2 independent practitioners with the Concordance, Validity, Safety, and Competency model.[23] ChatGPT-4 scored 23.5/34 (accurate rate: 69.1%) but did not reach the minimum passing score for the examination (70%). However, after providing further queries that explicitly focus on otolaryngology, ChatGPT-4 improved its score to reach an accurate rate of 75%, demonstrating the ChatGPT performance improvement after human feedback.[23] The accuracy of ChatGPT-3.5 was similarly observed in responding to questions related to tympanostomy.[24] Twenty responses from ChatGPT-3.5 matched with the recommendations of the American Academy of Otolaryngology—Head and Neck Surgery, which consisted of an accuracy of 95.7%.[24]

Patient information

Several studies have been conducted to evaluate the accuracy of AILM in providing patient information related to otolaryngologic diseases or surgeries. In the study of Zalzal and colleagues, 2 sets of 30 text-based questions related to surgical anatomy, otology, head and neck surgery, oncology, laryngology, rhinology, and fundamentals were input into the ChatGPT-3.5 API.[25] Two board-certified otolaryngologists independently rated the chatbot's responses and observed total and partial response accuracy in 56.7%, and 86.7% of the cases, respectively. Interestingly, the authors observed that the repeated inputs led to an improvement of total and partial accurate responses to 73.3%, and 96.7%, respectively, which corroborated the findings of

Long and colleagues who observed improvement of performance through regenerated questions and feedback.[23] In the study of Langlie and colleagues, 2 independent practitioners assessed the capability and accuracy of ChatGPT-3.5 in providing indications, procedures, and alternative therapeutic options for adenotonsillectomy, tympanoplasty, endoscopic sinus surgery, parotidectomy, and total laryngectomy.[26] To achieve its goal, the authors interrogated ChatGPT-3.5 with standardized questions (How do I know if I need [procedure]; What are treatment alternatives to [procedure]; What are the risks of [procedure]; How is a [procedure] performed; and What is the recovery process for [procedure]?) and they did not observe major errors in ChatGPT-3.5 responses. However, the chatbot reported difficulties when it needed to provide precision and details in the surgery steps, forgetting key surgical steps and major risks associated with several surgeries.[26] The high accuracy of ChatGPT in providing health information in otolaryngology was tempered by Nielsen and colleagues who reported an overall 5-point Likert scale score of 3.41 for the ChatGPT-4 information related to otitis, hearing impairment, vertigo, epistaxis, rhinosinusitis, pharyngitis, dysphonia, globus sensation, and conjunctivitis.[27] To date, most studies investigating the AILM potential in providing otolaryngology information for patients focused on ChatGPT. Only 2 investigations compared ChatGPT performance with other AILM or databases.[28,29] The first one was conducted by Ayoub and colleagues who evaluated the accuracy of the outputs of Google Search and ChatGPT-4 with several recommendations from clinical practice guidelines.[28] The authors reported that the mean patient education material assessment tool scores for medical advice were 68.2% versus 89.4% for ChatGPT-4 and Google Search, respectively, meaning that Google Search scored better than ChatGPT-4 for providing readable information. The findings of Ayoub and colleagues corroborated those of Bellinger and colleagues who showed that ChatGPT-4 and Google Search similarly scored for treating the urgency of some clinical situations.[29] Note that the only field where ChatGPT-4 scored better than Google Search was the patient education questions (general medical knowledge; 87% vs 78%) according to the patient education material assessment tool.

Clinical vignettes
One of the first studies assessing the performance of ChatGPT in the management of clinical cases was conducted to validate an instrument dedicated to evaluating the ChatGPT performance (artificial intelligence performance instrument; AIPI).[7] In this study, ChatGPT-4 was accurate in proposing adequate additional examinations, treatments, and diagnoses in 29%, 22%, and 56% to 71%, respectively.[7] However, the chatbot proposed a significantly higher number of additional examinations than practitioners and did not select the most appropriate ones.[7] The performance of ChatGPT-3.5 in managing clinical cases was similarly studied by Dallari and colleagues who presented 10 clinical theoretic vignettes of common otolaryngologic symptoms with 2 different scenarios per case to ChatGPT-3.5.[30] Five otolaryngologists rated the responses of ChatGPT-3.5 using a 5-point Likert scale for difficulty, correctness, and consistency outcomes. The ChatGPT-3.5 scores of correctness and consistency were 3.80 and 2.89, respectively, without being influenced by the difficulty of the clinical cases.[30] The lack of influence of case difficulty on the ChatGPT performances was similarly observed by Lechien and colleagues in laryngology and head and neck surgery clinical cases,[31] which corroborated the findings of Dallari. The lack of influence of the level of difficulty of clinical cases on the accuracy of ChatGPT-4 was similarly supported in 2 other studies including general otolaryngology[8] and laryngology clinical cases.[31] In the study of Qu and colleagues, the authors investigated the accuracy of ChatGPT-4 on 20 clinical theoretic vignettes in

general otolaryngology[8] and they observed high and significant agreements between ChatGPT-4 and attending physicians in the propositions of adequate differential diagnoses and treatment plans.[8] To date, only Karimov and colleagues compared the accuracy of ChatGPT-3.5 with another AILM (UpToDate) in providing management information and references for 25 clinical cases.[32] The authors observed that ChatGPT-3.5 did not give references in some clinical questions in contrast to UpToDate that supported the information with subheadings, tables, figures, and algorithms from scientific papers. According to the assessment of experts, UpToDate was found to be more useful and reliable than ChatGPT-3.5.[32]

Applications in Head and Neck Surgery

General information and knowledge

One hundred and fifty-four questions related to all head and neck cancer basic knowledge, diagnosis, and treatments were input into the application programming interface (API) of ChatGPT-4 by Kuscu and colleagues who reported correct, partially correct, and incorrect GPT-4 responses in 86.4%, 11%, and 2.6% of the cases, respectively.[33] ChatGPT-4 reported highest accuracy for prevention (100%), diagnosis (92.6%), treatment (88.9%), while the questions related to surgical management, for example, recovery, risks, complications and follow-up, reached 80% of accurate outputs. The authors observed a high stability of ChatGPT-4 throughout regenerated questions with 94.1% of response stability, which corroborated findings of other studies.[30,31,34] The accuracy of ChatGPT-4 was similarly investigated for 144 theoretic questions encompassing different subspecialties of head and neck or maxillofacial surgery in a cross-sectional study involving 18 experts subdivided into 8 working groups for the output analysis.[5] The authors reported an overall accuracy score of 5.43 (6-point Likert scale) and noted that there were no significant differences between the several subspecialty scores in terms of completeness and accuracy scores.[5]

Patient information

Chiesa-Estomba and colleagues interrogated ChatGPT-3.5 with the 5 most common questions of patients toward head and neck cancer and asked patients to compare the outputs of ChatGPT-3.5 versus practitioners.[35] In laryngeal and oropharyngeal cancers, patients reported significantly preferring the responses of practitioners compared to the ChatGPT-3.5 outputs, while there were no significant differences for salivary gland cancers.[35]

The accuracy of ChatGPT-3.5 in providing information on oropharyngeal cancer information was similarly evaluated by Davis and colleagues who introduced 15 common questions into the API, whereas the outputs of ChatGPT-3.5 were analyzed by 4 independent head and neck surgeons using a 5-point Likert scale.[36] Thus, experts reported average ChatGPT-3.5 accuracy, comprehensiveness, and similarity scores ranging from 3.67 to 3.88, corresponding to somewhat accurate responses.[36] The ChatGPT-3.5 responses were particularly accurate in post-treatment information and less accurate in diagnosis-related information.[36] Contrary to other studies, the findings of this study suggested that ChatGPT-3.5 could outright misinform patients and read at a more difficult grade level than is recommended for patient material. Lee and colleagues collected presurgical educational information (indications, risks, and recovery time) for 5 common head and neck surgeries from ChatGPT-3.5 and 5 experienced head and neck surgeons compared ChatGPT-3.5 outputs with the information available on the first publicly available website.[4] The authors reported that ChatGPT-generated pre-surgical information was comparable to websites in terms of readability, content of knowledge, accuracy, thoroughness, and numbers of medical errors, which corroborated the findings of some aforementioned studies.[4,24–26] In the field of endocrine surgery, Campbell and colleagues interrogated ChatGPT-3 for 30 questions related to thyroid nodule information and management.[37] Note that they input questions throughout 4 repeated sessions to assess the stability of the model. The authors observed an accurate rate of 69.2%, whereas 87.5% of the references provided by ChatGPT-3 were judged as legitimate citations, and 72.5% provided accurately reported information from the referenced publication.[37] The study, which was unique in the field of thyroid nodule information, supported a moderate-to-high accuracy of ChatGPT-3. Another original study was conducted in the sialendoscopy field by Chiesa-Estomba and colleagues who evaluated the accuracy of GPT-3.5 responses for providing clinical management of 6 salivary gland disorders and compared the ChatGPT-3.5 responses with those of 10 expert sialendoscopists.[38] The mean agreement score of experts was significantly higher compared to the ChatGPT-3.5 score (4.1 vs 3.4, 5-point Likert scale), while ChatGPT-3.5 and experts reported a comparable number of therapeutic alternatives. In this study, the authors observed that the expert treatment suggestions were rated higher than ChatGPT-3.5 suggestions in half of the clinical scenarios, whereas they were equal in the other half. Overall, the information provided by ChatGPT-3.5 was considered comprehensive and accurate.[38]

Clinical vignettes

A few studies investigated the accuracy of ChatGPT in managing clinical vignettes in head and neck surgery.[39–41] The accuracy of ChatGPT-3.5 was evaluated in recommending treatments for 727 head and neck cancer clinical vignettes through a comparison between ChatGPT-3.5 responses and the National Comprehensive Cancer Network Guidelines.[39] In this European cross-sectional study, the sensitivity and accuracy of ChatGPT-3.5 for primary treatments were 100% and 85.3%, respectively. The sensitivities for adjuvant treatments and follow-up indications wereboth 100%, whereas the accuracies were 95.6% and 94.1%, respectively. This study supported very high accuracy and sensitivity of ChatGPT-3.5 toward clinical vignettes of patients with head and neck cancer.[39] The findings of this study were corroborated in another European study where the findings of 20 medical records discussed in a multidisciplinary oncological board were input into the API to obtain cTNM explanations, and management propositions.[40] ChatGPT-4 was found to provide perfect explanations for cTNM staging in 19 cases (95%). In addition, ChatGPT-4 similarly indicated endoscopy-biopsy, human papilloma virus (HPV) research, ultrasonography, and PET-computed tomography (CT) to the oncological board. The therapeutic propositions of ChatGPT-4 were accurate in 13 cases (65%) but the number of proposed additional examinations was significantly higher compared to head and neck surgeons.[40] As found in other studies,[30,31,34] most additional examinations and primary treatment propositions were consistent throughout regenerated response process, which confirmed the high stability of ChatGPT-4. The last investigation conducted in head and neck oncology explored the ability of ChatGPT-4 to interpret confocal laser endomicroscopy images of normal versus cancerous oropharyngeal tissues.[41] In this study, the accuracy of ChatGPT-4 reached 71.2%, while the accuracy of the 3 experts, including 2 surgeons and 1 pathologist, was 88.5%.[41] This study is the only one that investigates the accuracy of ChatGPT-4 for analyzing clinical or histopathological images.

Laryngology and Broncho-Esophagology

Only 2 studies investigated the usefulness of ChatGPT in the field of laryngology and broncho-esophagology.[31,42] Then, the potential of ChatGPT-3.5 was investigated in dysphagia for generating research ideas in swallowing science. The study protocol involved 26 swallowing experts who rated a list of study ideas generated by ChatGPT-3.5 with a Likert-scale ranging from 1 to 5 according to feasibility, novelty, clinical implications, and relevance to current practice. Experts reported a mean rate of rankings of research ideas (/5) of 4.03 ± 0.17 for feasibility, 3.5 ± 0.17 for potential impact on the field, 3.84 ± 0.12 for clinical relevance, and 3.08 ± 0.36 for novelty and innovation, respectively.[42] Authors concluded that ChatGPT-3.5 offered promising findings in generating research ideas in swallowing, but it is still limited in innovation. From a clinical standpoint, s team explored the accuracy and performance of ChatGPT-4 in the management of clinical cases from the laryngology clinic.[31] In sum, the accuracy of ChatGPT-4 for indicating adequate additional examinations was lower (10% to 33%) compared to its accuracy for providing primary diagnosis (65%) and the most adequate treatment (60% to 79%). Similarly to other studies,[7,34] ChatGPT-4 proposed a significantly higher number of additional examinations per patient compared to practitioners. Interestingly, the accuracy of ChatGPT did not vary according to the level of clinical cases, which corroborated the findings of other studies.[7,30]

Rhinology, Allergy, and Facial and Plastic Surgery

Patient information

Two studies conducted in the facial and plastic surgery field are available in the literature.[43,44] The first study was conducted to investigate the accuracy of ChatGPT information in facial and plastic surgery.[43] In this study, Capelleras and colleagues focused on the information provided by ChatGPT (unspecified version) in postoperative guidance during rhinoplasty recovery, for example, pain management, swelling, bruising, or asymmetries. The authors reported high performance of ChatGPT in patient education, especially in general information related to the recovery step and reassurance.[43] Another team compared the performance of ChatGPT-3.5 versus that of an experienced surgeon in providing patient education in rhinoplasty.[44] In this cross-sectional study, 7 facial and plastic surgeons used a 5-point Likert scale assessment to show that ChatGPT-3.5 outperformed surgeon responses in 75% performance areas, earning significantly higher ratings in accuracy, completeness, and overall quality. Experts preferred the ChatGPT-3.5 responses to those of the practitioner in 80.95% of instances.[44]

Clinical vignettes

Radulesco and colleagues investigated the accuracy of ChatGPT-4 in the management of 40 rhinologic and allergic cases.[34] According to the artificial intelligence performance instrument (AIPI) scores, 3 blinded rhinologists judged the ChatGPT-4 performance as higher for primary and differential diagnosis propositions (63.3%) than in indicating pertinent and necessary additional examinations (15.8%) or pertinent and necessary treatments (16.7%).[34] The authors regenerated 5 times the outputs of ChatGPT-4 and reported significantly high stability, especially in proposing therapeutic approaches. Interestingly, some differential diagnoses changed from the first output to the regenerated second, making the stability variable. In this study, the authors observed that some additional examinations were found to be more variable from one output to another, that is, psychophysical olfactory testing, which corroborated the finding of other clinical studies.[7,34] The inability of ChatGPT-4 to reliably propose some unusual additional examinations such as psychophysical olfactory testing, and impedance-pH monitoring was similarly observed in other otolaryngologic subspecialties, such as laryngology.[31] Saibene and colleagues investigated the accuracy of

ChatGPT-3.5 and ChatGPT-4 in the management of theoretic odontogenic chronic rhinosinusitis clinical vignettes.[45] The analyses of the 8 experts involved in this study confirmed the better performance of ChatGPT-4 over ChatGPT-3.5 but there were substantial disagreements between experts and ChatGPT in the management of 91.3% of the cases.[45]

Sleep Disorders

Several studies have been conducted to evaluate the accuracy of ChatGPT in general sleep knowledge or information for patients.[46–49] Cheong and colleagues compared the accuracy of ChatGPT-3.5, ChatGPT-4.0, and Google Bard in responding to 301 text-based single-best-answer multiple choice questions (10 examination categories) from the American Sleep Medicine Certification Board Examination.[46] Considering a pass mark of 80% for the examination, the authors found that ChatGPT-4 successfully achieved the pass mark with 80% or above in 5/10 examination categories. In this study, ChatGPT-4 demonstrated superior performance in all examination categories (68.1%) compared to ChatGPT-3.5 (46.8%), and Google Bard (45.5%), respectively.[46] ChatGPT-3.5 and Google Bard similarly scored in this study. This high accuracy of ChatGPT in responding to theoretic sleep questions was similarly supported by Mira and colleagues who found that ChatGPT-3.5 shared 75% of the responses of 97 sleep practitioners in a virtual examination.[47] Another study of Cheong and colleagues reported that the understandability and actionability scores of the Patient Education Materials Assessment Tool—Printable for ChatgGPT-3.5 and Google Bard ranged from 46% to 92% and 20% to 80%, respectively,[48] concluding that, as for the American Sleep Medicine Certification Board Exam, ChatGPT-3.5 scored better than Google Bard in providing understandable and actionable information related to sleep disorders.[48] The quality of ChatGPT's sleep apnea syndrome outputs for patient education was similarly evaluated by Campbell and colleagues who introduced 24 questions into the API, which were regenerated 4 times.[49] The authors observed that 69 ChatGPT-3.5 responses were at least correct, which corresponded to an accurate rate of 71.9%, while ChatGPT-3.5 provided adequate outputs in 96.1% of the questions.[49]

Otology and Vertigo

Bellinger and colleagues collected the 5 most common patient questions about benign paroxysmal positional vertigo from Google. They introduced them in the API to assess the readability, quality, understandability, and actionability of ChatGPT responses (unspecified version).[29] They reported that ChatGPT had higher Flesch-Kincaid Grade Level and lower Flesch Reading Ease scores than Google, indicating lower readability. Similar findings were found for the quality of responses, which led the authors to conclude that Google information is still superior to those provided by ChatGPT.[29] From a clinical performance standpoint, Chee and colleagues input into the API 8 theoretic vignettes of vertigo including medical history, typos of prompts, or clinical pictures and reported that ChatGPT (unspecified version) succeeded in the diagnosis of 6/8 cases and differentiated well between vestibular and non-vestibular causes of dizziness.[50]

SUMMARY

The application of generative AI, particularly AILM, is booming in otolaryngology—head and neck surgery with ChatGPT as the main investigated model. The accuracy of ChatGPT appears high in providing general knowledge related to common otolaryngologic conditions for patients, students, and practitioners. However, its accuracy should be moderate overall as an adjunctive tool in managing clinical vignettes. The rapid evolution of models and the increasing number of published studies each week make the future unpredictable and exciting in the revolution of otolaryngology—head and neck surgery practices.

ACKNOWLEDGMENTS

None.

DISCLOSURE

Competing interest: None. Sponsorships: None. Funding source: None.

REFERENCES

1. Kedia N, Sanjeev S, Ong J, et al. ChatGPT and Beyond: An overview of the growing field of large language models and their use in ophthalmology. Eye 2024. https://doi.org/10.1038/s41433-023-02915-z.
2. Tahayori B, Chini-Foroush N, Akhlaghi H. Advanced natural language processing technique to predict patient disposition based on emergency triage notes. Emerg Med Australasia (EMA) 2021;33(3):480–4.
3. Venerito V, Bilgin E, Iannone F, et al. AI am a rheumatologist: a practical primer to large language models for rheumatologists. Rheumatology 2023;62(10):3256–60.
4. Lee JC, Hamill CS, Shnayder Y, et al. Exploring the Role of Artificial Intelligence Chatbots in Preoperative Counseling for Head and Neck Cancer Surgery. Laryngoscope 2023. https://doi.org/10.1002/lary.31243.
5. Vaira LA, Lechien JR, Abbate V, et al. Accuracy of ChatGPT-Generated Information on Head and Neck and Oromaxillofacial Surgery: A Multicenter Collaborative Analysis. Otolaryngol Head Neck Surg 2023. https://doi.org/10.1002/ohn.489.
6. Lechien JR, Briganti G, Vaira LA. Accuracy of ChatGPT-3.5 and -4 in providing scientific references in otolaryngology-head and neck surgery. Eur Arch Oto-Rhino-Laryngol 2024;281(4):2159–65.
7. Lechien JR, Maniaci A, Gengler I, et al. Validity and reliability of an instrument evaluating the performance of intelligent chatbot: the Artificial Intelligence Performance Instrument (AIPI). Eur Arch Oto-Rhino-Laryngol 2024;281(4):2063–79.
8. Qu RW, Qureshi U, Petersen G, et al. Diagnostic and Management Applications of ChatGPT in Structured Otolaryngology Clinical Scenarios. OTO Open 2023; 7(3):e67.
9. Lechien JR, Gorton A, Robertson J, et al. Is ChatGPT-4 Accurate in Proofread a Manuscript in Otolaryngology-Head and Neck Surgery? Otolaryngol Head Neck Surg 2023. https://doi.org/10.1002/ohn.526.
10. Salvagno M, Taccone FS, Gerli AG. Can artificial intelligence help for scientific writing? Crit Care 2023;27(1):75.
11. Chiesa-Estomba CM, Speth MM, Mayo-Yanez M, et al. Is the evolving role of artificial intelligence and chatbots in the field of otolaryngology embracing the future? Eur Arch Oto-Rhino-Laryngol 2024;281(4):2179–80.
12. Bur AM, Shew M, New J. Artificial Intelligence for the Otolaryngologist: A State of the Art Review. Otolaryngol Head Neck Surg 2019;160(4):603–11.
13. Panovski A. How Did Philosophy Help Develop Artificial Intelligence? The Collector 2023.

14. McCulloch WS, Pitts W. A logical calculus of the ideas immanent in nervous activity. Bull Math Biophys 1943;5:115–33.
15. Muthukrishnan N, Maleki F, Ovens K, et al. Brief History of Artificial Intelligence. Neuroimaging Clin N Am 2020;30(4):393–9.
16. Turing AMI. Computing machinery and intelli- gence. Mind 1950;LIX(236): 433–60.
17. McCorduck P. Machines who think. 2nd edition. Natick (MA): A K Peters, Ltd; 2004.
18. Briganti G. How ChatGPT works: a mini review. Eur Arch Oto-Rhino-Laryngol 2024;281(3):1565–9.
19. Tolsgaard MG, Boscardin CK, Park YS, et al. The role of data science and machine learning in Health Professions Education: practical applications, theoretical contributions, and epistemic beliefs. Adv Health Sci Educ Theory Pract 2020; 25(5):1057–86.
20. Alter IL, Chan K, Lechien JR, et al. ChatGPT, ENT, and Me: An Introduction to Artificial Intelligence and Machine Learning for Otolaryngologists. Eur Arch Oto-Rhino-Laryngol 2024;281(5):2723–31.
21. Hoch CC, Wollenberg B, Lüers JC, et al. ChatGPT's quiz skills in different otolaryngology subspecialties: an analysis of 2576 single-choice and multiple-choice board certification preparation questions. Eur Arch Oto-Rhino-Laryngol 2023; 280(9):4271–8.
22. Mahajan AP, Shabet CL, Smith J, et al. Assessment of Artificial Intelligence Performance on the OtolaryngologyResidency In-Service Exam. OTO Open 2023; 7(4):e98.
23. Long C, Lowe K, Zhang J, et al. A Novel Evaluation Model for Assessing ChatGPT on Otolaryngology-Head and Neck Surgery Certification Examinations: Performance Study. JMIR Med Educ 2024;10:e49970.
24. Moise A, Centomo-Bozzo A, Orishchak O, et al. Can ChatGPT Guide Parents on Tympanostomy Tube Insertion? Children 2023;10(10):1634.
25. Zalzal HG, Cheng J, Shah RK. Evaluating the Current Ability of ChatGPT to Assist in Professional Otolaryngology Education. OTO Open 2023;7(4):e94.
26. Langlie J, Kamrava B, Pasick LJ, et al. Artificial intelligence and ChatGPT: An otolaryngology patient's ally or foe? Am J Otolaryngol 2024;45(3):104220.
27. Nielsen JPS, von Buchwald C, Grønhøj C. Validity of the large language model ChatGPT (GPT4) as a patient information source in otolaryngology by a variety of doctors in a tertiary otorhinolaryngology department. Acta Otolaryngol 2023; 143(9):779–82.
28. Ayoub NF, Lee YJ, Grimm D, et al. Head-to-Head Comparison of ChatGPT Versus Google Search for Medical Knowledge Acquisition. Otolaryngol Head Neck Surg 2023. https://doi.org/10.1002/ohn.465.
29. Bellinger JR, De La Chapa JS, Kwak MW, et al. BPPV Information on Google Versus AI (ChatGPT). Otolaryngol Head Neck Surg 2023, https://doi.org/10.1002/ohn.506.
30. Dallari V, Sacchetto A, Saetti R, et al. Is artificial intelligence ready to replace specialist doctors entirely? ENT specialists vs ChatGPT: 1-0, ball at the center. Eur Arch Oto-Rhino-Laryngol 2024;281(2):995–1023.
31. Lechien JR, Georgescu BM, Hans S, et al. ChatGPT performance in laryngology and head and neck surgery: a clinical case-series. Eur Arch Oto-Rhino-Laryngol 2024;281(1):319–33.
32. Karimov Z, Allahverdiyev I, Agayarov OY, et al. ChatGPT vs UpToDate: comparative study of usefulness and reliability of Chatbot in common clinical presentations of

otorhinolaryngology-head and neck surgery. Eur Arch Oto-Rhino-Laryngol 2024; 281(4):2145–51.

33. Kuşcu O, Pamuk AE, Sütay Süslü N, et al. Is ChatGPT accurate and reliable in answering questions regarding head and neck cancer? Front Oncol 2023;13: 1256459.

34. Radulesco T, Saibene AM, Michel J, et al. ChatGPT-4 performance in rhinology: A clinical case series. Int Forum Allergy Rhinol 2024. https://doi.org/10.1002/alr. 23323.

35. Chiesa-Estomba CM, Urazan JD, Andueza M, et al. Comparative analysis of patient's perception between medical expert Vs chat-GPT advice for laryngeal, oropharyngeal, and salivary gland tumors. 2024. Scientific Presentation, San Sebastian Universty Hospital, Department of Otolaryngology, 2023.

36. Davis RJ, Ayo-Ajibola O, Lin ME, et al. Evaluation of Oropharyngeal Cancer Information from Revolutionary Artificial Intelligence Chatbot. Laryngoscope 2024; 134(5):2252–7.

37. Campbell DJ, Estephan LE, Sina E, et al. Evaluating ChatGPT responses on thyroid nodules for patient education. Thyroid 2024;34(3):371–7.

38. Chiesa-Estomba CM, Lechien JR, Vaira LA, et al. Exploring the potential of ChatGPT as a supportive tool for sialendoscopy clinical decision making and patient information support. Eur Arch Oto-Rhino-Laryngol 2024;281(4):2081–6.

39. Marchi F, Bellini E, Iandelli A, et al. Exploring the Landscape of AI-Assisted Decision-Making in Head and Neck Cancer Treatment: A Comparative Analysis of NCCN Guidelines and ChatGPT Responses. Eur Arch Oto-Rhino-Laryngol 2024; 281(4):2123–36.

40. Lechien JR, Chiesa-Estomba CM, Baudouin R, et al. Accuracy of ChatGPT in head and neck oncological board decisions: preliminary findings. Eur Arch Oto-Rhino-Laryngol 2024;281(4):2105–14.

41. Sievert M, Aubreville M, Muller S, et al. Confocal laser endomicroscopy, oropharyngeal squamous cell carcinoma, GPT, head and neck malignancies. Eur Arch Oto-Rhino-Laryngol 2024.

42. Nachalon Y, Broer M, Nativ-Zeltzer N. Using ChatGPT to Generate Research Ideas in Dysphagia: A Pilot Study. Dysphagia 2023. https://doi.org/10.1007/ s00455-023-10623-9.

43. Capelleras M, Soto-Galindo GA, Cruellas M, et al. ChatGPT and Rhinoplasty Recovery: An Exploration of AI's Role in Postoperative Guidance. Facial Plast Surg 2024. https://doi.org/10.1055/a-2219-4901.

44. Durairaj KK, Baker O, Bertossi D, et al. Artificial Intelligence Versus Expert Plastic Surgeon: Comparative Study Shows ChatGPT "Wins" Rhinoplasty Consultations: Should We Be Worried? Facial Plast Surg Aesthet Med 2023. https://doi.org/10. 1089/fpsam.2023.0224.

45. Saibene AM, Allevi F, Calvo-Henriquez C, et al. Reliability of large language models in managing odontogenic sinusitis clinical scenarios: a preliminary multidisciplinary evaluation. Eur Arch Oto-Rhino-Laryngol 2024;281(4):1835–41.

46. Cheong RCT, Pang KP, Unadkat S, et al. Performance of artificial intelligence chatbots in sleep medicine certification board exams: ChatGPT versus Google Bard. Eur Arch Oto-Rhino-Laryngol 2024;281(4):2137–43.

47. Mira FA, Favier V, Dos Santos Sobreira Nunes H, et al. Chat GPT for the management of obstructive sleep apnea: do we have a polar star? Eur Arch Oto-Rhino-Laryngol 2024;281(4):2087–93.

48. Cheong RCT, Unadkat S, Mcneillis V, et al. Artificial intelligence chatbots as sources of patient education material for obstructive sleep apnoea: ChatGPT versus Google Bard. Eur Arch Oto-Rhino-Laryngol 2024;281(2):985–93.
49. Campbell DJ, Estephan LE, Mastrolonardo EV, et al. Evaluating ChatGPT responses on obstructive sleep apnea for patient education. J Clin Sleep Med 2023;19(12):1989–95.
50. Chee J, Kwa ED, Goh X. "Vertigo, likely peripheral": the dizzying rise of ChatGPT. Eur Arch Oto-Rhino-Laryngol 2023;280(10):4687–9.

Autonomous Robotic Systems in Otolaryngology-Head and Neck Surgery

Shreya Sriram, BS[a,1], Francis X. Creighton Jr, MD[b,1],
Deepa Galaiya, MD[b,*,1]

KEYWORDS

- Artificial intelligence • Robotics • Otolaryngology-head and neck surgery • Haptics
- Autonomous systems • Force feedback

KEY POINTS

- It is increasingly important to characterize the current roles of robotic assistance in otolaryngology-head and neck surgery (OHNS) within modern definitions and identify sectors with potential for improved utilization.
- The goal of incorporating autonomous systems is not so much to create robots to replace surgeons, but rather to aid the surgeon by providing improved efficiency, consistency, safety, and outcomes.
- Semiautonomous guidance in surgery would rely on the operator to perform the task while augmenting and improving performance with artificial intelligence (AI)–guided identification of virtual fixtures, visual-tactile perception, and navigation.
- The role of an AI-guided robot is not solely mechanical with holding tools or increasing stability; rather, these systems can integrate information about the surgical field like anatomic location, feel, and compliance to enhance control of the robot—aspects that can be well developed within the field of skull base surgery.
- Cost to the health system should be considered, as robotic surgery is consistently more expensive than laparoscopic or open methods, as well as environmental impacts since minimally invasive procedures contribute to global carbon emissions more than laparoscopic or open methods.

 Video content accompanies this article at http://www.oto.theclinics.com.

INTRODUCTION

Surgery, one of the most ancient forms of medicine, is also at the forefront of technological development and possibility with the novel use of robotic systems in the last

[a] Johns Hopkins School of Medicine, Baltimore, MD, USA; [b] Department of Otolaryngology–Head and Neck Surgery, Johns Hopkins Hospital, Baltimore, MD, USA
[1] Present address: 101 North Wolfe Street, Apartment 470, Baltimore, MD 21231.
* Corresponding author. 601 North Caroline Street, Suite 6, Baltimore, MD 21287-0910.
E-mail address: Deepa.galaiya@jhmi.edu

Otolaryngol Clin N Am 57 (2024) 767–779
https://doi.org/10.1016/j.otc.2024.05.004   oto.theclinics.com
0030-6665/24/© 2024 Elsevier Inc. All rights reserved, including those for text and data mining, AI training, and similar technologies.

3 decades. The introduction of robotic assistance for medicine is seen in a variety of settings, from rehabilitation treatment to image guidance, to the operating theater.[1] In the field of otolaryngology-head and neck surgery (OHNS), transoral robotic surgery (TORS) with the da Vinci system has shown clear benefits in efficiency, patient outcomes, and expenditure compared to open methods and encouraged OHNS surgeons to incorporate these systems in their routine care.[2] As the interface between medicine and technology grows, and the burgeoning field of artificial intelligence (AI) crosses industry lines, surgeons are eager to understand what may be on the horizon in terms of robotic assistance in surgery. It is increasingly important to characterize the current roles of robotic assistance in OHNS within modern definitions and identify sectors with potential for improved utilization. This review will describe the current state of robotics in medicine and OHNS as well as future developments toward autonomous robotic systems.

BACKGROUND

The earliest record of a mechanical creation that could potentially step into a human role came with Leonardo da Vinci who drew metal-plated mechanical knights containing gears to create motion.[3] The term robot originated from the 1920s' Czech play entitled "Rossom's Universal Robots," morphing the Czech word "robota" meaning labor.[4] In 1972, robots were given a standardized definition by the Robot Institute of America as a "reprogrammable, multifunctional manipulator designed to move materials, parts, tools or specialized devices through variable programmed motions for the performance of a variety of tasks." In 1992, the MIT-Manus was unveiled as the first robotic device designed particularly for rehabilitation. Users place their arm into a brace and the machine will guide them to complete simple tasks with varying amounts of force depending on the patient's ability.[5,6]

Surgery presents the unique opportunity for a robot to combine the physical and mental acumen of a surgeon into automated actions. Nearly 2 decades ago, Dr Russ Taylor delineated the goals of surgical robots: to improve surgeons' technical capability and promote surgical safety.[7] Robotic assistance debuted in various fields in the 1980s starting with orthopedics (Arthrobot, 1983), neurosurgery (Programmable Universal Machine for Assembly, 1985), and urology (for transuretheral resection of prostate, 1988).[3] The introduction of more autonomous robotic systems began with the ROBODOC for orthopedics in 1992, which assisted the surgeon in planning their entry orientation.[8] In 1994, Computer Motion Inc, a group of researchers supported by a NASA grant, received Food and Drug Administration (FDA) approval for their Automated Endoscopic System for Optimal Positioning (AESOP) surgical system. The first of its kind to replace a human endoscope holder, it was controlled by foot pedals and voice commands and represented the true synergy that can be achieved between surgeons and robots in the operating room.[9] However, in 1998, Intuitive Surgery Inc introduced the current monolith of robotic surgery, the da Vinci surgical system.

Most recent da Vinci models are made of 3 surgical instrument arms and 1 camera arm. da Vinci understands that surgeons can only operate as well as they can see and expands the ability to operate around corners with a custom endoscope for full stereotactic vision and high resolution. Containing discrete channels of viewing for each eye and safety checks to prevent inappropriate manipulation, the da Vinci system debuted in cardiothoracic surgery.[10] In the following 2 years, da Vinci was applied to all general surgery procedures and received FDA approval.[11] The precise wrist movement with 7° of freedom, or axes of motion, encouraged OHNS surgeons at the University of

Pennsylvania to pilot da Vinci for the first otolaryngologic procedure in 2005, termed TORS.[12] TORS utilizes da Vinci's visualization abilities to access structures deep in the pharynx through the natural oral orifice. Since 2005, TORS has helped with oropharyngeal, laryngeal, and tongue base tumor resections; surgeries for obstructive sleep apnea; thyroid resections; neck and salivary gland dissections, and even select neuro-otologic applications.[13,14]

The da Vinci system has since grown to be the standard of care in high-volume hospital systems; however, as an assistive robot, it cannot complete surgical tasks autonomously. Beyaz and colleagues[8] described a distinction between the array of robotic systems currently available for surgical use: haptic versus active. Haptic systems are surgeon-guided and still require the mastery of a trained surgeon; like da Vinci, they are meant to improve surgical performance. Active systems can be considered autonomous and can follow a preset plan of operations executed by the robot with minimal to no input from a surgeon. These robots still require the surgeon to direct advancement from one stage of surgery to the next, identify target tissue, and distinguish between diseased and healthy anatomy. It is in this sphere that robotic systems have the greatest potential to grow into being a fully functioning, autonomous system.

LEVELS OF SURGICAL AUTONOMY

Current development of surgical robots focuses on creating semiautonomous machines that can independently perform discrete tasks under the purview and guidance of the surgeon, ultimately to enhance, not replace, the surgeon's existing capability. The field of surgery is nascent in incorporating autonomous systems. There is a level of hesitancy from surgeons and patients with the concept of a robot stepping into the role of a surgeon.[15] A recently published survey of American Rhinologic Society members found that over 80% of respondents would involve AI for clinical decision-making and diagnostics, such as using AI to analyze radiographic images. The use of AI for direct treatments like surgery was polarizing for the cohort, with only 50% interested in even exploring this possibility. However, select surgeons indicated their interest in using AI for preoperative planning and surgical navigation by segmenting images and recognition of tumor tissue and anatomy.[16,17]

Analogous developments in the motor vehicle industry can demonstrate how AI could be used in surgery to improve efficiency and safety. For autonomous driving, there exist multiple levels of human versus machine control, ranging from the driver in full control of the car to a fully autonomous car requiring neither human hands nor vision, a level that has not yet been achieved. Within that spectrum, there are a variety of automated tools we have become accustomed to, such as lane assistance, which automatically detects roadway lanes and provides feedback to the car and driver to course-correct. Our representation of corollary levels of autonomy for robotic surgery in inspired by Yang and colleagues[18], where level 1 is manual surgery, level 3 is the ability to complete tasks without direct surgeon intervention, and level 5 is a fully autonomous robotic surgeon—the material of science fiction (**Fig. 1**). At this stage, research and development of surgical robots remains at levels 2 to 3.

Like lane assistance technology in motor vehicles, semiautonomous guidance in surgery would rely on the operator to perform the task while augmenting and improving performance through AI-guided identification of virtual fixtures, visual-tactile perception, and navigation. A semiautonomous system thereby requires less infrastructure and provides flexibility, as not every outcome needs to be programmed and individualized to each patient and procedure. Finally, if semiautonomous robotic guidance proves to be more acceptable to the general population, patient hesitance

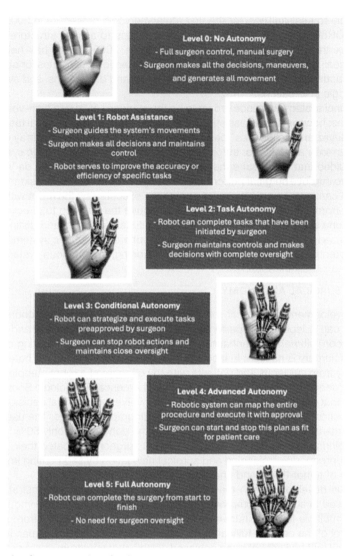

Fig. 1. Levels of autonomy in robotic surgery.

around surgical robots would be mitigated by the knowledge that the surgeon is the primary controller.

ARTIFICIAL INTELLIGENCE AND ROBOTICS IN OTOLARYNGOLOGY

For otolaryngology, the current state of AI is mainly split between oncologic, laryngologic, and neuro-otologic applications. A recent systematic review found that AI applications for head and neck cancer surgery primarily involved surgical margin assessment, complications assessment, and salvage surgery.[19] The studies used machine learning to intraoperatively identify accurate margins to improve surgical efficiency or analyze large datasets to predict common postoperative adverse events and oncologic risk factors. Bur and colleagues[20] suggest implementing machine learning in high-stakes skull base surgery to label critical structures such as the carotid artery and optic nerve. In 2016, Carlson and colleagues[21] used machine learning techniques to visualize glottic opening, eventually used in endotracheal intubation for real-time feedback to physicians. The AESOP surgical robot was the first AI platform that integrated the surgeon's voice to control the position of a camera for endoscopic procedures.[22,23] Despite use in a variety of surgical procedures requiring endoscopy, including otolaryngology, widespread utilization is hindered by the need to constantly readjust the endoscope's view.[24–26]

Autonomous robots could alleviate this stress by having an intuition to follow the surgeon's workflow and focus the camera on the appropriate area. In order for the AESOP to be incorporated with AI, the endoscope should be able to optimize the viewpoint without any guidance or readjustments from the surgeon. In 2008, the AutoLap (MST, Israel) system, which uses image analysis and computer-based instrument recognition to tag the surgeon's instrument and shift the view based off the surgeon's movement, was piloted for clinical use as the first foray into AI integration.[27] In 2020, a joint group from Italy and Johns Hopkins introduced the System for Camera Autonomous Navigation (SCAN) ability which tracks the tools and adjusts the endoscope position independent of surgeon guidance.[28,29] The researchers compared SCAN's autonomous to manual camera control modalities, and found shorter task times with autonomous camera control mode and surgeons reported greater ease of use. As such, it appears that the future of automated endoscopic manipulation might be on the horizon.

ROSA machines (Medtech) are a series of platforms for orthopedic surgery that are seen as more autonomous extensions of the original ROBODOC for an arthroplasty and can perform the entire procedure without direct surgeon guidance.[30] Succeeding versions of this technology include the Robotic Arm Interactive Orthopedic System (RIO) (MAKO Surgical Corp), CASPAR, and NAVIO which all act as active-autonomous systems that are still controlled by the surgeon and have been documented to improve surgical outcomes.[31–34] The ROSA robot took these a step further as a semiautonomous system, FDA-approved in 2019, which calibrates itself to the femoral and tibial landmarks and identifies a "best scenario" surgical plan based on intraoperative measurements.[35] The ROSA confirms these measurements and proceeds with the planned incisions, all independently.[36] ROSA is a newer technology which has shown both improved patient outcomes with reduced operative time, yet still with dissatisfying accuracy in surgical planning.[36,37]

ROSA ONE (Zimmer Biomet) is a stereotactic robot for neurosurgery that has been proven successful and comprises a robotic arm, touchscreen, robot stand, and navigating telescope arm.[38–40] The ROSA ONE uses preoperative images to register the surgical field and plan for multiple surgical paths. According to Zimmer Biomet, the ROSA ONE can ensure "instruments are placed in the planned area while avoiding critical structures."[41] They have developed robotic systems for both the brain and spine with the purpose of functional and stereotactic endoscopic open skull procedures or pedicle screw placement, respectively.[41,42] While the ROSA ONE effectively implements the concepts of registration and virtual fixtures, this does not qualify as an AI-driven surgical robot.

Applications of active-autonomous systems into otolaryngology are mainly in the field of cochlear implant (CI) insertion. The majority of CI surgery is vastly successful and follows a manual approach with a mastoidectomy bordering the facial nerve. Minimally invasive robotic assistance can minimize risks with the mastoid approach while preserving optimal outcomes seen with the traditional method.[43] The first robotic-assisted CI insertion used image guidance from a preoperative computed tomography

(CT) scan for segmentation and path planning to facilitate stereotactic drilling. Labadie and colleagues[43] present the novel use of this robot on 7 patients with 6 successful insertions. Two years later, Caversaccio and colleagues[44] presented HEARO, a robotic platform with an arm as the first semiautonomous drill, for CI insertion. It is capable of segmenting critical anatomy and registration of surgical plan using surgical screws as references, and plan execution. Preoperative imaging was used to guide the robot and the safety of the drilling path was verified with intraoperative imaging and various sensors ensuring safe drilling. This system has since been proven as feasible and efficacious for CI insertion in patients, even those with complications.[45–47]

iotaMotion (Iowa City, IA, USA) created the iotaSOFT Insertion System for electrode array insertions in CI surgeries consisting of a single-use sterile drive unit. iotaSOFT can help in preserving the delicate inner ear structures and minimizing damage to anatomy crucial for optimal hearing after insertion.[48,49] This robot has been especially helpful in inserting the electrode array at a slow and steady pace, something human surgeons are physiologically incapable of. iotaSOFT, however, requires significant surgeon involvement in locking the drive head tip to a location within 5 to 10 mm of the round window. The subsequent movement direction and speed in the inner ear is controlled entirely by a foot pedal operated by the surgeon, emphasizing the lack of robotic autonomy.[50]

ARTIFICIAL INTELLIGENCE–DRIVEN ROBOTICS

The role of an AI-guided robot is not solely mechanical; rather, these systems can integrate information about the surgical field like anatomic location, feel, and compliance to enhance control of the robot. Machine learning algorithms have been developed to identify structures (image segmentation) for intraoperative guidance (image navigation) and improve haptic feedback to improve surgeon drilling ability.[51–53]

It can be argued that the skull base is the ideal surgical field for the development of autonomous robotic tools. The skull base is difficult to access, containing important neurovascular and neurologic structures separated by mere millimeters, and pathologies in this space often require long surgeries and extensive training for competency. The potential consequences of a complication in skull base surgery that may arise from an injury are very high.[54] In comparison to other anatomic areas, the skull base is entirely fixed in bone, and anatomic structures do not move relative to one another, making surgical scene segmentation and image navigation easier to accomplish than in soft tissue surgery. In this space, we can independently address several problems in parallel to create a full robotic system for surgery.

Haptics is one of these problems. Robotics has resulted in haptic feedback being largely diminished or entirely removed from the hands of the surgeon. Haptics encompasses a number of different sensory inputs, including "kinesthetic sensation," that is, where the body is relative to itself with (for example, joint angles in limb movement), and "tactile sensation," which is information about the physical characteristics of objects outside of the body. In contrast to vision, haptic information regarding an object's physical properties requires the body to come into contact with the object. Research has been focusing on restoring haptic information sensing that can detect tool to tissue forces and tissue deformation, augmenting the human ability to sense this information (for example, with a force sensor that is more sensitive to compliance changes than the human hand), and then presenting this information to a surgeon in real time without temporal delay. Robotic systems must be able to provide kinematic precision (tools move to the surgeon's command accurately), kinetic fidelity (haptic information is accurately measured), and with minimal temporal lag. When this is achieved, we may be able to do force scaling and augment sensory information to feel, for example, the force involved in causing tip foldover in a CI electrode. We can also apply force limits to avoid errors, protect sensitive tissue, and alert a surgeon when critical thresholds are approached. We can also generate higher fidelity surgical simulators for training that can feel more like real surgery.

Largely regarded as one of the pitfalls of robotic-assisted surgery, lack of tactile and haptic sensation can result in tissue damage and comorbidities. Visual cues can only partially compensate for the reduction in kinetics.[55] Laparoscopic surgeons use visual cues in the absence of haptic feedback to estimate force on tissue. Endoscopic surgeons subconsciously estimate depth with small motions of the hand and camera despite a monocular field of view. In the field of orthopedics, it took nearly 15 years of development before introducing RIO , which was equipped with advanced haptic technology using tactile feedback from the robot to the surgeon. RIO has grown to be the most widely used robot for certain orthopedic procedures.[56] The RIO system uses preoperative CT to create a 3-dimensional model of the target bone and set a preset cutting zone for the robot. As such, final manipulation and actions are still determined by the surgeon who operates the robot. This preoperative planning ensures that the surgeon stays within the boundaries of the surgical zone while maintaining complete control over the tool. The haptic feedback allows the surgeon to use the robot as they would use a regular drill with the added advantage of having these preset anatomic guard rails. The robot can identify in real time where the surgeon is operating and will constrain the force-controlled tip of the instrument to only function within the predefined drilling zone or resection limits.[57,58] The concept of "no-go zones" is not novel for autonomous robots and has been discussed for nearly 2 decades.[7]

For otolaryngology, a combined engineering-OHNS team at the start-up Galen Robotics has developed a cooperative control robot platform that provides surgeons with a steady hand known as the robotic ENT microsurgery system (REMS).[59] The Galen REMS has 5° of freedom. Unlike the da Vinci system, which uses teleoperation with manual surgeon manipulation of the robotic arms outside the surgical field; cooperative control platforms like the REMS or RIO allow the surgeon to hold and operate with their instrument of choice in tandem with the robot. REMS can augment surgeon control with hand tremor cancellation, which can be crucial for the tight anatomic regions otolaryngologists operate in.[60] REMS also uses virtual fixtures to define the surgical space and prevent the surgeon from moving beyond that. Studies have demonstrated novices successfully performing a mastoidectomy in 5 trials using anatomic virtual fixtures enforced by REMS, with no training or coaching, in a mean time to completion of ~3.6 minutes.[61] This was a great step toward the implementation of semiautonomous robotic systems in surgery, as the operative time with fully autonomous procedures was reported to be around 90 minutes.[62] A force-sensing drill has also been developed that can be used in conjunction with a cooperative robot such as REMS.[63] Force information can be integrated with positional data to enforce force thresholds that the surgeon cannot exceed when touching critical structures with haptic feedback.[64]

In addition to providing safety barriers, another crucial area for AI-guided robotics is accurate and automated image segmentation using computer vision. Manually segmented imaging studies are used to train machine learning algorithms to automatically segment, localize, and track anatomy and objects on scans and video streams of surgery. The goal of an automated robot is to register imaging to anatomic structures accurately and consistently while quickly adjusting to new structures uncovered as the surgical view changes. Sinha and colleagues[65] presented an algorithm using AI machine learning techniques to register surrounding anatomy to submillimeter accuracies while conducting an active clinical endoscopy. This potentiates applications for structures without a reference preoperative CT scan.

Ding and colleagues[66] report a novel method for automated registration-based segmentation of temporal bone anatomy without the need for a preoperative CT scan. They created a standard template for the average temporal bone after compiling standard temporal bone CTs with salient anatomy labeled. Their findings presented a more rapid, automated process for segmentation of the temporal bone. Thus, patient outcomes benefit from the use of segmentation to develop virtual fixtures and protect vulnerable middle and inner ear structures. One year later, the same group published findings supporting the use of deep learning networks to autonomously segment temporal bone anatomy to expedite the preoperative planning process. The utilized deep learning neural network, nnU-Net, resulted in submillimeter accuracy for manual versus automated labeled structures of interest.[67] Automatic registration has since expanded to other fields using neural network–produced anatomic annotation. Intraoperative landmark localization was achieved for fluoroscopic navigation of the hip, suggesting that this technology, with further research and surgical validation studies to refine registration techniques can be used for image-guided otolaryngologic surgery in the skull base.[68,69]

OTHER CONSIDERATIONS

With all these areas of burgeoning research, robotic surgery and semiautonomous systems can provide new tools on the horizon to enhance a surgeon's performance. Ideally these advancements would also optimize efficiency in the operation room and reduce costs. A major consideration before implementing any robotic system is the cost to the health system, as robotic surgery is consistently more expensive than laparoscopic or open methods.[70] However, robotic assistance has proved its worth and established itself as a standard of care for certain centers. These hubs have welcomed the use of robots and found that for high case volumes, robotic assistance can improve postoperative quality of life with increased cost-effectiveness.[71] For example, the cost of RIO orthopedic robot as a barrier to adoption. Although robotic hip and knee arthroplasty had higher fixed costs and longer operative times, a Medicare analysis showed cost-effectiveness when considering the lower revision rate, shorter length of stay, and fewer complications when compared to open surgery with implementation at high-volume centers.[72]

In addition to cost, the environmental effects of robotic systems should be considered. Minimally invasive procedures contribute to global carbon emissions more than laparoscopic or open methods. Recent analyses show that robotic gynecologic procedures have around 40% greater greenhouse gas (GHG) emissions and create nearly 25% more waste than laparoscopic procedures.[73] The reimbursement model for many medical device companies in high-income countries relies on single-use instruments that contribute to a high carbon footprint. Robotic systems also use single-use instruments, yet costs can be higher due to the complexity of these instruments.[74] Analyses of cost-effectiveness and environmental impacts for autonomous procedures are still insufficient due to low surgical volumes, and research in this area is limited. A 2022 study analyzing potential GHG emissions for an AI diabetic eye examination found an 80% expense reduction as opposed to in-person eye examinations. The implications for surgery are vastly different; however, machine learning can be utilized to encourage the autonomous system to choose environmentally efficient options while still upholding a high quality of patient care. Furthermore, part of the purpose of implementing autonomous systems is to improve operative efficiency and patient outcomes, which can significantly reduce travel-related or complication-related carbon emissions.[75]

SUMMARY

Semiautonomous robotic systems are an emerging technology with a potential for augmenting a surgeon's capabilities. AI is being integrated into these robotic platforms to help perform higher level tasks. Several critical components of surgery are being simultaneously automated and refined, including surgical field segmentation, image segmentation, navigation and registration, tool tracking, and tool-to-tissue force sensing. These elements can enforce virtual boundaries, provide enhanced force sensing, and allow for customized, high-fidelity surgical simulations for planning and training. As these systems are increasingly refined, the machine-physician interface can become more seamless to enhance a surgeon's abilities.

Fig. 1 and Video 1 detail the different stages that an autonomous surgical robot would progress through. Level 0 represents the lowest level of autonomy where the robot has no intrinsic ability to enhance the procedure outside of its mechanical purpose. Level 5 represents the highest level achievable for an autonomous system where the robot essentially does take the place of a surgeon. Current AI-driven robotics for surgery sit at level 1 or 2.

CLINICS CARE POINTS

- Including AI into surgery is not meant to replace the surgeon but enhance the surgeon's skill and support achievement of efficient and effective methods for optimal patient outcomes.

- Haptic feedback, virtual fixtures, force-feedback, tremor control, and automated image segmentation are all existing starting points for AI-driven robotics in OHNS, which serve to improve surgical outcomes.

- The current state of autonomous systems in surgery is far from being entirely independent. Rather, these machines are just starting to broach the level of being semiautonomous. This means the surgeon initiates and oversees the robot actions, which are limited to smaller tasks that it may have been instructed to do. The surgeon also maintains complete control over these actions and can take over or terminate the process at any time.

DISCLOSURE

The authors have nothing to disclose.

FUNDING

This work was supported in part by a research contract from Galen Robotics, by NIDCD K08 Grant DC019708, by a research agreement with the Hong Kong Multi-Scale Medical Robotics Centre, and by Johns Hopkins University internal funds. These have been reviewed, approved and are in accordance with Johns Hopkins University conflict of interest policies.

SUPPLEMENTARY DATA

Supplementary data to this article can be found online at https://doi.org/10.1016/j.otc.2024.05.004.

REFERENCES

1. Morgan AA, Abdi J, Syed MAQ, et al. Robots in Healthcare: a Scoping Review. Curr Robot Rep 2022;3(4):271–80.
2. Niewinski P, Golusiński W. Current indications and patient selection for transoral roboticsurgery in head and neck cancer: a brief review. Współczesna Onkol 2022;26(2):91–6.
3. Yates DR, Vaessen C, Roupret M. From Leonardo to da Vinci: the history of robot-assisted surgery in urology. BJU Int 2011;108(11):1708–13, discussion 1714.
4. Marino MV, Shabat G, Gulotta G, et al. From Illusion to Reality: A Brief History of Robotic Surgery. Surg Innov 2018;25(3):291–6.
5. Hogan N, Krebs HI, Charnnarong J, et al. MIT-MANUS: a workstation for manual therapy and training. I. In: [1992] Proceedings IEEE International Workshop on Robot and Human Communication. IEEE; 1992. p. 161–5. https://doi.org/10.1109/ROMAN.1992.253895.
6. Payedimarri AB, Ratti M, Rescinito R, et al. Effectiveness of platform-based robot-assisted rehabilitation for musculoskeletal or neurologic injuries: a systematic review. Bioeng Basel Switz 2022;9(4):129.
7. Taylor RH. A perspective on medical robotics. Proc IEEE 2006;94(9):1652–64.
8. Beyaz S. A brief history of artificial intelligence and robotic surgery in orthopedics & traumatology and future expectations. Jt Dis Relat Surg 2020;31(3):653–5.
9. Shah J, Vyas A, Vyas D. The history of robotics in surgical specialties. Am J Robot Surg 2014;1(1):12–20.
10. Rivero-Moreno Y, Echevarria S, Vidal-Valderrama C, et al. Robotic Surgery: A Comprehensive Review of the Literature and Current Trends. Cureus 2023. https://doi.org/10.7759/cureus.42370.
11. George EI, Brand TC, LaPorta A, et al. Origins of robotic surgery: from skepticism to standard of care. J Soc Laparoendosc Surg 2018;22(4):e201800039. https://doi.org/10.4293/JSLS.2018.00039.
12. Garas G, Arora A. Robotic Head and Neck Surgery: History, Technical Evolution and the Future. ORL (Oto-Rhino-Laryngol) (Basel) 2018;80(3–4):117–24.
13. Fonseca AS. Transoral robotics in otolaryngology: a new frontier to be conquered. Braz J Otorhinolaryngol 2022;88(6):821–2.
14. Cammaroto G, Stringa LM, Zhang H, et al. Alternative Applications of Trans-Oral Robotic Surgery (TORS): A Systematic Review. J Clin Med 2020;9(1):201.
15. Chappell AG, Teven CM. How Should Surgeons Consider Emerging Innovations in Artificial Intelligence and Robotics? AMA J Ethics 2023;25(8):E589–97.
16. Asokan A, Massey CJ, Tietbohl C, et al. Physician views of artificial intelligence in otolaryngology and rhinology: A mixed methods study. Laryngoscope Investig Otolaryngol 2023;8(6):1468–75.
17. Andras I, Mazzone E, van Leeuwen FWB, et al. Artificial intelligence and robotics: a combination that is changing the operating room. World J Urol 2020;38(10):2359–66.
18. Yang GZ, Cambias J, Cleary K, et al. Medical robotics—Regulatory, ethical, and legal considerations for increasing levels of autonomy. Sci Robot 2017;2(4):eaam8638. https://doi.org/10.1126/scirobotics.aam8638.
19. Loperfido A, Celebrini A, Marzetti A, et al. Current role of artificial intelligence in head and neck cancer surgery: a systematic review of literature. Explor Target Antitumor Ther 2023;4(5):933–40.
20. Bur AM, Shew M, New J. Artificial intelligence for the otolaryngologist: a state of the art review. Otolaryngol–Head Neck Surg 2019;160(4):603–11.

21. Carlson JN, Das S, De la Torre F, et al. A novel artificial intelligence system for endotracheal intubation. Prehosp Emerg Care 2016;20(5):667–71.
22. Li Z, Chiu PWY. Robotic endoscopy. Visc Med 2018;34(1):45–51.
23. Healy DA, Murphy SP, Burke JP, et al. Artificial interfaces ("AI") in surgery: Historic development, current status and program implementation in the public health sector. Surg Oncol 2013;22(2):77–85.
24. Nathan CA, Chakradeo V, Malhotra K, et al. The voice-controlled robotic assist scope holder aesop for the endoscopic approach to the sella. Skull Base 2006;16(03):123–31.
25. Alessandrini M, De Padova A, Napolitano B, et al. The AESOP robot system for video-assisted rigid endoscopic laryngosurgery. Eur Arch Oto-Rhino-Laryngol 2008;265(9):1121–3.
26. Mettler L, Ibrahim M, Jonat W. One year of experience working with the aid of a robotic assistant (the voice-controlled optic holder AESOP) in gynaecological endoscopic surgery. Hum Reprod 1998;13(10):2748–50.
27. Wijsman PJM, Broeders IAMJ, Brenkman HJ, et al. First experience with THE AUTOLAP™ SYSTEM: an image-based robotic camera steering device. Surg Endosc 2018;32(5):2560–6.
28. Mariani A, Colaci G, Da Col T, et al. An experimental comparison towards autonomous camera navigation to optimize training in robot assisted surgery. IEEE Robot Autom Lett 2020;5(2):1461–7.
29. Col TD, Mariani A, Deguet A, et al. SCAN: system for camera autonomous navigation in robotic-assisted surgery. In: 2020 IEEE/RSJ International conference on intelligent robots and systems (IROS). IEEE; 2020. p. 2996–3002. https://doi.org/10.1109/IROS45743.2020.9341548.
30. Bullock E, Brown M, Clark G, et al. Robotics in total hip arthroplasty: current concepts. J Clin Med 2022;11(22):6674.
31. Kalavrytinos D, Koutserimpas C, Kalavrytinos I, et al. Expanding robotic arm-assisted knee surgery: the first attempt to use the system for knee revision arthroplasty. Case Rep Orthop 2020;2020:1–5.
32. Batailler C, Hannouche D, Benazzo F, et al. Concepts and techniques of a new robotically assisted technique for total knee arthroplasty: the ROSA knee system. Arch Orthop Trauma Surg 2021;141(12):2049–58.
33. Hampp E, Chughtai M, Scholl L, et al. Robotic-arm assisted total knee arthroplasty demonstrated greater accuracy and precision to plan compared with manual techniques. J Knee Surg 2019;32(03):239–50.
34. Ofa SA, Ross BJ, Flick TR, et al. Robotic total knee arthroplasty vs conventional total knee arthroplasty: a nationwide database study. Arthroplasty Today 2020;6(4):1001–8.e3.
35. Demirtas Y, Emet A, Ayik G, et al. A novel robot-assisted knee arthroplasty system (ROSA) and 1-year outcome: A single center experience. Medicine (Baltim) 2023;102(42):e35710. https://doi.org/10.1097/MD.0000000000035710.
36. Shin C, Crovetti C, Huo E, et al. Unsatisfactory accuracy of recent robotic assisting system ROSA for total knee arthroplasty. J Exp Orthop 2022;9(1):82.
37. Bolam SM, Tay ML, Zaidi F, et al. Introduction of ROSA robotic-arm system for total knee arthroplasty is associated with a minimal learning curve for operative time. J Exp Orthop 2022;9(1):86.
38. Brandmeir NJ, Savaliya S, Rohatgi P, et al. The comparative accuracy of the ROSA stereotactic robot across a wide range of clinical applications and registration techniques. J Robot Surg 2018;12(1):157–63.

39. González-Martínez J, Bulacio J, Thompson S, et al. Technique, results, and complications related to robot-assisted stereoelectroencephalography. Neurosurgery 2016;78(2):169–80.
40. Lefranc M, Capel C, Pruvot-Occean AS, et al. Frameless robotic stereotactic biopsies: a consecutive series of 100 cases. J Neurosurg 2015;122(2):342–52.
41. Nelson JH, Brackett SL, Oluigbo CO, et al. Robotic stereotactic assistance (ROSA) for pediatric epilepsy: a single-center experience of 23 consecutive cases. Children 2020;7(8):94.
42. Hsu BH, Liu HW, Lee KL, et al. Learning Curve of ROSA ONE Spine System for Transpedicular Screw Placement. Neurospine 2022;19(2):367–75.
43. Labadie RF, Balachandran R, Noble JH, et al. Minimally invasive image-guided cochlear implantation surgery: First report of clinical implementation. Laryngoscope 2014;124(8):1915–22.
44. Caversaccio M, Gavaghan K, Wimmer W, et al. Robotic cochlear implantation: surgical procedure and first clinical experience. Acta Otolaryngol (Stockh) 2017;137(4):447–54.
45. Auinger AB, Riss D, Baumgartner W, et al. Robot-assisted cochlear implant surgery in a patient with partial ossification of the basal cochlear turn: A technical note. Clin Otolaryngol 2022;47(3):504–7.
46. Auinger AB, Dahm V, Liepins R, et al. Robotic cochlear implant surgery: imaging-based evaluation of feasibility in clinical routine. Front Surg 2021;8:742219. https://doi.org/10.3389/fsurg.2021.742219.
47. Topsakal V, Heuninck E, Matulic M, et al. First study in men evaluating a surgical robotic tool providing autonomous inner ear access for cochlear implantation. Front Neurol 2022;13:804507. https://doi.org/10.3389/fneur.2022.804507.
48. Gantz JA, Gantz BJ, Kaufmann CR, et al. A steadier hand: the first human clinical trial of a single-use robotic-assisted surgical device for cochlear implant electrode array insertion. Otol Neurotol 2023;44(1):34–9.
49. Kaufmann CR, Henslee AM, Claussen A, et al. Evaluation of insertion forces and cochlea trauma following robotics-assisted cochlear implant electrode array insertion. Otol Neurotol 2020;41(5):631–8.
50. Henslee AM, Kaufmann CR, Andrick MD, et al. Development and characterization of an electrocochleography-guided robotics-assisted cochlear implant array insertion system. Otolaryngol Neck Surg 2022;167(2):334–40.
51. Chatterjee S, Das S, Ganguly K, et al. Advancements in robotic surgery: innovations, challenges and future prospects. J Robot Surg 2024;18(1):28.
52. Tomihama RT, Dass S, Chen S, et al. Machine learning and image analysis in vascular surgery. Semin Vasc Surg 2023;36(3):413–8.
53. Unberath M, Gao C, Hu Y, et al. The impact of machine learning on 2D/3D registration for image-guided interventions: a systematic review and perspective. Front Robot AI 2021;8:716007. https://doi.org/10.3389/frobt.2021.716007.
54. Liu JK, Saedi T, Delashaw JB, et al. Management of complications in neurotology. Otolaryngol Clin North Am 2007;40(3):651–67, x-xi.
55. Oliveira CM, Nguyen HT, Ferraz AR, et al. Robotic surgery in otolaryngology and head and neck surgery: a review. Minim Invasive Surg 2012;2012:1–11.
56. Jahng KH, Kamara E, Hepinstall MS. Haptic robotics in total hip arthroplasty. In: Scuderi GR, Tria AJ, editors. Minimally invasive surgery in orthopedics. Springer International Publishing; 2015. p. 1–15. https://doi.org/10.1007/978-3-319-15206-6_131-1.
57. Li T, Badre A, Alambeigi F, et al. Robotic systems and navigation techniques in orthopedics: a historical review. Appl Sci 2023;13(17):9768.

58. Chen X, Deng S, Sun ML, et al. Robotic arm-assisted arthroplasty: The latest developments. Chin J Traumatol Zhonghua Chuang Shang Za Zhi 2022;25(3): 125–31.
59. Akst LM, Olds KC, Balicki M, et al. Robotic microlaryngeal phonosurgery: Testing of a "steady-hand" microsurgery platform. Laryngoscope 2018;128(1):126–32.
60. Feng AL, Razavi CR, Lakshminarayanan P, et al. The robotic ENT microsurgery system: A novel robotic platform for microvascular surgery. Laryngoscope 2017;127(11):2495–500.
61. Ding AS, Capostagno S, Razavi CR, et al. Volumetric accuracy analysis of virtual safety barriers for cooperative-control robotic mastoidectomy. Otol Neurotol 2021;42(10):e1513–7.
62. Razavi CR, Wilkening PR, Yin R, et al. Image-guided mastoidectomy with a cooperatively controlled ENT microsurgery robot. Otolaryngol Neck Surg 2019;161(5): 852–5.
63. Chen Y, Goodridge A, Sahu M, et al. A force-sensing surgical drill for real-time force feedback in robotic mastoidectomy. Int J Comput Assist Radiol Surg 2023;18(7):1167–74.
64. Ishida H, Sahu M, Munawar A, et al. Haptic-assisted collaborative robot framework for improved situational awareness in skull base surgery. arXiv 2024. https://doi.org/10.48550/ARXIV.2401.11709.
65. Sinha A, Ishii M, Hager GD, et al. Endoscopic navigation in the clinic: registration in the absence of preoperative imaging. Int J Comput Assist Radiol Surg 2019; 14(9):1495–506.
66. Ding AS, Lu A, Li Z, et al. Automated registration-based temporal bone computed tomography segmentation for applications in neurotologic surgery. Otolaryngol Neck Surg 2022;167(1):133–40.
67. Ding AS, Lu A, Li Z, et al. A self-configuring deep learning network for segmentation of temporal bone anatomy in cone-beam CT imaging. Otolaryngol Neck Surg 2023;169(4):988–98.
68. Grupp RB, Unberath M, Gao C, et al. Automatic annotation of hip anatomy in fluoroscopy for robust and efficient 2D/3D registration. Int J Comput Assist Radiol Surg 2020;15(5):759–69.
69. Cho SM, Grupp RB, Gomez C, et al. Visualization in 2D/3D registration matters for assuring technology-assisted image-guided surgery. Int J Comput Assist Radiol Surg 2023;18(6):1017–24.
70. Gkegkes ID, Mamais IA, Iavazzo C. Robotics in general surgery: A systematic cost assessment. J Minimal Access Surg 2017;13(4):243–55.
71. Rajan PV, Khlopas A, Klika A, et al. The cost-effectiveness of robotic-assisted versus manual total knee arthroplasty: a markov model-based evaluation. J Am Acad Orthop Surg 2022;30(4):168–76.
72. Sousa PL, Sculco PK, Mayman DJ, et al. Robots in the operating room during hip and knee arthroplasty. Curr Rev Musculoskelet Med 2020;13(3):309–17.
73. Papadopoulou A, Kumar NS, Vanhoestenberghe A, et al. Environmental sustainability in robotic and laparoscopic surgery: systematic review. Br J Surg 2022; 109(10):921–32.
74. Chan KS, Lo HY, Shelat VG. Carbon footprints in minimally invasive surgery: Good patient outcomes, but costly for the environment. World J Gastrointest Surg 2023;15(7):1277–85.
75. Wolf RM, Abramoff MD, Channa R, et al. Potential reduction in healthcare carbon footprint by autonomous artificial intelligence. Npj Digit Med 2022;5(1):62.

The Application of Artificial Intelligence to Acoustic Data in Otolaryngology

Anthony Law, MD, PhD

KEYWORDS

- Artificial intelligence • Laryngology • Dysphonia • Acoustic data • Otology

KEY POINTS

- Artificial intelligence (AI) has become nearly synonymous with deep learning, a subset of machine learning characterized by the use of deep neural networks (DNNs).
- AI applied to acoustic data is an exhilarating field with numerous high-quality proof-of-concept studies.
- It holds the potential to transform health care delivery in laryngology and otology fundamentally.

INTRODUCTION

Artificial intelligence (AI) has undergone a renaissance over the past decade and now permeates into many aspects of daily life.[1–3] The term AI is somewhat nebulous but generally refers to any attempt to use computers to complete a task traditionally done by humans. In contemporary usage, AI has become nearly synonymous with deep learning, a subset of machine learning characterized by the use of deep neural networks (DNNs). It is deep learning that has demonstrated high accuracy in various complex and noisy systems, from autonomous vehicles to object identification to language translation. In many areas, deep learning now achieves or even surpasses human accuracy in specific tasks underscoring the transformative impact of this technique in modern applications.

Given the ability of deep learning models to robustly capture complex system, many are seeing an opportunity in the medical field to leverage these models in the care of patients. There has been exponential growth in research related to health care applications of deep learning models. In the medical domain, subspecialists with a dependence on digital data such as pathology[4] and radiology[5] have been first movers for the introduction of deep learning into their practice.

Department of Otolaryngology/Head & Neck Surgery, Emory University, Winship Cancer Institute, 550 Peachtree Street, Atlanta, GA 30308, USA
E-mail address: anthony.law@emory.edu

Otolaryngol Clin N Am 57 (2024) 781–789
https://doi.org/10.1016/j.otc.2024.06.011
oto.theclinics.com

Otolaryngology, similar to radiology and pathology, has a strong history of the digitally archiving patient data and integrating digital data into clinical practice. From recorded videolaryngoscopy to the acoustic recordings of patients with dysphonia to the use electronic health records, digital data are essential to the clinical care within many subspecialities of otolaryngology. These rich databases built by otolaryngologist are ripe for exploration by DNNs. Unique to otolaryngology, however, is the use and digital archiving of sound and acoustic data in the care of patients.

Here, we review investigations that apply deep learning to acoustic data in the subspecialties of laryngology and otology. Given the rapid advancements in AI, we specifically explore the use of DNNs as these represent the state-of-the-art models. We discuss the most significant challenges in these "twin subdisciplines" with regards to the manipulation and analysis of sound and discuss how deep learning is beginning to advance the field.

DEEP LEARNING BACKGROUND

Traditional approaches to modeling rely on combining a series of human-selected features in specific ways that allow accurate predictions within a desired system. Deep learning turns this paradigm on its head; the features (or parameters) of the model are defined by data alone and human intuition has no role in defining the system. In the training deep models, input and output are known, and technique referred as back-propagation learns the details of the model by iteratively tuning with each new piece of data. Once model-training process is complete, new inputs may be applied to the model and novel predictions are made.

For robust and accurate predictions, several key principles must be followed. First, the accuracy of deep learning models tends to improve with larger datasets.[6,7] Extremely large datasets help mitigate overfitting during the computational optimization of the millions of parameters in each network. Second, the dataset must be properly labeled. During the training phase of a DNN, each input must correspond to an accurate output, enabling the network to learn the relationship between the two. For example, if we are training a network to identify different animals, an image of a giraffe should be labeled as "giraffe." Lastly, the quality of the dataset is crucial. High-quality, well-curated data are essential, as noise in the input (such as audio files with acoustic interference or blurry images) and labeling errors (mislabels) can significantly reduce the accuracy and reliability of the predictions.[6,8] High-quality datasets also ensure that data are diverse and adequately represent the population the model is intended to be used for. Failure to build deep learning models on diverse and representative data can result in poor accuracy, biases, and, most concerning for medicine, a lack of fairness for minority and underrepresented populations.

Acoustics, Laryngology, and Deep Learning

Acoustic analysis in laryngology

Acoustic analysis of voice has become standard practice for many multidisciplinary laryngology and speech-language pathology clinics. It provides objective metrics to longitudinally track voice progress and infer specific deficits in voice. Measures such as cepstral peak prominence (CPP), cepstal spectral index of dysphonia (CSID), and other indices offer insights into the acoustic abnormalities heard in dysphonic voices.[9,10] While understanding a constellation of these values provides some macroscopic view of disease severity or specific pathologies, the correlation between these measures and clinical outcomes is generally modest.[11–13] This limitation stems partly from the fact that the limited number of acoustic variables available in practice are likely insufficient to fully capture the complexity of the human voice. The variability within normal human voices is broad, and an accurate representation likely requires analyzing a large number of variables combined in a nonlinear manner.

As a result, research groups are now turning to deep learning to provide a more complete mathematical understanding of voice. Deep learning approaches consider millions of features (or parameters) in various combinations thus offers the potential for a more accurate capture of voice characteristics. Researchers have utilized datasets such as the Saarbrücken Voice Database,[14] the Massachusetts Eye and Ear Infirmary database,[15] and the Arabic Voice Pathology Database, in house-build database and refine their models.

Pathology Classification Through Deep Learning

There are overall over 50 distinct diseases that have voice change as a clinical sign of pathology. Further, dysphonia often presents as an early sign of disease[16] underscoring the importance of both subjective and objective voice analyses in clinical settings. Thus, the use of voice as a biomarker is a compelling means for early detection and improvement of diagnostic accuracy for a number of diseases. The idea is further bolstered by the fact that voice analysis is traditionally noninvasive and easily scalable to nonclinical settings. Considerable efforts have thus been invested in developing objective methods to diagnose disease from vocal acoustics. Historically, acoustic features of voice such as jitter, shimmer, signal-to-noise ratio, and CPP have been used to attempt to predict specific laryngeal pathology. While some success has been achieved in distinguishing normal from pathologic voices,[17,18] robust classification of pathologies with dysphonic cohorts based on voice alone has proved challenging.[19,20]

Deep learning mitigates many of the limitations of traditional machine learning techniques. Deep learning facilitates the accurate prediction of highly complex systems by considering an extremely large number of variables that are inform only by the data and not the limits of human intuition. To date, several groups have successfully utilized deep learning to identify laryngeal pathology using voice alone. The investigations overwhelmingly take similar approaches. Acoustic data are transformed into a visual representation of voice as a spectrogram; labeled spectrograms are used to train a specific kind of DNN referred to as convolution neural network, which are particularly apt at modeling image inputs. The investigations differ in the size and source of the dataset, quality of the input, type of classification, and methods of validation.

For instance, Alhussein and colleagues[21] in 2019 built a deep learning model based on the SVD dataset (~2000 samples of sustained vowel /a/) and found an accuracy of greater than 90% accuracy for the identification of vocal fold cyst, polyp, paralysis versus normal voice. Also in 2019, Powell and colleagues[22] fine-tuned a previous trained model with a dataset of voice samples collected from clinic. Datasets include 8 total groups, normal and 7 pathologic states, with 10 subjects in each groups. Given the smaller nature of the dataset, a pairwise comparison of pathologic groups was validated using cross-validation, where accuracy was testing in small random subsets, and the results were averaged to ensure accuracy. The study demonstrated accuracy in successful diagnosis ranging from 50% to 90%. Finally, Chen and colleagues trained a DNN on approximately 500 subject clinic collected dataset where approximately half of the subjects had dysphonic voice. Binary classification resulted in an accuracy of approximately 95%.[23]

These investigations show promise and represent a proof of concept for the use of voice as a biomarker for pathology. Yet, it is imperative to note that reported accuracy in silico often is a more optimistic picture than the same model in clinic. A known issue is the significant drop in model accuracy when moving from in silico platforms to real-world applications due to environmental noise, nonstandardized data collection, and variable hardware. Additionally, the clinical utility of these models must be validated, ensuring that they improve patient outcomes. One of the most significant barriers to improved models, model accuracy and clinical utility are driven by the lack of a large, well-labeled, and standardized dataset. Collaboration and cooperation from multiple institutions and patient groups are necessary for a clinical utility of deep learning models.

Severity Classification and Objective Assessment

The accurate and reproducible assessment of dysphonia severity presents a significant challenge in otolaryngology. Traditional practices rely heavily on subjective evaluations such as the Consensus Auditory-Perceptual Evaluation of Voice (CAPE-V) and the GRBAS scale. Despite their widespread use, these methods are prone to considerable interrater variability, which complicates the consistent monitoring of a patient's voice quality over time.

To address this issue, many researchers have sought more objective and reproducible assessments. Deep learning approaches to assessing dysphonia severity often mirror the workflow used to classify pathologies by voice. Voice samples are labeled, converted into spectrograms, and then fed into a convolutional neural network (CNN) for training. Sample labels reflect the severity of dysphonia as defined by the GRBAS scale, which rates voice on a 0 to 3 severity scale across 5 domains: G—grade, R—roughness, B—breathiness, A—asthenia, and S—strain.

Using this approach, Garcia and Rosset built a deep learning model that attempted to grade voice severity using the GRBAS scale. The model was trained on a cohort of 296 audio files from the Perceptual Voice Qualities Database that contains voices with a wide range of severity of dysphonia. The model demonstrated modest accuracy in initial models highlighting the difficulty of capturing and classifying voice severity.[24] Improvements have been made; however, accuracy remains modest. For instance, Aziz and David[25] used multitask learning and deep learning to both classify voice samples into functional voice disorders, organic voice disorders, or normal voice and rate the severity of dysphonia. The accuracy of the classification task was approximately 90% and a correlation with human scored severity of 88%. Difficulty in using deep learning to assess dysphonia severity likely lies in the complexity of the problem and the difficulty in obtaining a well-standardized dataset.

An interesting alternative application of this model is its use in distinguishing between male and female voices, leveraging objective measures to enhance gender classification with a CNN trained on a specific dataset. Bensoussan and Johns[26] trained a DNN to distinguish between a traditional male and a traditional female voice. They deploy this model in assessing the progress of voice feminization or masculinization in transgender populations.

Voice Generation and Rehabilitation

Deep learning may not only help with the interpretation and classification of voice but also serve as an alternative means for voice production. Traditional methods for voice restoration, like the use of an electrolarynx, tracheal/esophageal puncture or esophageal speech, allow speech production; however, they often result in a voice that lacks the natural tonal qualities of the patient's original voice. This disconnect can be isolating for patients, as the voice constitutes a core part of an individual's identity.

Enter generative deep learning models—these sophisticated algorithms do not merely predict or classify; they have the capacity to generate. By leveraging techniques such as generative adversarial networks, deep learning synthesizes voices that not only resemble natural speech but also echo the unique vocal characteristics of the individual. This means that patients who have undergone laryngectomy might one day have the opportunity to speak in a voice that closely resembles their own presurgery voice, a significant stride toward improving their quality of life. Research in this field is nascent but evolving rapidly, suggesting a future where the artificial production of personalized voices might become a transformative tool in voice rehabilitation therapy.

DEEP LEARNING ON ACOUSTIC DATA IN OTOLOGY

Deep learning offers the promise of early diagnosis and improved diagnostic accuracy within laryngology. In the domain of otology, deep learning on acoustic data offers the possibility of personalized medicine. Deep learning techniques are allowing patients to have more personalized optimization of their hearing rehabilitation devices.

Optimization of Hearing Aids

With a globally aging population, the optimization of hearing aids has become increasingly important. Untreated hearing loss often leads to isolation and depression.[27] Despite these risks, it is estimated that over 80% of individuals who could benefit from a hearing aid choose not to use one.[28] The reluctance to adopt hearing aids frequently stems from issues with sound quality, system optimization, localization, and signal-to-noise ratios.

Understanding the role of AI and deep learning in enhancing hearing aids requires a basic knowledge of how conventional hearing aids function. Contrary to a simple sound amplification, hearing aids must also compress audio signals and suppress unwanted sounds or "noise." AI has fostered significant advancements in both amplification and noise suppression.

For patients with hearing loss, frequency-based gain (selective amplification) derived from user's pure tone threshold must be compressed into the range of residual hearing frequency for patients. One central challenge is that the act of compression narrows the tolerable sound pressure level (SPL), window and boundary between audible and uncomfortable narrows.[29] Typically, compression settings based on aggregate data are employed to guide patients in selecting the most suitable compression strategy for various environments. However, studies suggest that as many as half of the users prefer amplification or compression settings that deviate from standard presets.[30,31]

A study by Alamdari and Kehtarnavaz[32] in 2020 explored a deep learning approach known as reinforcement deep learning in optimizing compression strategies. This method allows an algorithm to employ trial-and-error learning alongside pattern recognition capabilities inherent in deep learning, enabling the program to learn and perform complex tasks autonomously. The study highlighted a strong user preference for personalized settings derived from this model over the conventional Desired Sensation Level (DSL v5) settings.

While amplification and compression are fundamental to hearing aid functionality, they are not solely sufficient for auditory rehabilitation. Various studies have shown that noisy environments can significantly diminish speech intelligibility for those with hearing impairments. Traditional noise suppression methods, like beamforming and postfiltering, though beneficial, are known to introduce undesirable artifacts. For instance, adaptive beamforming may lead to excessive signal removal, causing users to feel isolated. Postfiltering, which focuses on eliminating unwanted frequencies, needs constant adjustment to suit different acoustic environments.

Deep learning approaches have made significant progress in the domain of noise suppression. These methods rapidly classify environmental noise type and then suppress the identified background noise without distorting speech. This approach results in improved intelligibility in noisy environments when compared to traditional approaches.[33] These and other approaches continue to push the boundaries of intelligibility is noisy environments for hearing aid patients.

Optimization of Cochlear Implant

Optimization of cochlear implant (CI) via deep learning approaches has taken a similar path as that of hearing aids. CI sound processing is increasingly adopting deep learning techniques. Multiple studies have demonstrated theoretic and clinical improvements in speech intelligibility using deep learning over traditional methods.[34–36] Further, music remixing based via deep learning approaches has resulted in improved enjoyment of music for CI users.[37,38] These techniques allow efficient source separation and sound augmentation without artifact introduction. Finally, speech in noise algorithms based on deep learning models have also been highly effective in improving the efficacy of CIs. Multiple groups have demonstrated that deep learning-based indication and subsequent suppression of noise results in improved intelligibility scores over traditional techniques.[39–41]

Taken collectively, deep learning approaches have shown potential in enhancing speech recognition amid noise, sound localization,[42] and audio processing for both CIs and hearing aids. Advances in these areas continue to drive increased sophistication and potential future adoption. Moreover, these advancements enhance our understanding of the auditory perception system as a whole.

FUTURE

Deep learning, synonymous with advanced AI, has made remarkable strides over the past decade. Deep learning now provides accurate and robust predictions for highly complex issues in the fields of otolaryngology, particularly otology and laryngology, where acoustic data play a pivotal role. Therefore, the application of deep learning to quantify, classify, or generate acoustic data introduces several promising avenues for enhancing patient care.

One significant obstacle to continued progress is the challenge of acquiring and maintaining a high-quality database for model training. The accuracy of a model is inherently tied to the quality of input data and the precision of the associated labels. Currently, laryngology, in particular, faces suboptimal rates of data interoperability. Acoustic data are collected using various equipment, with differing prompts, and rarely are datasets enriched with associated demographic data. A concerted effort across multiple institutions to standardize voice collection, storage, and the labeling of patient demographics and pathologies related to voice files is paramount. Without such standardization, acquiring datasets robust and generalizable enough for routine clinical use may remain elusive.

Moreover, advancing algorithmic development is crucial. In studies concerning both laryngology and otology, predictions are often limited to a single diagnosis. However, it is common for patients, especially those with voice disorders, to present with multiple diagnoses. A patient might exhibit a laryngeal mass alongside compensatory supraglottic hyperfunction or have Reinke's edema with areas that mimic mass-like behavior. Algorithmic enhancements need to accommodate such complexities.

Perhaps, the most impactful development would be the adoption of multimodal models. With new deep learning architectures continuing to evolve, multimodal methodologies are now more feasible and typically offer end-to-end solutions. In otology, integrating audiograms, tympanic membrane imagery, and patient demographics may significantly enhance prediction accuracy beyond what audiograms can achieve alone. A similar integrative approach in laryngology—incorporating voice data, demographic information, and laryngoscopic imagery—could substantially improve diagnostic accuracy.

However, arguably the most crucial focus should be on the clinical testing of these models in relevant settings. As is standard for any medical tool under consideration, carefully designed and executed prospective clinical trials are essential. This is especially pertinent for deep learning models for 2 reasons: models often exhibit a marked reduction in accuracy when moving from in silico environments to real-world applications. For instance, in our laboratory, voice prediction accuracy drops from 95% to 83% when applied in a clinical setting—where factors like ambient noise and user error come into play. Furthermore, the clinical utility of deep learning models remains to be validated. Despite their impressive predictive accuracy with complex problems, no study to date has demonstrated improved patient outcomes, resource optimization, or a reduction in physician workload.

SUMMARY

In conclusion, AI applied to acoustic data is an exhilarating field with numerous high-quality proof-of-concept studies. It holds the potential to transform health care delivery in laryngology and otology fundamentally. Ongoing research will determine how we integrate this powerful tool into clinical practice in order to maximally benefit our patients.

CLINICS CARE POINTS

- Deep learning shows potential to aid in the treatment and diagnosis of voice and hearing disease.
- The majority of current deep learning models are proof-of-concept and require clinical testing to understand their performance in a clinical setting.

REFERENCES

1. He K, Zhang X, Ren S, et al. Deep Residual Learning for Image Recognition. 2016. 770–778 Available at: http://image-net.org/challenges/LSVRC/2015/.
2. Vaswani A, et al. Attention is All you Need. Adv Neural Inf Process Syst 2017;30.
3. Krizhevsky A, Sutskever I, Hinton GE. ImageNet Classification with Deep Convolutional Neural Networks. Adv Neural Inf Process Syst 2012;25.
4. van der Laak J, Litjens G, Ciompi F. Deep learning in histopathology: the path to the clinic. Nat Med 2021;27(5):775–84.
5. Aggarwal R, et al. Diagnostic accuracy of deep learning in medical imaging: a systematic review and meta-analysis. npj Digital Medicine 2021;1–23.
6. Gütter J, Kruspe A, Zhu XX, et al. Impact of Training Set Size on the Ability of Deep Neural Networks to Deal with Omission Noise. Frontiers in Remote Sensing 2022;3:932431.
7. Althnian A, AlSaeed D, Al-Baity H, et al. Impact of Dataset Size on Classification Performance: An Empirical Evaluation in the Medical Domain. Appl Sci 2021;11: 796–811.

8. Hasebe K, Kojima T, Fujimura S, et al. The Effect of Noise on Deep Learning for Classification of Pathological Voice. Laryngoscope 2024. https://doi.org/10.1002/LARY.31303.

9. Awan S, Roy N, Jetté M, et al. G. M.-C. linguistics & & 2010, undefined. Quantifying dysphonia severity using a spectral/cepstral-based acoustic index: Comparisons with auditory-perceptual judgements from the CAPE-V. Clin Linguist Phon 2010;24:742–58.

10. Awan SN, Roy N, Dromey C. Estimating dysphonia severity in continuous speech: Application of a multi-parameter spectralcepstral model estimating dysphonia severity in continuous speech. Clin Linguist Phon 2009;23:825–41.

11. Eadie TL, Doyle PC. Classification of dysphonic voice: Acoustic and auditory-perceptual measures. J Voice 2005;19:1–14.

12. Malyska N, Quatieri TF, Sturim D. Automatic dysphonia recognition using biologically-inspired amplitude-modulation features. Philadelphia, PA: Institute of Electrical and Electronics Engineers Inc; 2005.

13. Martin D, Fitch J, Wolfe V. Pathologic Voice Type and the Acoustic Prediction of Severity. J Speech Lang Hear Res 1995;38:765–71.

14. Saarbrücken Voice Database. Available at: http://www.stimmdatenbank.coli.uni-saarland.de/help_en.php4. [Accessed 21 October 2022].

15. MEEI Database. Massachusetts Eye and ear infirmary voice and speech lab, Boston, MA. &. KayPENTAX, Kay Elemetrics Disordered Voice Database, Model 4337. 1994.

16. Pylypowich A, Duff E. Differentiating the symptom of dysphonia. J Nurse Pract 2016;12:459–66.

17. Roy N, Barkmeier-Kraemer J, Eadie T, et al. Evidence-based clinical voice assessment: a systematic review. Am J Speech Lang Pathol 2013;22:212–26.

18. Ma EPM, Yiu EML. Multiparametric evaluation of dysphonic severity. J Voice 2006;20:380–90.

19. Carding PN, Steen IN, Webb A, et al. The reliability and sensitivity to change of acoustic measures of voice quality. Clin Otolaryngol Allied Sci 2004;29:538–44.

20. Awan SN, Roy N. Outcomes measurement in voice disorders: application of an acoustic index of dysphonia severity. J Speech Lang Hear Res 2009;52:482–99.

21. Alhussein M, Muhammad G. Voice pathology detection using deep learning on mobile healthcare framework. IEEE Access 2018;6:41034–41.

22. Powell ME, Rodriguez Cancio M, Young D, et al. Decoding phonation with artificial intelligence (DeP AI): Proof of concept. Laryngoscope Investig Otolaryngol 2019;4:328–34.

23. Chen L, Chen J. Deep neural network for automatic classification of pathological voice signals. J Voice 2022;36:288.e15–24.

24. Garcia M.A., Rosset A.L., Deep neural network for automatic assessment of dysphonia. ArXiv, 2022. abs/2202.12957.

25. Aziz D, David S. Multitask and transfer learning approach for joint classification and severity estimation of dysphonia. IEEE J Transl Eng Health Med 2024;12:233–44.

26. Bensoussan Y, Pinto J, Crowson M, et al. Deep learning for voice gender identification: proof-of-concept for gender-affirming voice care. Laryngoscope 2021;131:E1611–5.

27. Huang AR, Reed NS, Deal JA, et al. Depression and health-related quality of life among older adults with hearing loss in the achieve study. J Appl Gerontol 2023;550–61.

28. McCormack A, Fortnum H. Why do people fitted with hearing aids not wear them? Int J Audiol 2013;52:360–8.
29. Plomp R. Auditory handicap of hearing impairment and the limited benefit of hearing aids. J Acoust Soc Am 1978;63(2):533–49.
30. Keidser G, Alamudi K. Real-Life efficacy and reliability of training a hearing aid. Ear Hear 2013;34:619–29.
31. Wong LLN. Evidence on self-fitting hearing aids. Trends Amplif 2012;15:215–25.
32. Alamdari N, Lobarinas E, Kehtarnavaz N. Personalization of hearing aid compression by human-in-the-loop deep reinforcement learning. IEEE Access 2020;8: 203503–15.
33. Park G, Cho W, Kim KS, et al. Speech enhancement for hearing aids with deep learning on environmental noises. Appl Sci 2020;10:6077–110.
34. Goehring T, Bolner F, Monaghan JJM, et al. Speech enhancement based on neural networks improves speech intelligibility in noise for cochlear implant users. Hear Res 2017;344:183.
35. Mamun N, Khorram S, Hansen JHL. Convolutional Neural Network-based Speech Enhancement for Cochlear Implant Recipients. Interspeech 2019;2019:4265.
36. (PDF) ElectrodeNet – A Deep Learning Based Sound Coding Strategy for Cochlear Implants. Available at: https://www.researchgate.net/publication/358805808_ElectrodeNet_-_A_Deep_Learning_Based_Sound_Coding_Strategy_for_Cochlear_Implants.
37. Gajęcki T, Nogueira W. Deep learning models to remix music for cochlear implant users. J Acoust Soc Am 2018;143:3602–15.
38. Pons J, Janer J, Rode T, et al. Remixing music using source separation algorithms to improve the musical experience of cochlear implant users. J Acoust Soc Am 2016;140:4338–49.
39. Lai YH, Tsao Y, Lu X, et al. Deep learning-based noise reduction approach to improve speech intelligibility for cochlear implant recipients. Ear Hear 2018;39: 795–809.
40. Vivek VS, Vidhya S, Madhanmohan P. Acoustic Scene Classification in Hearing aid using Deep Learning. Proceedings of the 2020 IEEE International Conference on Communication and Signal Processing, ICCSP 2020;2020:695–9.
41. Diehl PU, Singer Y, Zilly H, et al. Restoring speech intelligibility for hearing aid users with deep learning. Sci Rep 2023;13:1–12.
42. Goli P, Van De Par S. Deep Learning-Based Speech Specific Source Localization by Using Binaural and Monaural Microphone Arrays in Hearing Aids. IEEE/ACM Trans Audio Speech Lang Process 2023;31:1652–66.

APPLICATIONS OF AI WITHIN SUBSPECIALTIES

Artificial Intelligence in Otology and Neurotology

Nicholas Rapoport, BS[a], Cole Pavelchek, MD[b],
Andrew P. Michelson, MD[c,d], Matthew A. Shew, MD[e,*]

KEYWORDS

- Artificial intelligence • Machine learning • Hearing aids • Cochlear implant
- Hearing wearables • Audiogram

KEY POINTS

- Artificial intelligence (AI) in Otology & Neurotology can enhance patient care through improved diagnostics, personalized treatment, and hearing health care access and delivery.
- Current AI applications within Otology & Neurotology include optimizing hearing aid settings, streamlining cochlear implant care delivery models, predicting cochlear implant outcomes, improving audiogram efficiency and delivery, objectifying various electrophysiology measures, and improving personalized diagnosis for various hearing-related pathologies.
- Challenges include small datasets, ethical issues around implementation and need for human verification, and the need for explainable models with clinical sensibility; careful integration into workflows and accountability will be crucial.
- While AI promises transformative advancements in Otology & Neurotology, collaboration between clinicians and data scientists will be essential for responsible and effective integration.

INTRODUCTION

In an era of increasing computational power and Big Data, applications of Artificial intelligence (AI) have grown exponentially. It is a contemporary focal point of innovative research and offers seemingly unlimited possibilities. Data rich fields, such as Otology

[a] Washington University School of Medicine in St. Louis, 660 South Euclid Avenue, PO Box 8115, St Louis, MO 63110, USA; [b] Oregon Health & Science University, 3181 SW Sam Jackson Park Road, Portland, OR 97239-3098, USA; [c] Department of Pulmonary Critical Care, Washington University School of Medicine, 660 South Euclid Avenue, PO Box 8052-43-14, St Louis, MO 63110, USA; [d] Institute for Informatics, Washington University School of Medicine, St Louis, MO, USA; [e] Otology & Neurotology, Department of Otolaryngology–Head and Neck Surgery, Washington University School of Medicine in St. Louis, 660 South Euclid Avenue, PO Box 8115, St Louis, MO 63110, USA
* Corresponding author.
E-mail address: mshew@wustl.edu
Twitter: @MatthewShewMD (M.A.S.)

Otolaryngol Clin N Am 57 (2024) 791–802
https://doi.org/10.1016/j.otc.2024.04.009
0030-6665/24/© 2024 Elsevier Inc. All rights reserved.

and Neurotology, are increasingly interested in its potential applications. AI is an umbrella term for multiple tasks (eg, machine learning, deep learning, natural language processing [NLP], and so forth.) that mimic humanlike intelligence such as reasoning, problem solving, and knowledge presentation, performed by machines at higher speeds and greater depth than human capabilities.[1]

The power and utility of AI is intrinsically linked to both the quality and quantity of data provided. While there is a dearth of high quality and high quantity datasets in Otolaryngology as a whole, recent initiatives such as Reg-ENT, an otolaryngology-specific clinical registry, and multi-institutional collaborations to pool data have begun to expand the authors' ability to properly utilize AI.[2–4] Despite this, Otolaryngology is several steps behind many medical specialties in understanding how AI can help augment clinical decision making and improve precision medicine delivery because of the lack of large and high-quality datasets. Currently, AI has the most impact in high-income settings, or in institutions on the cutting edge of research.[5] However, with advances in information technology infrastructure and mobile computing power, AI is becoming more accessible for areas or institutions with lower resources.[6] This is important not only for health equity and equality, but also for the advancement and future power of AI. Increasing both the amount of data and heterogeneity of contexts data are presented; it will increase the adaptability of AI and allow users to customize its usage for specific purposes, ranging from specific individuals to specific communities with unique needs.

There are important pitfalls to be wary of, for example, feeding AI poor or inaccurate data can lead to incorrect conclusions or analysis. It must be trained and used judiciously, and critically assessed to ensure its conclusions fit within clinical plausibility. Most importantly, it must be incorporated as an aid or adjunct to clinical decision making, rather than a fully autonomous clinical entity. This article focuses on AI applications within Otology and Neurotology and the authors would encourage readers to keep several key concepts in mind to understand and maximize its utilization: (1) the need to hold AI to human verification; (2) embracing the benefit of AI while simultaneously developing rules for accountability; and (3) investing in open AI and maximizing transparency and collaboration.

DISCUSSION
Goals and Current Implementations

The goal of AI in Otology and Neurotology, and medicine in general, is to enhance patient care by advancing research techniques, improving health care delivery, personalizing technology and treatments, and optimizing diagnostic accuracy. AI has received plenty of media attention for its potential applications in ophthalmology and radiology, enabled by the large amount of image data generated, but any data-rich field or technology has potential to utilize AI for improvements. AI utilization within Otology and Neurotology is still in its infancy, but its future utilization will be directly linked to the development of larger, richer, and higher quality data repositories. One common format is structured tabular data, often sourced from clinical databases or repositories, insurance claims databases, and electronic medical records. Images and unstructured texts represent other data rich formats, and are particularly amenable to AI-based approaches such as convolutional neural networks and NLP, respectively. There has also been a tremendous rise in health care wearables, such as smart watches or Holter monitors, which allow access to tremendous amount of personalized data.[7] Within hearing health sciences, there are large opportunities with hearing wearables including both hearing aids and cochlear implants (CI).[8,9] Finally, there are exciting uses for AI in imaging specific to Otology and Neurotology, and also the research of personalized biomarkers and revolutionary health care delivery (**Table 1**).

Hearing wearables – hearing aids

Hearing loss is estimated to impact over 1.5 billion worldwide and hearing aids are the first-line therapy for many patients.[10] They increase quality of life for patients and there is growing evidence they may have protective effects against cognitive decline.[11] However, the ability of hearing aids to restore natural sound and speech perception, particularly in complex listening environments, have their limitations. Hearing aids replace the natural role of outer hair cells by artificially compressing and amplifying sound through multichannel wide dynamic range compression. However, they fail to improve the natural speech perception mechanisms that require complex non-linear temporal and spatial neuronal activity patterns. AI based approaches have helped revolutionize how the authors study these evasive problems through its ability to analyze enormous amounts of data and understand complex patterns unrestricted by the data-source type or scale. Researchers are looking at the use of deep neural networks to more accurately learn and recreate the complex auditory pathway to restore "natural" speech perception.[12] This would improve restoration of normal hearing perception as opposed to the current restoration of simple sensitivity, and especially improve hearing in noisy environments. AI also has been used to study personal, behavioral, and environmental factors to optimize both fitting and user utilization of hearing aids.[13] Fitting is done in a sterile, relatively standard acoustic environment such as a hearing clinic, which differs significantly from normal environments of daily life. To account for this, hearing aids typically have several specific modes for different environments that are manually selected by the wearer. Patients must actively switch hearing aid settings and modes to the environment they are in at that very moment. This process can be cumbersome, and often leads to frustration and underperformance of hearing aids in certain listening environments. AI has been able to leverage large complex datasets that accurately recreate different listening environments to adjust hearing aid settings in real time, leading to improved patient experience.[14]

The variety of acoustic environments also greatly influences the effectiveness of hearing aids. Hearing aids can have difficulty accurately classifying certain acoustic environments, typically those with strong reverberations and tonal or fluctuating noises.[15]

Table 1	
Summary of current implementations of artificial intelligence in Otology and Neurotology	
Implementation	**Summary**
Hearing aids	Improved speech perception and streamlined setting selection
Cochlear implants	Decreased CI programming time, increase CI health care access to CI in areas with limited resources, leveraging heterogenous biomarkers to predict outcomes
Audiograms	Lower number of datapoints required and quicker to obtain with similar accuracy to clinicians
Imaging	Expand utility of electrocochleography, accurate diagnosis of middle ear pathology, expand access to remote health care, and enhance counseling on complex topics such as vestibular schwannomas
Personalized medicine and "omics"	Prediction of disease probability based on molecular analysis and anticipating need for multi-disciplinary care

For these "challenging" acoustic environments, some AI features, such as Starkey's Edge Mode, allow for users to inform the hearing aid of the environment through a simple gesture picked up by the hearing aid, which will then take a "snapshot" of the environment and optimize the hearing settings in real time. These on-demand and independently computed adjustments have demonstrated improvement in several key challenging environments, such as restaurants, automobiles, and reverberant environments.[16] Overall, AI has shown the ability to improve recognition of and adaptation to traditionally challenging environments for hearing aid users, improve the customizability of their devices, and has the potential to transform hearing aid output to a more "normal" signal to the brain.

Cochlear implants

CI are another example of health care wearables, and through their daily use there are plethora of data available. Promising avenues within AI based CI care include optimizing clinical efficiency and CI care delivery models, CI programming, CI speech perception outcome prediction modeling, and ultimately improve overall CI outcomes.

As CI market penetration is currently lacking, with fewer than 2% of CI candidates receiving therapy, there is a need for improved clinical efficiencies both in the ability to see and evaluate potential CI candidates and to streamline post-operative care.[17] Pre-operative speech perception testing and audiometric evaluation is both time consuming and resource intensive. By leveraging large scale multi-center datasets, investigators have shown the ability to accurately impute a full 11-frequency audiogram using 3 to 4 thresholds.[4] This has the potential to drastically cut down on the time required to obtain an audiogram. Similarly, it has been shown one can impute different speech perception tests from one another (ie, Consonant nucleus consonant [CNC] words, AzBio sentences in quiet, and AzBio sentences in varying levels of background noise) with mean absolute error below 10%.[3] For example, clinicians may only need to obtain CNC words and AzBio sentences at +10 dB in the clinic and simply impute AzBio sentences in quiet. In a full clinic day, this can significantly improve patients' access to testing.

CI programming is another time-consuming process. Programming primarily relies on subjective feedback and objective measures. Some investigators hypothesize the lack of standardization in programming may contribute to variation in outcomes and performance.[18] A study comparing clinician programmed implants using patient feedback to AI programmed implants leveraging objective data from prior patients showed no significant differences.[19] Despite no clinical improvement in CI outcomes based on different programming options, the creation of a standardized AI approach could revolutionize how performance measures are studied and improved upon, and improve CI care access to otherwise less experienced CI centers.[19] Similarly, as AI based programming was found to be non-inferior, AI based programming could free up CI audiology clinicians appointment times. While the prior study demonstrated non-inferiority, there are studies that indicate utilizing AI as an adjunct tool for clinicians can improve auditory results when compared with manual fitting alone.[20] Finally, in the process of CI mapping, AI has demonstrated the ability to improve CI speech intensity and perception outcomes by modifying parameters that are often not typically addressed.[21] With similar outcomes to manual programming, it is likely that AI will continue to improve and be utilized as a tool to trained clinicians. The ability of AI to support standardization of CI programming across centers could lead to more powerful research studies, enable larger data collections, improve precision medicine mapping, increase clinical efficiency and productivity, and improve CI access and utilization across institutions with less experience in CI.

Post-operative computed tomography (CT) analysis has also drastically improved the authors' understanding of final electrode position and structural preservation, and there is a growing interest in utilizing this technology to better apply personalized anatomy-based tonotopic mapping. An opportunity many researchers are actively investigating is CI electrode frequency-to-place mismatch. Additionally, there are studies assessing how image and anatomy-based mapping for electrode frequency allocation may improve outcomes.[22,23] One limitation with conventional post-operative CT imaging and implementing anatomy-based fitting is fully visualizing critical structures like the basilar membrane, scala positioning, and the spiral ganglion. Recent developments in synchrotron radiation phase-contrast imaging have allowed researchers to make accurate 3-dimensional tonotopic mapping of the basilar membrane and spiral ganglion beyond traditional histology and temporal bone specimen approaches; this demonstrates a landmark breakthrough in the feasibility of image-guided surgical approaches.[24] This technology has already revolutionized how the authors understand electrode positioning within Scala compartments, different electrode types and their relationship to the basilar membrane, and complex cochlear anatomy, and electrode relationships. Investigators are exploring how these technologies can validate electrode positioning and ultimately create customized anatomy-based frequency allocation maps. However, 1 limitation is that it requires manual tracing and labeling; manual inputs of these data are too onerous for realistic use. AI has revolutionized the ability to perform accurate and individual segmentation of a patient's cochlea, thereby, making these approaches more feasible. AI-based techniques have allowed not only this auto-segmentation process to be seamless for everyday clinical use, but have allowed augmentation of regular CT scan images to provide high quality and granular information based on the data rich synchrotrons and micro-CT based libraries.

Finally, AI offers novel approaches to prediction modeling, with the potential to improve diagnosis and management of various diseases. Cochlear implantation is an ideal setting for such approaches given the significant variability in speech perception outcomes and the authors' current limitations of traditional regression approaches to accurately capture CI performance trajectory.[25] Most studies to date looking at machine learning based prediction models have been severely hampered by inadequate sample size, non-relevant datasets, and poor or non-transparent methodology that has led to severely overfit models with no clinical viability.[26,27] This highlights the need for more rigorous evaluation and transparency. One of the best studies to date leveraged over 2489 patients across 3 institutions across 2 countries; investigators demonstrated how machine learning models can outperform traditional linear regression models by decreasing mean absolute error from 21.8% to 17.9%.[8] However, while the prediction performance is statistically significant, the authors acknowledge the limited clinical utility. These findings fit within clinical reasoning given the limited prognostic value of traditional clinical variables (ie, audiogram, age, and duration of hearing loss). Nonetheless, this does highlight future opportunity to improve AI-based prediction modeling as a decision support tool by feeding It better biomarkers for CI speech perception performance. For example, researchers recently demonstrated the potential to improve speech perception performance prediction using deep learning to analyze preoperative MRI data and other patient-related comorbid factors.[28–30] The aforementioned imaging studies have analyzed pre-surgical neuroanatomical MRIs of CI recipients compared with normal hearing patients and found that certain areas in multiple structures, such as the bilateral auditory cortex, right cerebellum, and left superior and middle gyrus, and less consistently the occipital lobe, inferior frontal gyrus and cingulate gyrus, predicted speech-perception development, and CI outcomes. However, these are limited by small sample sizes; AI-based techniques ultimately depend on big data. It is critical for the authors to start somewhere and build upon these valuable preliminary findings by improving data harmonization and funding for future lines of investigation.

Overall, health care wearables offer a unique opportunity at the intersection of precision medicine and AI because of the large amount of data generated for any one single individual. However, progress within this realm will rely heavily on collaboration between industry and clinicians. This rich source of data will need to be leveraged in a manner allowing AI to analyze it and create actionable items.

Audiogram

Audiograms are currently the gold standard of measuring hearing capabilities. Audiologists test a single frequency at a time, with pure tones delivered manually at each new frequency for a sequence of ascending or descending sound levels. Machine learning based approaches have the potential to revolutionize efficiency and access. For example, by leveraging a novel nonparametric approach using Bayesian estimation and machine learning, investigators have shown the ability to obtain a full audiogram in a much more efficient, reliable, and accurate manner.[31] Online machine learning audiometry has shown equivalent results to manual audiometry performed by an audiologist, with short acquisition times; it can also be easily adapted to other hearing tests, such as bone conduction, masking, or speech perception, which provides an efficient and unified test of overall hearing ability.[9] Further studies have supported these results, with a meta-analysis including 29 studies indicating that automated audiometry provides accurate measurements of hearing thresholds.[32] Automated audiometry, which utilizes machine learning algorithms, also requires significantly fewer samples, as conventional approaches must query frequencies individually, follow rigorous rules for selecting tone intensities, and depend upon multiple variables; this leads to collection of a significant amount of uninformative data.[31] These machine learning algorithms are faster because they utilize uncertainty sampling, allowing for rapid accumulation of relevant information.

Unstructured data (image and text) analysis using deep learning

Some of the most innovative approaches within AI include deep-learning and NLP. Deep-learning and NLP have been a revolution with AI-based technologies because of their unique ability to breakdown granular pixels within images or words within texts, understand complex patterns and contextual references, and ultimately offer novel prediction or language models not previously possible. An exciting avenue within deep-learning is improving generalizability of electrocochleography (ECochG). ECochG is increasingly being used across CI centers as a strong prognostic marker for both CI performance and residual hearing by measuring electric potentials in response to various acoustic stimuli. However, the current gold standard relies on experienced audiologists and clinicians that can understand the complex electrophysiologic signals and distinguish them from the noise floor. This has limited generalizability of this technology both in its utilization and reproducibility. Deep-learning offers the novel ability to interpret complex ECochG signals and images based on pixel patterns, which can bring this tool to non-electrophysiologic experts. One study demonstrated that deep learning algorithms have equivalent accuracy to ECochG experts. The objectification and reproducibility conferred by this method would alleviate concerns of generalizability and enable comparison of longitudinal outcomes.[33] Similar to ECochG, auditory brainstem response (ABR) testing may be used to diagnose hearing dysfunction and is useful because of its ability to diagnose dysfunction without patients' active cooperation. However, ABR tests also rely on experienced clinicians to interpret output. Automated interpretation with deep-learning has been shown to aid identification of characteristic wave forms and can perceive subtle parameters, allowing for deeper data collections and avoiding subjective error in manual identification.[34,35]

Otoscope images and radiographic imaging, such as MRI or CT, often have information or patterns that are not discernible to humans and could provide valuable information. Researchers have begun to study how pre-operative brain MRIs of pediatric patients receiving CI can predict language outcomes. This not only offers novel opportunities for CI prediction modeling but deep-learning insights within poor CI performers also will help us uncover novel areas of investigation that were not previously identified using conventional methods.[36] With otoscope images, investigators are looking at ways to improve diagnosis of variable middle ear conditions across general practitioners or rural clinics without easy access to Otolaryngologists.[37] A recent meta-analysis demonstrated how machine learning has shown robust competency at diagnosis middle ear pathologies, possibly at equivalent or superior accuracy to current standards of clinicians.[38] Along similar lines, remote health care has exploded because of the coronavirus disease 2019 pandemic, however, pitfalls include limited physical examinations, visibility, and a lack of point-of-care treatment. A recent study used images from a home otoscope and AI to automize the diagnosis of acute otitis media, and found some models accurately diagnosed greater than 80% of cases, comparable to otolaryngologists and superior to family medicine practitioners.[39] This demonstrates AI's potential to alleviate one of the biggest drawbacks of remote health care, namely the restricted diagnostic ability of diseases that require visualization.

The use of AI in imaging can also improve patient care beyond accurate diagnosis, but also disease monitoring. AI has also been used for calculating both the volume and recurrence chance of vestibular schwannoma. Counseling and management of vestibular schwannoma is complex, but having accurate estimates of these variables that are otherwise logistically time-consuming, challenging, or simply unfeasible could revolutionize how schwannomas are treated.[39,40] However, while preliminary data is exciting, future studies will need to closely scrutinize generalizability of these models and biologic sensibility to ensure data are not overfitted. One challenge moving forward to improve generalizability and accuracy of deep-learning diagnostic tools within health care will be standardization of imaging.

"Omics" and personalized medicine

AI has tremendous potential to elucidate complex or subtle patterns in data that are typically difficult to analyze with more traditional computing methods. The predicted panacea of "personalized medicine" will likely heavily rely on AI for this very reason. Data often have "hidden" patterns, but AI has shown the ability to bring these patterns into practical use. This is particularly prevalent in the "omics" fields, such as genomics or proteomics, which have incredible potential for personalized care. The inner ear is difficult to study; there is currently no biopsy equivalent to study, and it is difficult to ascertain what is occurring on a molecular level. Analysis of perilymph miRNA samples utilizing machine learning has been shown to predict not only presence or absence of hearing loss, but also severity.[41] Similarly, perilymph proteomic studies have identified disease-specific protein profiles in Meniere's disease, enlarged vestibular aqueducts, and otosclerosis.[42] These successes indicate untapped potential for studying inner ear pathologies. Harnessing AI to develop reliable and accurate biomarkers for these processes would be revolutionary for patient care, as well as a breakthrough in the overall research of inner ear pathology and physiology. However, current utilization is severely limited by sample size.

Personalized medicine entails more than recognition and analysis of phenotypes and genotypes, but also addressing personal changes of complications or circumstances. Early recognition of medical problems can lead to disease prevention, but also provides logistical advantages for both patients and clinicians, such as early coordination of care.[43] For example, machine learning algorithms have shown promise in predicting hearing loss in patients with head and neck cancer receiving chemotherapy, and pre-treatment recognition of this debilitating condition would allow for clinicians to coordinate specialty care with audiologists and otologists before initiation of chemotherapy.[44] In summary, personalized medicine is a complex idea with many moving parts, and AI will likely play an important role in its realization going forward.

Current challenges

The future of AI applications is not without drawbacks and limitations. Current datasets for wearable health care devices are still relatively small datasets for AI. Datasets sizes are relatively smaller concern for image-based data, as CT and MRI scans have hundreds of data points per scan (eg, pixels), but standardization is an issue. . Finally, within personalized medicine there is still a significant gap between identifying individual's genotype or phenotype and actually delivering care to these individuals. Other fields, such as oncology, have utilized "omic" data to start molecular tumor boards (MTB), which attempt to treat cancers based on specific mutations or susceptibilities. MTBs aim to identify potential treatment options based on genetic analysis but currently, fewer than 20% of patients discussed at MTBs receive immunotherapies.[45] The sources of data can also affect generalizability; for example, it has been well-documented that many available genomic datasets are composed mainly of individuals of European ancestry.[46] Ultimately, the foundation for any AI-based bedside tool is data-quality; generalizability is a widespread challenge, as there is inevitably bias from different environments and manual human input or interpretation.

There has been understandable hesitancy to adopt complex machine learning or AI in health care, partially due to misconceptions about AI or general mistrust in clinical relevance. Explainable models, which essentially show the models' reasoning, would allow the clinician to determine if the model is clinically sound.[47] However, AI input can also lead to anchoring bias in clinicians; when an automated diagnosis is incorrect, physicians may be more likely to agree with the diagnosis than when interpreting independently.[48] Nonetheless, AI in health care is inevitable. It will be critical providers closely evaluate the clinical relevance of AI findings. For example, any CI provider should know that the authors cannot predict word recognition scores within 6%; if AI may be able to predict within 5%, it is likely not a valuable improvement.[49] Finally, AI presents significant economic and legal implications; the effect on the health care workforce, insurance reimbursement, regulation, and generalizability are complex. Legally, there will be need for a clear and ironclad guidance and laws regarding malpractice insurance coverage, and liability will be a complex issue.[50]

Overall, there are practical concerns regarding the use of AI in medicine. Proper development of clinically relevant models, integration into workflow, and realistic assessments of the value provided by these models must have careful oversight, and ideally long-term studies of prototype systems before widespread adoption. It will be imperative clinicians and data-scientists are at the center of these conversations with the goal of maximizing data quality, reproducibility of equitable models, and ultimately hold models accountable so that they can reach their full potential for improving patient care and augmenting provider decision making.

SUMMARY

AI has is being actively explored and leveraged cross multiple disciplines within Otology and Neurotology. It has demonstrated the ability to improve currently used wearable hearing devices, and the potential to revolutionize how these technologies work. It will likely be used as an adjunct to multiple hearing related measures (eg, audiogram, ECochG, ABRs), similar to how current electrocardiograms are read with a computer-based diagnosis before it is seen by a human. AI will lead to crucial breakthroughs in predicting outcomes, recognition of risk factors or trends, development of new treatments or techniques, and improve how care is delivered.

AI will revolutionize many aspects of medicine. In many cases, it is still in the proof-of-concept phase, and has many hurdles left to face. However, the future of integrating AI into Otology and Neurotology, and medicine as a whole, is bright and exciting. As the authors move forward, it is critical as a specialty; they are open to its use with a skeptical eye in how it can augment clinical care and are actively involved with conversations on its utilization and implementation.

CLINICS CARE POINTS

- AI can optimize hearing aid fitting, allow for patient customization, and improve performance in difficult hearing environments.
- AI can streamline auditory evaluation and CI mapping, freeing up audiologist resources and increasing accessibility to CIs.
- Pre-operative imaging of CI recipients can predict outcomes and inform optimal CI electrode placement.
- Providing data that are difficult to procure to accurately inform and counsel patients on treatment options for otherwise challenging diagnoses, such as vestibular schwannoma.
- Expand use of "omic" data for personalized medicine, including prognostic outcomes and coordinating health care in advance.
- Irreplaceable research tool that enables the study of massive datasets or data that are too complex for human analysis.

DISCLOSURE

N. Rapoport, C. Pavelchek, and A.P. Michelson have no conflicts of interest to disclose. M.A. Shew – consultant for Cochlear l td; Triological Society Research Career Development Award.

REFERENCES

1. Stead WW. Clinical implications and challenges of artificial intelligence and deep learning. JAMA 2018;320(11):1107–8.
2. American Academy of Otolaryngology–Head and Neck Surgery. Reg-ent ENT clinical data registry. Available at: https://www.entnet.org/quality-practice/reg-ent-clinical-data-registry/. [Accessed 8 January 2024].

3. Pavelchek C, Lee DS, Walia A, et al. Responsible imputation of missing speech perception testing data & analysis of 4,739 observations and predictors of performance. Otol Neurotol 2023;44(6):e369–78.

4. Pavelchek C, Michelson AP, Walia A, et al. Imputation of missing values for cochlear implant candidate audiometric data and potential applications. PLoS One 2023;18(2):e0281337.

5. Schwalbe N, Wahl B. Artificial intelligence and the future of global health. Lancet 2020;395(10236):1579–86.

6. Wahl B, Cossy-Gantner A, Germann S, et al. Artificial intelligence (AI) and global health: how can AI contribute to health in resource-poor settings? BMJ Glob Health 2018;3(4):e000798.

7. Dunn J, Runge R, Snyder M. Wearables and the medical revolution. Per Med 2018;15(5):429–48.

8. Shafieibavani E, Goudey B, Kiral I, et al. Predictive models for cochlear implant outcomes: Performance, generalizability, and the impact of cohort size. Trends Hear 2021;25. 23312165211066174.

9. Barbour DL, Howard RT, Song XD, et al. Online machine learning audiometry. Ear Hear 2019;40(4):918–26.

10. Deafness and hearing loss. World Health Organization. Available at: https://www.who.int/health-topics/hearing-loss#tab=tab_2. [Accessed 5 March 2024].

11. Lin FR, Pike JR, Albert MS, et al. Hearing intervention versus health education control to reduce cognitive decline in older adults with hearing loss in the USA (ACHIEVE): a multicentre, randomised controlled trial. Lancet 2023;402(10404): 786–97.

12. Lesica NA. Why Do Hearing Aids Fail to Restore Normal Auditory Perception? Trends Neurosci 2018;41(4):174–85.

13. Iliadou E, Su Q, Kikidis D, et al. Profiling hearing aid users through big data explainable artificial intelligence techniques. Front Neurol 2022;13:933940.

14. Balling LW, Mølgaard LL, Townend O, et al. The collaboration between hearing aid users and artificial intelligence to optimize sound. Semin Hear 2021;42(3): 282–94.

15. Buchler M, Allegro S, Launer S, et al. Sound classification in hearing aids inspired by auditory scene analysis. EURASIP J Appl Signal Process 2005;(18):2991–3002.

16. Fabry DA, Bhowmik AK. Improving speech understanding and monitoring health with hearing aids using artificial intelligence and embedded sensors. Semin Hear 2021;42(3):295–308.

17. Nassiri AM, Sorkin DL, Carlson ML. Current estimates of cochlear implant utilization in the United States. Otol Neurotol 2022;43(5):e558–62.

18. Vaerenberg B, Smits C, De Ceulaer G, et al. Cochlear implant programming: a global survey on the state of the art. Sci World J 2014;2014:501738.

19. Waltzman SB, Kelsall DC. The use of artificial intelligence to program cochlear implants. Otol Neurotol 2020;41(4):452–7.

20. Wathour J, Govaerts PJ, Deggouj N. From manual to artificial intelligence fitting: Two cochlear implant case studies. Cochlear Implants Int 2020;21(5):299–305.

21. Wathour J, Govaerts PJ, Lacroix E, et al. Effect of a CI programming fitting tool with artificial intelligence in experienced cochlear implant patients. Otol Neurotol 2023;44(3):209–15.

22. Oxenham AJ, Bernstein JG, Penagos H. Correct tonotopic representation is necessary for complex pitch perception. Proc Natl Acad Sci USA 2004;101(5): 1421–5.

23. Jiam NT, Gilbert M, Cooke D, et al. Association between flat-panel computed tomographic imaging-guided place-pitch mapping and speech and pitch perception in cochlear implant users. JAMA Otolaryngol Head Neck Surg 2019;145(2):109–16.

24. Li H, Helpard L, Ekeroot J, et al. Three-dimensional tonotopic mapping of the human cochlea based on synchrotron radiation phase-contrast imaging. Sci Rep 2021;11(1):4437.

25. Moberly AC, Bates C, Harris MS, et al. The enigma of poor performance by adults with cochlear implants. Otol Neurotol 2016;37(10):1522–8.

26. Guerra-Jiménez G, Ramos De Miguel Á, Falcón González JC, et al. Cochlear implant evaluation: prognosis estimation by data mining system. J Int Adv Otol 2016;12(1):1–7.

27. Ramos-Miguel A, Perez-Zaballos T, Perez D, et al. Use of data mining to predict significant factors and benefits of bilateral cochlear implantation. Eur Arch Oto-Rhino-Laryngol 2015;272(11):3157–62.

28. Feng G, Ingvalson EM, Grieco-Calub TM, et al. Neural preservation underlies speech improvement from auditory deprivation in young cochlear implant recipients. Proc Natl Acad Sci USA 2018;115(5):E1022–31.

29. Tan L, Holland SK, Deshpande AK, et al. A semi-supervised Support Vector Machine model for predicting the language outcomes following cochlear implantation based on pre-implant brain fMRI imaging. Brain Behav 2015;5(12):e00391.

30. Dang S, Kallogjeri D, Dizdar K, et al. Individual patient comorbidities and effect on cochlear implant performance. Otol Neurotol 2024;45(4):e281–8.

31. Song XD, Wallace BM, Gardner JR, et al. Fast, continuous audiogram estimation using machine learning. Ear Hear 2015;36(6):e326–35.

32. Mahomed F, Swanepoelde W, Eikelboom RH, et al. Validity of automated threshold audiometry: a systematic review and meta-analysis. Ear Hear 2013; 34(6):745–52.

33. Schuerch K, Wimmer W, Dalbert A, et al. Objectification of intracochlear electrocochleography using machine learning. Front Neurol 2022;13:943816.

34. Chen C, Zhan L, Pan X, et al. Automatic recognition of auditory brainstem response characteristic waveform based on bidirectional long short-term memory. Front Med 2021;7:613708.

35. McKearney RM, Bell SL, Chesnaye MA, et al. Auditory brainstem response detection using machine learning: a comparison with statistical detection methods. Ear Hear 2022;43(3):949–60.

36. Wilson BS, Tucci DL, Moses DA, et al. Harnessing the power of artificial intelligence in otolaryngology and the communication sciences. J Assoc Res Otolaryngol 2022;23(3):319–49.

37. Ezzibdeh R, Munjal T, Ahmad I, et al. Artificial intelligence and tele-otoscopy: A window into the future of pediatric otology. Int J Pediatr Otorhinolaryngol 2022; 160:111229.

38. Cao Z, Chen F, Grais EM, et al. Machine learning in diagnosing middle ear disorders using tympanic membrane images: a meta-analysis. Laryngoscope 2023; 133(4):732–41.

39. Cass ND, Lindquist NR, Zhu Q, et al. Machine learning for automated calculation of vestibular schwannoma volumes. Otol Neurotol 2022;43(10):1252–6.

40. Abouzari M, Goshtasbi K, Sarna B, et al. Prediction of vestibular schwannoma recurrence using artificial neural network. Laryngoscope Investig Otolaryngol 2020;5(2):278–85.

41. Shew M, New J, Wichova H, et al. Using machine learning to predict sensorineural hearing loss based on perilymph micro RNA expression profile. Sci Rep 2019;9(1):3393.
42. Schmitt HA, Pich A, Prenzler NK, et al. Personalized proteomics for precision diagnostics in hearing loss: disease-specific analysis of human perilymph by mass spectrometry. ACS Omega 2021;6(33):21241–54.
43. JaKa MM, Beran MS, Andersen JA, et al. The role of care coordination: a qualitative study of care coordinator perceptions. J Nurs Care Qual 2024;39(1):44–50.
44. Abdollahi H, Mostafaei S, Cheraghi S, et al. Cochlea CT radiomics predicts chemoradiotherapy induced sensorineural hearing loss in head and neck cancer patients: A machine learning and multi-variable modelling study. Phys Med 2018;45:192–7.
45. Luchini C, Lawlor RT, Milella M, et al. Molecular tumor boards in clinical practice. Trends Cancer 2020;6(9):738–44.
46. Martin AR, Kanai M, Kamatani Y, et al. Clinical use of current polygenic risk scores may exacerbate health disparities [published correction appears in Nat Genet. 2021 May;53(5):763]. Nat Genet 2019;51(4):584–91.
47. Kurant DE. Opportunities and challenges with artificial intelligence in genomics. Clin Lab Med 2023;43(1):87–97.
48. Lehman CD, Wellman RD, Buist DS, et al. Diagnostic accuracy of digital screening mammography with and without computer-aided detection. JAMA Intern Med 2015;175(11):1828–37.
49. Kim H, Kang WS, Park HJ, et al. Cochlear implantation in postlingually deaf adults is time-sensitive towards positive outcome: prediction using advanced machine learning techniques. Sci Rep 2018;8(1):18004.
50. Yu KH, Beam AL, Kohane IS. Artificial intelligence in healthcare. Nat Biomed Eng 2018;2(10):719–31.

Artificial Intelligence in Head and Neck Surgery

Jamie Oliver, MD[a], Rahul Alapati, MD[a], Jason Lee, MD, PhD[a],
Andrés Bur, MD[a],*

KEYWORDS

- Artificial intelligence • Machine learning • Head and neck cancer
- Squamous cell carcinoma • Histopathology image analysis • Radiomics
- Prognostication • Treatment response

KEY POINTS

- This article examines artificial intelligence's (AI's) impact on diagnosing and managing head and neck cancers, emphasizing early detection, prognostication, and treatment planning.
- This article highlights AI-driven image analysis's high accuracy in identifying head and neck cancer through clinical, endoscopic, and histopathologic images.
- The role of radiomics in diagnosis, nodal metastasis prediction, and evaluating treatment response in head and neck cancer is discussed.
- The study recognizes AI's potential while addressing limitations and emphasize the importance of clinician-data scientist collaboration to bring these promising AI tools into clinical practice.

INTRODUCTION

Artificial intelligence (AI) is a rapidly expanding field of computer and data science encompassing a wide range of technologies that aim to emulate the decision-making capabilities of the human mind. One of the greatest strengths of AI is its ability to recognize patterns within data. As the quantity of collected and aggregated electronic health data increases, so does the potential to develop AI tools using these data. There has been considerable interest in applying these technologies to aid otolaryngologists in improving care and outcomes for head and neck cancer patients.

Funding/Support: No funding sources to disclose.
[a] Department of Otolaryngology–Head and Neck Surgery, University of Kansas School of Medicine, 3901 Rainbow Boulevard M.S. 3010, Kansas City, KS, USA
* Corresponding author. Department of Otolaryngology–Head and Neck Surgery, University of Kansas School of Medicine, 3901 Rainbow Boulevard M.S. 3010, Kansas City, KS.
E-mail address: abur@kumc.edu

Common applications of AI and machine learning (ML) have included tools to aid in cancer diagnosis, prognostication, and evaluation of treatment response. In particular, deep convolutional neural networks (CNNs) have been frequently employed in cancer research and achieved particularly strong performance on visual tasks such as identifying malignancy on radiographic or histopathologic images. More than most, otolaryngology-head and neck surgery is a particularly visual field, and many head and neck cancers are initially diagnosed through physical examination, either through direct visualization in the oral cavity/oropharynx or endoscopic nasopharyngolaryngoscopy. As such, there has also been interest in developing otolaryngology-specific tools to aid in detecting malignancy based on endoscopic or direct visualization of tumors.

Due to its rapid and ongoing development, it is vital for otolaryngologists and, in particular, head and neck oncologists to be aware of recent technological advances that have the potential to impact head and neck cancer patient care.

CLINICAL AND ENDOSCOPIC IMAGE ANALYSIS

Early detection of oral cavity squamous cell carcinoma (SCC) improves overall survival.[1,2] However, a significant number of oral cavity SCC patients are diagnosed at an advanced stage. As a result, there is strong clinical interest in developing reliable and noninvasive screening methods to detect these cancers using AI. Early attempts at AI automated detection of oral cancer focused on using specialized images, such as autofluorescence or spectroscopy. For instance, in the early 2000s, a research group from Taiwan demonstrated that premalignant and malignant tissues could be differentiated from benign tissue based on fluorospectrometer readings using a partial least-squares and artificial neural network classification algorithm. This algorithm achieved a high sensitivity of 0.81 and a specificity of 0.96.[3] Similarly, around that time, a research group from India showed that early-stage oral cancer could be distinguished from healthy mucosa by using the Bayesian ML framework of statistical pattern recognition, achieving 0.91 sensitivity and 0.96 specificity.[4] Similar efficacy in automated detection was also demonstrated by other investigators using other ML approaches.[5,6]

More recently, plain clinical photographs have been investigated as a source of rapid screening to eliminate the need for specialized equipment.[7–9] Using a CNN approach, researchers were able to show that simple images captured using a smartphone could be readily classified into suspicious or not suspicious with great sensitivity (85%) and specificity (88%).[7] Another large research group in China utilized an impressive dataset of 44,000 clinical images obtained from 11 hospitals around China over a 15-year period to develop their deep learning algorithm.[8] After training on a large subset of this dataset, their AI system achieved an area under the curve of receiver operating characteristic curve (AUC) of 0.983 on their internal validation dataset and an AUC of 0.935 on an external validation dataset (published clinical photographs from dentistry and oral surgery journals). Diagnostic accuracy was similar between the algorithm and oral cancer experts reviewing the same images (92% vs 92%) and superior to the average medical student (87%). Such algorithms may benefit primary care physicians or other providers with limited experience evaluating oral cavity lesions to determine whether a lesion warrants referral for further evaluation and, if so, what the relative urgency of that referral should be. It is important to note that while the algorithm developed by Fu and colleagues[8] performed similarly to oral surgeons in their research testing, photographic evaluation is significantly limiting to surgeons as it does not allow for other components of the physical examination (eg, palpation) or consideration of clinical history. It is likely that oral cancer surgeon malignancy detection would be significantly higher if not tested in this artificial research setting. This is important to note when considering the results of this study, as well as many other studies that also use a similar approach to compare AI and human performance.

It is important to consider that variability in photography techniques can impact the applicability of the algorithms in the studies mentioned earlier, particularly when considering some of the challenges in obtaining pictures from the oral cavity. Systemic approaches are recommended to ensure high-quality photos are obtained based on oral cavity subsites (retractors, lighting, mirrors, and so forth).[10] These techniques are essential for providers clinically evaluating patients and researchers developing computer vision algorithms. Insufficient field-of-view, lighting, shadowing, and focus can all significantly impact the quality of photographs and subsequently limit the ability of an algorithm to be effectively applied.

Several AI algorithms have been developed to assist in identifying and diagnosing nasopharyngeal carcinoma using transnasal endoscopic images. Such algorithms have produced promising results with model accuracy ranging from 88% to 96%.[11–13] One algorithm, by oncologists at the Department of Nasopharyngeal Carcinoma at Sun Yat-Sen University Cancer Center in China, was developed using a fully convolutional network based on the inception architecture and trained on a training dataset of 19,000 biopsy-proven images from 5557 patients.[11] It was then tested on an independent prospective dataset and shown to outperform fully trained physicians with a diagnostic accuracy of 88.0% (compared to 80.5%). The differences in performance were unsurprisingly greater when the algorithm was compared to residents (72.8% accuracy) and interns (66.5% accuracy). This performance is impressive and suggests that these tools may have the ability to aid clinicians in diagnosing nasopharyngeal carcinoma.

There has also been interest in developing algorithms to identify and classify lesions on laryngeal endoscopy. Such algorithms have shown promising diagnostic accuracy in classifying benign and malignant lesions (83%–93%).[14–16] Beyond single-frame image analysis, researchers have also explored utilizing AI to analyze endoscopic video data, termed videomics.[17] In particular, this is a technique that is well suited for laryngeal examinations given the relatively standardized views that are obtained when visualizing the larynx through a transnasal approach. One research group from the Netherlands recently developed an algorithm capable of localizing and classifying benign and malignant laryngeal lesions on video endoscopy in real time.[18] During endoscopy, this algorithm processed video at a frame rate of 63 frames per second and made predictions in just 16 milliseconds per frame. Malignancy detection sensitivity ranged between 71% and 78%, and benign lesion detection ranged between 70% and 82%. There is room for improvement in performance, but the potential utility of such algorithms to support clinicians in identifying malignancy on endoscopy is significant.

Recently, a research group in Munich developed a statistical model that utilizes computer analysis of high-speed laryngeal videos to measure the characteristics of vocal cord dynamics.[19] While limited to a cohort of just 30 patients, this phonovibrographic analysis was able to discriminate precancerous lesions and T1a glottic carcinoma with very high performance (sensitivity 100%, specificity 100%). This will need to be further developed and tested using larger scale datasets, but it is an exciting avenue of study. Intuitively, capturing data from both the appearance and vibration dynamics of vocal cord lesions should allow algorithms to better identify malignancies that are, by definition, invasive and extend below the vocal fold epithelium.

HISTOPATHOLOGY IMAGE ANALYSIS

There has also been significant interest in utilizing AI to aid in diagnosing head and neck cancers through histopathologic analysis. The majority of these applications have used a technique called whole slide imaging. In this technique, conventional glass histopathologic slides are scanned to generate digital slides, which form the basis of large histopathologic image sets.[20] This provides AI algorithms with the maximum available data and requires the model to identify relevant areas of interest.

Numerous AI models have been developed to identify head and neck cancers on histopathologic slides, typically achieving diagnostic accuracy rates greater than 90%.[20] The vast majority of applications have focused on identifying SCC, with the oral cavity being the most commonly investigated subsite.[20,21–24] However, other research groups have specifically investigated laryngeal SCC, nasopharyngeal SCC, or included all head and neck subsites.[23,25–29]

In general, algorithms trained with larger data sets perform better. One standout study from China developed an AI algorithm with an extensive dataset of 3458 pathologic images from 1228 patients.[27] This study specifically investigated laryngeal biopsy specimens and obtained impressive diagnostic accuracy in identifying malignancy on both internal test data (AUC = 0.981) and independent external test data (AUC = 0.982). Another study investigating nasopharyngeal SCC found that after being exposed to 1856 images from 618 patients, an AI algorithm was able to distinguish between cases of inflammation, lymphoid hyperplasia, and nasopharyngeal carcinoma with a mean AUC of 0.936 on a test set of 114 images (114 patients).[28] This significantly exceeded the mean diagnostic accuracy of a junior (AUC = 0.903) and intermediate experienced pathologist (AUC = 0.909) but had lower diagnostic accuracy compared to the senior pathologist in the study (>10 years of experience, AUC = 0.956). A second study investigating nasopharyngeal carcinoma produced an algorithm with an AUC of 0.985 for slide-level identification of nasopharyngeal carcinoma.[29] This algorithm performed better than 2 pathology residents in training but was less accurate than all 4 attending pathologists and a pathology chief resident it was compared with.

Another pathology group from China created an AI algorithm to diagnose oral cavity SCC with the aim of exploring how pathologists might benefit from access to an AI assistant.[30] Trained using a dataset of 1925 pathology images, the algorithm was able to diagnose cancers on a separate test dataset with an F1 score of 0.951. This performance was greater than that of 2 of the 3 junior pathologists in the study. Importantly, when given access to the deep learning algorithm for assistance, the 3 junior pathologists in the study were significantly more efficient, requiring an average of 11.2 minutes to diagnose oral cavity SCC (vs 17.5 minutes per case without the AI algorithm). The diagnostic accuracy of junior pathologists also improved when given access to the deep learning model. However, senior pathologists were not significantly impacted by the access to the AI tool either in terms of diagnostic speed or accuracy.

Results such as this are impressive and suggest that access to AI tools can be of significant value to pathologists, particularly those with less experience. Such tools may be of particular value in instances where faster pathology evaluation has the potential to reduce anesthesia time (frozen pathology) or in situations where the pathologist reviewing a case has less familiarity with head and neck cancer (on-call pathologists, hospitals with low volumes of head and neck cancer surgery). Additionally, these technologies could help health care institutions support their existing pathologists, who are under increasing demands due to a growing shortage of new pathologists.[31]

VOICE ANALYSIS AND CANCER SCREENING

There are many exciting applications of AI-assisted diagnosis of head and neck cancer that do not rely on clinical images or histopathology. Voice analysis is another data source well suited for AI analysis and unique to otolaryngology. Since voice changes are the most strongly associated symptom with laryngeal malignancies, it stands to reason that AI could be trained to diagnose laryngeal cancer via voice analysis.[32] Utilizing a CNN, researchers from Korea developed an algorithm that analyzed voice samples of the sustained phonated vowel sound /a:/ (over 4 seconds) to identify patients with laryngeal malignancy.[33] In their cohort of 95 exclusively male patients (50 had laryngeal cancer—mostly T1–T2, 45 normal healthy subjects), the binary classification algorithm was able to achieve a diagnostic accuracy of 85% in identifying dysphonia in patients with cancers. This accuracy was significantly greater than the performance of 2 laryngologists listening to the same voice samples (69.9%) and greatly exceeded the accuracy of non-experts (62.8%). While formal voice recording is required to perform this analysis, it is conceivable that such an algorithm could be utilized to screen high-risk patients (such as long-standing smokers who present for lung cancer screening computed tomography scans) and identify high-risk individuals who might warrant referral for laryngoscopy evaluation. Further training and validation would be required as such populations would also have a considerably higher incidence of dysphonia that is not cancer-related. This is a particularly salient point; to be clinically valuable, such tools will need to be able to classify populations of dysphonic patients and distinguish between those who have voices concerning benign and malignant etiologies of dysphonia.

There are additional AI tools that attempt to identify patients with oral cancer without using a computer vision approach. In patients with symptoms of oral cancer, researchers from India developed a neural network that utilizes clinical symptoms and history to classify patient histories and distinguish between malignant and nonmalignant cases.[34] Overall classification accuracy of this neural network was 80%. While this accuracy lags behind what can be achieved through image or pathologic analysis of oral lesions, there is still potential utility for tools like this in environments where oral cancers are frequently diagnosed at advanced stages. Lastly, there has also been interest in utilizing data from salivary samples to diagnose oral cancer. One study from Germany developed a ML algorithm that was able to utilize specific mid-infrared spectral signatures from oral cavity salivary exosomes to accurately differentiate saliva samples from patients with oral cavity malignancies compared to healthy individuals (classification accuracy 89%–95%).[35] These tools may similarly allow for earlier diagnosis of oral cancer or potentially be honed to identify oral lesions with the potential for malignant transformation.

RADIOLOGICAL IMAGE ANALYSIS

Otolaryngology has seen significant advances through the application of AI in the analysis of radiologic images, termed radiomics. This technique involves extracting and analyzing quantitative features from radiographic images, translating qualitative differences into measurable data. These features encompass various image characteristics, including pixel quality, density, color, and arrangement, which can be quantitatively assessed to gain insights from imaging studies.

One of the primary applications of radiomics in otolaryngology has been identifying and predicting nodal metastases in head and neck cancers. For example, one research group from China developed a radiomics model to predict lymph node metastasis in thyroid cancer with an accuracy of 78%.[36] Similarly, other studies have successfully predicted nodal metastases in oral cavity, oropharynx, larynx, and nasopharyngeal cancers with accuracies ranging from 76% to 92%.[36–59] This is important as the presence of nodal metastases significantly impacts stage, prognosis, and treatment decision-making. Early and accurate prediction of nodal status may guide the extent of surgery or radiotherapy and the need for adjuvant therapies, thereby potentially improving survival and reducing morbidity.

Interestingly, a research group from Japan performed a study where an AI model was evaluated against the diagnostic performance of 2 experienced radiologists and a dentist in identifying cervical nodal metastases in oropharyngeal SCC.[51] With final pathology used as the ground truth, the AI model performed significantly better than each of the readers at identifying nodal metastases in levels I and II (AUC 0.820 vs 0.798–0.816). The AI model's superior accuracy emphasizes its potential in clinical settings, thereby enhancing the precision of medical prognostication. This is particularly true in cases of human papillomavirus (HPV)–related cancers, which can be managed both surgically and medically, and where estimates concerning the number of involved lymph nodes preoperatively may impact the decision to pursue surgical treatment. AI tools also have the capability of predicting HPV status based on imaging, though this is a clinical question that is typically answered definitively using pathology before treatment.[60,61]

Delta radiomics, a type of radiomics that analyzes quantitative changes between serial radiologic images, has proven useful in evaluating treatment response, tumor progression, and recurrence. Several studies have demonstrated the effectiveness of radiomics models in monitoring responses to treatment in various head and neck cancers with accuracies ranging between 65% and 92%.[62–65] These models have been refined for specific cancer subtypes, improving the predictability of treatment outcomes, recurrence, and overall survival.[66–75] The capacity to predict such outcomes has significant clinical importance, as it could potentially guide therapeutic decisions, tailor follow-up protocols, and facilitate patient counseling regarding prognosis. In particular, delta radiomics has been utilized to predict the likelihood of xerostomia following radiotherapy with up to 92% precision.[76–81] Xerostomia can severely impact a patient's quality of life, leading to difficulties in speaking and eating, as well as an increased risk of dental disease and oral infections. The high predictive accuracy of the delta radiomics model allows for proactive interventions, enabling clinicians to preemptively address xerostomia, optimizing treatment regimens and mitigating xerostomia's impact on the quality of life.

In head and neck cancer patient care, radiomics has had the potential to impact radiation oncology treatment significantly. Radiation oncologists have used radiomics to predict gross tumor volumes, thereby assisting with image contouring.[82–85] Furthermore, efforts have been made to refine models that enhance image segmentation and create automated radiation treatment plans with accuracies ranging from 68% to 95%.[86–104] These advances in image segmentation are not specific to radiation oncology and have also led to the development of models that automatically segment and contour images, which can potentially aid in the diagnosis of nasopharyngeal carcinoma.[105–127] Building upon this, additional research has yielded accurate radiomics models that use imaging for prognostication of patients with nasopharyngeal carcinoma with accuracies around 90%.[73,128–135]

In addition to increasing radiation oncologist efficiency and prognostication, radiomics has also been explored to minimize morbidity and optimize functional outcomes following radiotherapy completion. For instance, the Involved Nodal Radiotherapy using AI-based Radiomics (INRT-AIR) study demonstrated that INRT-AIR yielded dosimetric benefits for head and neck SCC over elective neck irradiation, allowing for more selective radiation treatments to suspicious lymph nodes, which correlated with improved swallowing function given the higher MD Anderson Dysphagia Index scores at the 1-year follow-up.[136] Other radiomics applications have been developed to predict radiation-related fibrosis, provide early detection of temporal lobe injury, and assist with treatment planning to reduce risk of post-treatment trismus.[86,88,98] While not yet standard of care, such tools provide promise for improving radiation therapy outcomes.

CLINICAL PREDICTIONS AND PROGNOSTICATION

Some researchers have explored developing ML algorithms to analyze clinical and pathologic data from early-stage clinically node-negative oral cancers and predict pathologic nodal status. These algorithms have achieved performance that significantly exceeds estimates based on depth of invasion, a frequent parameter used to estimate the risk of nodal involvement and clinically decide when to perform elective neck dissection (AUC 0.840 vs 0.657).[137] Other researchers have expanded the data utilized to create such models to additionally incorporate molecular biomarkers to aid in predictions of nodal disease.[138,139] One such algorithm utilized the biomarkers CD31 and PROX1 in addition to other relevant clinical and pathologic factors and achieved an AUC of 0.89 at classifying node-negative and node-positive patients.[139] Importantly, the authors' random forest model achieved an accuracy of 88% while maintaining a high negative predictive value (>95%).

Another common application of ML is the prognostication of head and neck cancer patients. Similar to the studies that sought to predict nodal status, researchers have created ML algorithms to predict oral cancer survival using clinical and pathologic data.[140–145] In general, these algorithms perform quite well at predicting survival and estimating the likelihood of recurrence. Other researchers have additionally used molecular biomarker data in their predictions and demonstrated increased accuracy when these data are utilized.[144,145] Such research is not limited to oral cavity cancers, and numerous other studies have been performed to similarly estimate recurrence risk and survival for cancers of other head and neck subsites.[146–148]

LIMITATIONS

Though many of the AI studies mentioned in this review show exciting and promising results, it is important to refrain from sensationalizing the performance of AI. In general, many algorithms create AI models that perform very well in the setting in which they were trained but have the potential to decline substantially in performance when tested on patient populations or in settings that vary significantly from the patient population used to train the algorithm. Thus, without validation using external data sets, such AI models' external validity is likely lower than what has been reported using internal test data.

Conversely, in many instances, the head-to-head comparisons between clinicians and AI models likely underestimate clinicians' performance. As an example, while oral surgeons performed similarly to an AI algorithm at identifying images of oral cancers (92% vs 92%) in the study by Fu and colleagues[8], the true in-office diagnostic accuracy of oral surgeons is likely considerably higher than 92% when surgeons can physically palpate and examine lesions as well as consider a patient's clinical history and risk factors. Cancer evaluations are not typically performed in a telehealth setting for this reason. While AI tools may show considerable promise at triaging patients and identifying cancers on imaging, there is no substitute for an in-office evaluation by a head and neck cancer surgeon.

Beyond this, several additional barriers limit the implementation of many of the aforementioned AI tools into clinical practice. One key limitation is the black box nature of AI predictions and the need for easy interpretability regarding how AI tools arrive at their conclusions. In particular, when it comes to care for cancer patients, errors in diagnosis or treatment have the potential to be life altering. In certain instances, data used to create algorithms have been accidently biased, such as when an algorithm developed to predict malignancy on dermatoscopic images was unintentionally influenced by the presence or absence of a ruler (malignancy was highly associated with images containing rulers).[149] While most AI tools are hopefully developed to avoid such biases, even just a few reports of instances like these generate justifiable hesitancy. Rigorous clinical testing on external data sets that include diverse patient populations is critical to developing accurate and robust AI systems. While considerable progress has been made in this direction, this has been a particular challenge in health care compared to other fields due to the inherent regulatory barriers limiting data sharing and accumulation.

SUMMARY

As the field of AI rapidly expands, there are many potential avenues through which AI systems may impact the field of head and neck oncology. It is up to the physicians caring for these patients to seek opportunities to collaborate with data scientists and ensure that the right clinical data are collected to address clinically meaningful questions. Through effective collaboration, AI provides many exciting opportunities to develop algorithms that may significantly benefit head and neck cancer patient care.

CLINICS CARE POINTS

- Standardization of Imaging Techniques: Increasing standardization of imaging techniques for capturing clinical, endoscopic, and histopathologic images will enhance the applicability and accuracy of AI algorithms across different settings and populations.
- Integration with Clinical Workflow: Integrate AI tools into existing clinical workflows to enhance efficiency, particularly in areas like radiology and pathology evaluation where AI assistance may improve diagnostic speed and accuracy.
- Interpretation Considerations: Recognize the limitations of AI algorithms in replacing comprehensive clinical evaluation, including patient history and physical exam, particularly in settings where factors like palpation are crucial for accurate diagnosis.
- Validation and External Testing: Prioritize validation of AI algorithms using external datasets to assess their performance across diverse patient populations and clinical settings, ensuring robustness and generalizability of results.
- Collaborative Approach: Foster collaboration between clinicians and data scientists to address clinically relevant questions and develop AI tools tailored to specific clinical needs, optimizing their impact on head and neck cancer care.

ACKNOWLEDGMENTS

The authors are grateful for the contributions of Atharva Desai, BA, without whom this work would not have been possible.

DISCLOSURE

No conflicts of interest to disclose.

FUNDING

Funding from NIGMS P20GM130423 and NCI R03CA253212 should be acknowledged.

REFERENCES

1. Markopoulos AK. Current aspects on oral squamous cell carcinoma. Open Dent J 2012;6:126–30.
2. Zini A, Czerninski R, Sgan-Cohen HD. Oral cancer over four decades: epidemiology, trends, histology, and survival by anatomical sites. J Oral Pathol Med 2010;39(4):299–305.
3. Wang CY, Tsai T, Chen HM, et al. PLS-ANN based classification model for oral submucous fibrosis and oral carcinogenesis. Laser Surg Med 2003;32(4): 318–26.
4. Majumder SK, Ghosh N, Gupta PK. Relevance vector machine for optical diagnosis of cancer. Laser Surg Med 2005;36(4):323–33.
5. Chan CH, Huang TT, Chen CY, et al. Texture-Map-Based Branch-Collaborative Network for Oral Cancer Detection. IEEE transactions on biomedical circuits and systems 2019;13(4):766–80.
6. Aubreville M, Knipfer C, Oetter N, et al. Automatic Classification of Cancerous Tissue in Laserendomicroscopy Images of the Oral Cavity using Deep Learning. Sci Rep 2017;7(1):11979.
7. Uthoff RD, Song B, Sunny S, et al. Point-of-care, smartphone-based, dual-modality, dual-view, oral cancer screening device with neural network classification for low-resource communities. PLoS One 5 2018;13(12):e0207493.
8. Fu Q, Chen Y, Li Z, et al. A deep learning algorithm for detection of oral cavity squamous cell carcinoma from photographic images: A retrospective study. EClinicalMedicine 2020;27:100558.
9. Welikala RA, Remagnino P, Lim JH, et al. Automated Detection and Classification of Oral Lesions Using Deep Learning for Early Detection of Oral Cancer. IEEE Access 2020;8:132677–93.
10. Lin I, Datta M, Laronde DM, et al. Intraoral Photography Recommendations for Remote Risk Assessment and Monitoring of Oral Mucosal Lesions. Int Dent J 2021;71(5):384–9.
11. Li C, Jing B, Ke L, et al. Development and validation of an endoscopic images-based deep learning model for detection with nasopharyngeal malignancies. Cancer Commun 2018;38(1):59.
12. Mohammed MA, Abd Ghani MK, Arunkumar N, et al. A real time computer aided object detection of nasopharyngeal carcinoma using genetic algorithm and artificial neural network based on Haar feature tear. Future Generat Comput Syst 2018;89:539–47.
13. Mohammed MA, Abd Ghani MK, Arunkumar N, et al. Trainable model for segmenting and identifying Nasopharyngeal carcinoma. Comput Electr Eng 2018; 71:372–87.
14. Esmaeili N, Sharaf E, Gomes Ataide EJ, et al. Deep convolution neural network for laryngeal cancer classification on contact endoscopy-narrow band imaging. Sensors 2021;21(23):8157.
15. Bur AM, Zhang T, Chen X, et al. Interpretable computer vision to detect and classify structural laryngeal lesions in digital flexible laryngoscopic images. Otolaryngology–Head and Neck Surgery 2023;169(6):1564–72.

16. Nakajo K, Ninomiya Y, Kondo H, et al. Anatomical classification of pharyngeal and laryngeal endoscopic images using artificial intelligence. Head Neck 2023;45(6):1549–57.

17. Paderno A, Holsinger FC, Piazza C. Videomics: bringing deep learning to diagnostic endoscopy. Curr Opin Otolaryngol Head Neck Surg 2021;29(2):143–8.

18. Wellenstein DJ, Woodburn J, Marres HAM, et al. Detection of laryngeal carcinoma during endoscopy using artificial intelligence. Head Neck 2023;45(9): 2217–26.

19. Unger J, Lohscheller J, Reiter M, et al. A noninvasive procedure for early-stage discrimination of malignant and precancerous vocal fold lesions based on laryngeal dynamics analysis. Cancer Res 2015;75(1):31–9.

20. Bassani S, Santonicco N, Eccher A, et al. Artificial Intelligence in head and neck cancer diagnosis. J Pathol Inf 2022;13. https://doi.org/10.1016/j.jpi.2022. 100153.

21. Das DK, Bose S, Maiti AK, et al. Automatic identification of clinically relevant regions from oral tissue histological images for oral squamous cell carcinoma diagnosis. Tissue Cell 2018;53:111–9.

22. Das DK, Bose S, Kumar A, et al. Tissue and cell automatic identification of clinically relevant regions from oral tissue histological images for oral squamous cell carcinoma diagnosis. Tissue Cell 2018;53(May):111–9.

23. Rahman TY, Mahanta LB, Chakraborty C, et al. Textural pattern classification for oral squamous cell carcinoma. J Microsc 2017;1–9.

24. Rahman TY, Mahanta LB, Das AK, et al. Automated oral squamous cell carcinoma identification using shape, texture and color features of whole image strips. Tissue Cell 2020;63:101322.

25. Halicek M, Shahedi M, Little JV, et al. Head and neck cancer detection in digitized wholeslide histology using convolutional neural networks. Sci Rep 2019;1–11.

26. Mavuduru A, Halicek M, Shahedi M, et al. Using a 22-Layer U-Net to perform segmentation of squamous cell carcinoma on digitized head and neck histological images. Proc SPIE Int Soc Opt Eng 2020;1–14.

27. He Y, Cheng Y, Huang Z, et al. A deep convolutional neural network-based method for laryngeal squamous cell carcinoma diagnosis. Ann Transl Med 2021;9(24):1797.

28. Diao S, Hou J, Yu H, et al. Computer-aided pathologic diagnosis of nasopharyngeal carcinoma based on deep learning. Am J Pathol 2020;190(8):1691–700.

29. Chuang WY, Chang SH, Yu WH, et al. Successful identification of nasopharyngeal carcinoma in nasopharyngeal biopsies using deep learning. Cancers 2020;12(2):507.

30. Yang SY, Li SH, Liu JL, et al. Histopathology-based diagnosis of oral squamous cell carcinoma using deep learning. J Dent Res 2022 Oct;101(11):1321–7.

31. Prajapati PR, Wells A, Tyler A, et al. Pathologists Shortage in United States of America (USA) - How Academic Centers and Private Laboratories Can Play an Effective Role in Recruiting Qualified Future Pathology Residents from Pool of United States (US) and International Medical Graduates (IMGs). Am J Clin Pathol 2023;160(Issue Supplement_1):S65–6.

32. Shephard EA, Parkinson MA, Hamilton WT. Recognising laryngeal cancer in primary care: a large case-control study using electronic records. Br J Gen Pract 2019;69(679):e127–33.

33. Kim H, Jeon J, Han YJ, et al. Convolutional neural network classifies pathological voice change in laryngeal cancer with high accuracy. J Clin Med 2020; 9(11):3415.

34. Sharma N, Om H. Usage of probabilistic and general regression neural network for early detection and prevention of oral cancer. TheScientificWorldJOURNAL 2015;2015:234191.

35. Zlotogorski-Hurvitz A, Dekel BZ, Malonek D, et al. FTIR-based spectrum of salivary exosomes coupled with computational-aided discriminating analysis in the diagnosis of oral cancer. J Cancer Res Clin Oncol 2019;145(3):685–94.

36. Wang Y-W, Wu C-S, Zhang G-Y, et al. Can parameters other than minimal axial diameter in MRI and PET/CT further improve diagnostic accuracy for equivocal retropharyngeal lymph nodes in nasopharyngeal carcinoma? PLoS One 2016; 11(10):e0163741.

37. Forghani R, Chatterjee A, Reinhold C, et al. Head and neck squamous cell carcinoma: prediction of cervical lymph node metastasis by dual-energy CT texture analysis with machine learning. Eur Radiol 2019;29(11):6172–81.

38. Liu T, Zhou S, Yu J, et al. Prediction of lymph node metastasis in patients with papillary thyroid carcinoma: a radiomics method based on preoperative ultrasound images. Technol Cancer Res Treat 2019;18. 1533033819831713.

39. Lu W, Zhong L, Dong D, et al. Radiomic analysis for preoperative prediction of cervical lymph node metastasis in patients with papillary thyroid carcinoma. Eur J Radiol 2019;118:231–8.

40. Romeo V, Cuocolo R, Ricciardi C, et al. Prediction of tumor grade and nodal status in oropharyngeal and oral cavity squamous-cell carcinoma using a radiomic approach. Anticancer Res 2020;40(1):271–80.

41. Lee JH, Ha EJ, Kim D, et al. Application of deep learning to the diagnosis of cervical lymph node metastasis from thyroid cancer with CT: external validation and clinical utility for resident training. Eur Radiol 2020;30(6):3066–72.

42. Lee JH, Ha EJ, Kim JH. Application of deep learning to the diagnosis of cervical lymph node metastasis from thyroid cancer with CT. Eur Radiol 2019;29(10): 5452–7.

43. Kann BH, Aneja S, Loganadane GV, et al. Pretreatment identification of head and neck cancer nodal metastasis and extranodal extension using deep learning neural networks. Sci Rep 2018;8(1):14036.

44. Dohopolski M, Chen L, Sher D, et al. Predicting lymph node metastasis in patients with oropharyngeal cancer by using a convolutional neural network with associated epistemic and aleatoric uncertainty. Phys Med Biol 2020;65(22): 225002.

45. Kawauchi K, Furuya S, Hirata K, et al. A convolutional neural network-based system to classify patients using FDG PET/CT examinations. BMC Cancer 2020; 20(1):227.

46. Chen L, Zhou Z, Sher D, et al. Combining manyobjective radiomics and 3D convolutional neural network through evidential reasoning to predict lymph node metastasis in head and neck cancer. Phys Med Biol 2019;64(7).

47. Ariji Y, Fukuda M, Kise Y, et al. Contrast-enhanced computed tomography image assessment of cervical lymph node metastasis in patients with oral cancer by using a deep learning system of artificial intelligence. Oral surgery, Oral Medicine, Oral Pathology and Oral Radiology 2019;127(5):458–63.

48. Romeo V, Cuocolo R, Ricciardi C, et al. Prediction of tumor grade and nodal status in oropharyngeal and oral cavity squamous-cell carcinoma using a radiomic approach. Anticancer Res 2020;40:271–80.

49. Bardosi ZR, Dejaco D, Santer M, et al. Benchmarking Eliminative Radiomic Feature Selection for Head and Neck Lymph Node Classification. Cancers 2022;14:477.

50. Onoue K, Fujima N, Andreu-Arasa VC, et al. Cystic cervical lymph nodes of papillary thyroid carcinoma, tuberculosis and human papillomavirus positive oropharyngeal squamous cell carcinoma: Utility of deep learning in their differentiation on CT. Am J Otolaryngol 2021;42:103026.

51. Tomita H, Yamashiro T, Heianna J, et al. Nodal-based radiomics analysis for identifying cervical lymph node metastasis at levels I and II in patients with oral squamous cell carcinoma using contrast-enhanced computed tomography. Eur Radiol 2021;31:7440–9.

52. Chen L, Dohopolski M, Zhou Z, et al. Attention Guided Lymph Node Malignancy Prediction in Head and Neck Cancer. Int J Radiat Oncol Biol Phys 2021;110: 1171–9.

53. Kann BH, Hicks DF, Payabvash S, et al. Multi-Institutional Validation of Deep Learning for Pretreatment Identification of Extranodal Extension in Head and Neck Squamous Cell Carcinoma. J Clin Oncol 2020;38:1304–11.

54. Seidler M, Forghani B, Reinhold C, et al. Dual-Energy CT Texture Analysis With Machine Learning for the Evaluation and Characterization of Cervical Lymphadenopathy. Comput Struct Biotechnol J 2019;17:1009–15.

55. Ariji Y, Sugita Y, Nagao T, et al. CT evaluation of extranodal extension of cervical lymph node metastases in patients with oral squamous cell carcinoma using deep learning classification. Oral Radiol 2020;36:148–55.

56. Zhou Z, Chen L, Sher D, et al. Predicting Lymph Node Metastasis in Head and Neck Cancer by Combining Many-objective Radiomics and 3-dimensioal Convolutional Neural Network through Evidential Reasoning. Annu Int Conf IEEE Eng Med Biol Soc 2018;2018:1–4.

57. Chen L, Zhou Z, Sher D, et al. Combining many-objective radiomics and 3D convolutional neural network through evidential reasoning to predict lymph node metastasis in head and neck cancer. Phys Med Biol 2019;64:075011.

58. Ariji Y, Fukuda M, Kise Y, et al. Contrast-enhanced computed tomography image assessment of cervical lymph node metastasis in patients with oral cancer by using a deep learning system of artificial intelligence. Oral Surg Oral Med Oral Pathol Oral Radiol 2019;127:458–63.

59. Kann BH, Aneja S, Loganadane GV, et al. Pretreatment Identification of Head and Neck Cancer Nodal Metastasis and Extranodal Extension Using Deep Learning Neural Networks. Sci Rep 2018;8:14036.

60. Haider SP, Mahajan A, Zeevi T, et al. PET/CT radiomics signature of human papillomavirus association in oropharyngeal squamous cell carcinoma. Eur J Nucl Med Mol Imaging 2020;47(13):2978–91.

61. Fujima N, Andreu-Arasa VC, Meibom SK, et al. Prediction of the human papillomavirus status in patients with oropharyngeal squamous cell carcinoma by FDG-PET imaging dataset using deep learning analysis: a hypothesis-generating study. Eur J Radiol 2020;126:108936.

62. Tran WT, Suraweera H, Quiaoit K, et al. Quantitative ultrasound delta-radiomics during radiotherapy for monitoring treatment responses in head and neck malignancies. Future Sci OA 2020;6:FSO624.

63. Morgan HE, Wang K, Dohopolski M, et al. Exploratory ensemble interpretable model for predicting local failure in head and neck cancer: The additive benefit of CT and intra-treatment cone-beam computed tomography features. Quant Imaging Med Surg 2021;11:4781–96.

64. Sellami S, Bourbonne V, Hatt M, et al. Predicting response to radiotherapy of head and neck squamous cell carcinoma using radiomics from cone-beam CT images. Acta Oncol 2022;61:73–80.

65. Vallie'res M, Kay-Rivest E, Perrin LJ, et al. Radiomics strategies for risk assessment of tumour failure in head-and-neck cancer. Sci Rep 2017;7(1):10117.

66. Fatima K, Dasgupta A, DiCenzo D, et al. Ultrasound delta-radiomics during radiotherapy to predict recurrence in patients with head and neck squamous cell carcinoma. Clin. Transl. Radiat Oncol 2021;28:62–70.

67. Xi Y, Ge X, Ji H, et al. Prediction of Response to Induction Chemotherapy Plus Concurrent Chemoradiotherapy for Nasopharyngeal Carcinoma Based on MRI Radiomics and Delta Radiomics: A Two-Center Retrospective Study. Front Oncol 2022;12:824509.

68. Corino VDA, Bologna M, Calareso G, et al. Refining Tumor Treatment in Sinonasal Cancer Using Delta Radiomics of Multi-Parametric MRI after the First Cycle of Induction Chemotherapy. J Imaging 2022;8:46.

69. Kumdee O, Bhongmakapat T, Ritthipravat P. Prediction of nasophar- yngeal carcinoma recurrence by neuro-fuzzy techniques. Fuzzy Sets Syst 2012;203:95–111.

70. Haider SP, Sharaf K, Zeevi T, et al. Prediction of post-radiotherapy locoregional progression in HPV-associated oropharyngeal squamous cell carcinoma using machine-learning analysis of baseline PET/CT radiomics. Transl Oncol 2021;14(1):100906.

71. Haider SP, Zeevi T, Baumeister P, et al. Potential added value of PET/CT radiomics for survival prognostication beyond AJCC 8th edition staging in oropharyngeal squamous cell carcinoma. Cancers 2020;12(7):1–16.

72. Folkert MR, Setton J, Apte AP, et al. Predictive modeling of outcomes following definitive chemoradiotherapy for oropharyngeal cancer based on FDG-PET image characteristics. Phys Med Biol 2017;62(13):5327–43.

73. Peng H, Dong D, Fang M-J, et al. Prognostic value of deep learning PET/CT-based radiomics: potential role for future individual induction chemotherapy in advanced nasopharyngeal carcinoma. Clin Cancer Res 2019;25(14):4271–9.

74. Fujima N, Andreu-Arasa VC, Meibom SK, et al. Deep learning analysis using FDG-PET to predict treatment outcome in patients with oral cavity squamous cell carcinoma. Eur Radiol 2020;30(11):6322–30.

75. Wang C, Liu C, Chang Y, et al. Dose-distributiondriven PET image-based outcome prediction (DDD-PIOP): a deep learning study for oropharyngeal cancer IMRT application. Front Oncol 2020;10:1592.

76. van Dijk LV, Brouwer CL, van der Laan HP, et al. Geometric Image Biomarker Changes of the Parotid Gland Are Associated With Late Xerostomia. Int J Radiat Oncol Biol Phys 2017;99:1101–10.

77. van Dijk LV, Langendijk JA, Zhai TT, et al. Delta-radiomics features during radiotherapy improve the prediction of late xerostomia. Sci Rep 2019;9:12483.

78. Wu H, Chen X, Yang X, et al. Early Prediction of Acute Xerostomia During Radiation Therapy for Head and Neck Cancer Based on Texture Analysis of Daily CT. Int J Radiat Oncol Biol Phys 2018;102:1308–18.

79. Rosen BS, Hawkins PG, Polan DF, et al. Early Changes in Serial CBCT-Measured Parotid Gland Biomarkers Predict Chronic Xerostomia After Head and Neck Radiation Therapy. Int J Radiat Oncol Biol Phys 2018;102:1319–29.

80. Liu Y, Shi H, Huang S, et al. Early prediction of acute xerostomia during radiation therapy for nasopharyngeal cancer based on delta radiomics from CT images. Quant Imaging Med Surg 2019;9:1288–302.

81. Berger T, Noble DJ, Shelley LEA, et al. Predicting radiotherapy-induced xerostomia in head and neck cancer patients using day-to-day kinetics of radiomics features. Phys Imag Radiat Oncol 2022;24:95–101.

82. Huang B, Chen Z, Wu P-M, et al. Fully automated delineation of gross tumor volume for head and neck cancer on PET-CT using deep learning: a dual-center study. Contrast Media Mol Imaging 2018;2018:8923028.

83. Moe Y.M., Groendahl A.R., Mulstad M., et al., Deep learning for automatic tumour segmentation in PET/CT images of patients with head and neck cancers. arXiv preprint arXiv:1908.00841. 2019. https://doi.org/10.48550/arXiv.1908.00841.

84. Guo Z, Guo N, Gong K, et al. Gross tumor volume segmentation for head and neck cancer radiotherapy using deep, dense multimodality network. Phys Med Biol 2019;64(20):205015.

85. Park Y-I, Kang S-W, Kim K-H, et al. Feasibility study of deep learning tumor segmentation for a merged tumor dataset: head & neck and limbs. J Korean Phys Soc 2020;77(11):1049–54.

86. Wang J, Liu R, Zhao Y, et al. A predictive model of radiation-related fibrosis based on the radiomic features of magnetic resonance imaging and computed tomography. Transl Cancer Res 2020;9(8):4726–38.

87. Yang X, Li X, Zhang X, et al. Segmentation of organs at risk in nasopharyngeal cancer for radiotherapy using a self-adaptive Unet network. Nan Fang Yi Ke Da Xue Xue Bao 2020;40(11):1579–86.

88. Zhang B, Lian Z, Zhong L, et al. Machine-learning based MRI radiomics models for early detection of radiation-induced brain injury in nasopharyngeal carcinoma. BMC Cancer 2020;20(1):502.

89. Wen D-W, Lin L, Mao Y-P, et al. Normal tissue complication probability (NTCP) models for predicting temporal lobe injury after intensity-modulated radiotherapy in nasopharyngeal carcinoma: a large registry-based retrospective study from China. Radiother Oncol 2021;157:99–105.

90. Chen X, Yang J, Yi J, et al. Quality control of VMAT planning using artificial neural network models for nasopharyngeal carcinoma. Chin J Radiol Med Prot 2020;40(2):99–105.

91. Bai P, Weng X, Quan K, et al. A knowledge-based intensity-modulated radiation therapy treatment planning technique for locally advanced nasopharyngeal carcinoma radiotherapy. Radiat Oncol 2020;15(1):188.

92. Jiao S-X, Chen L-X, Zhu J-H, et al. Prediction of dose-volume histograms in nasopharyngeal cancer IMRT using geometric and dosimetric information. Phys Med Biol 2019;64(23):23NT04.

93. Men K, Chen X, Zhang Y, et al. Deep deconvolutional neural network for target segmentation of nasopharyngeal cancer in planning computed tomography images. Front Oncol 2017;7:315.

94. Olin AB, Hansen AE, Rasmussen JH, et al. Feasibility of multiparametric positron emission tomography/magnetic resonance imaging as a one-stop-shop for radiation therapy planning for patients with head and neck cancer. Int J Radiat Oncol Biol Phys 2020;108(5):1329–38.

95. Chen X, Sun S, Bai N, et al. A deep learning-based autosegmentation system for organs-at-risk on whole-body computed tomography images for radiation therapy. Radiother Oncol 2021;160:175e84.

96. van Rooij W, Dahele M, Ribeiro Brandao H, et al. Deep learning-based delineation of head and neck organs at risk: geometric and dosimetric evaluation. Int J Radiat Oncol Biol Phys 2019;104(3):677e84.

97. Aliotta E, Nourzadeh H, Choi W, et al. An automated workflow to improve efficiency in radiation therapy treatment planning by prioritizing organs at risk. Adv Radiat Oncol 2020;5(6):1324e33.

98. Thor M, Iyer A, Jiang J, et al. Deep learning auto-segmentation and automated treatment planning for trismus risk reduction in head and neck cancer radiotherapy. Phys Imaging Radiat Oncol 2021;28(19):96e101.

99. McIntosh C, Welch M, McNiven A, et al. Fully automated treatment planning for head and neck radiotherapy using a voxel-based dose prediction and dose mimicking method. Phys Med Biol 2017;62(15):5926e44.

100. Babier A, Boutilier JJ, McNiven AL, et al. Knowledge-based automated planning for oropharyngeal cancer. Med Phys 2018;45(7):2875e83.

101. Cornell M, Kaderka R, Hild SJ, et al. Noninferiority study of automated knowledge-based planning versus humandriven optimization across multiple disease sites. Int J Radiat Oncol Biol Phys 2020;106(2):430e9.

102. Cilla S, Ianiro A, Romano C, et al. Templatebased automation of treatment planning in advanced radiotherapy: a comprehensive dosimetric and clinical evaluation. Sci Rep 2020;10(1):423.

103. Sher DJ, Godley A, Park Y, et al. Prospective study of artificial intelligence-based decision support to improve head and neck radiotherapy plan quality. Clin Transl Radiat Oncol 2021;20(29):65e70.

104. Miki K, Kusters M, Nakashima T, et al. Evaluation of optimization workflow using custom-made planning through predicted dose distribution for head and neck tumor treatment. Phys Med 2020;80:167e74.

105. Tang P, Zu C, Hong M, et al. DA-DSUnet: dual attention-based dense SU-net for automatic head-and-neck tumor segmentation in MRI images. Neurocomputing 2021;435:103–13.

106. Cai M, Wang J, Yang Q, et al. Combining images and t-staging information to improve the automatic segmentation of nasopharyngeal carcinoma tumors in MR images. IEEE Access 2021;9:21323–31.

107. Bai X, Hu Y, Gong G, et al. A deep learning approach to segmentation of nasopharyngeal carcinoma using computed tomography. Biomed Signal Process 2021;64:102246.

108. Wu B, Khong PL, Chan T. Automatic detection and classification of nasopharyngeal carcinoma on PET/CT with support vector machine. Int J Comput Assist Radiol Surg 2012;7:635–46.

109. Mohammed MA, Abd Ghani MK, Hamed RI, et al. Artificial neural networks for automatic segmentation and identification of nasopharyngeal carcinoma. J Comput Sci 2017;21:263–74.

110. Li S, Xiao J, He L, et al. The tumor target segmentation of nasopharyngeal cancer in CT images based on deep learning methods. Technol Cancer Res Treat 2019;18. 1533033819884561.

111. Liang S, Tang F, Huang X, et al. Deep-learning-based detection and segmentation of organs at risk in nasopharyngeal carcinoma computed tomographic images for radiotherapy planning. Eur Radiol 2019;29(4):1961–7.

112. Lin L, Dou Q, Jin Y-M, et al. Deep learning for automated contouring of primary tumor volumes by MRI for nasopharyngeal carcinoma. Radiology 2019;291(3):677–86.

113. Liu Z, Fan J, Li M, et al. A deep learning method for prediction of three-dimensional dose distribution of helical tomotherapy. Med Phys 2019;46(5):1972–83.

114. Ma Z, Zhou S, Wu X, et al. Nasopharyngeal carcinoma segmentation based on enhanced convolutional neural networks using multi-modal metric learning. Phys Med Biol 2019;64(2):025005.

115. Zhong T, Huang X, Tang F, et al. Boostingbased cascaded convolutional neural networks for the segmentation of CT organs-at-risk in nasopharyngeal carcinoma. Med Phys 2019;46(12):5602–11.

116. Zou M, Hu J, Zhang H, et al. Rigid medical image registration using learning-based interest points and features. Comput Mater Continua (CMC) 2019; 60(2):511–25.

117. Chen H, Qi Y, Yin Y, et al. MMFNet: a multi-modality MRI fusion network for segmentation of nasopharyngeal carcinoma. Neurocomputing 2020;394: 27–40.

118. Wu X, Dong D, Zhang L, et al. Exploring the predictive value of additional peri-tumoral regions based on deep learning and radiomics: a multicenter study. Med Phys 2021;48(5):2374–85.

119. Wong LM, King AD, Ai QYH, et al. Convolutional neural network for discriminating nasopharyngeal carcinoma and benign hyperplasia on MRI. Eur Radiol 2021;31(6):3856–63.

120. Wong LM, Ai QYH, Mo FKF, et al. Convolutional neural network in nasopharyngeal carcinoma: how good is automatic delineation for primary tumor on a non-contrast-enhanced fat-suppressed T2-weighted MRI? Jpn J Radiol 2021;39(6): 571–9.

121. Xue X, Qin N, Hao X, et al. Sequential and iterative auto-segmentation of high-risk clinical target volume for radiotherapy of nasopharyngeal carcinoma in planning CT images. Front Oncol 2020;10:1134.

122. Xue X, Hao X, Shi J, et al. Auto-segmentation of high-risk primary tumor gross target volume for the radiotherapy of nasopharyngeal carcinoma. J Image Graph 2020;25(10):2151–8.

123. Wang X, Yang G, Zhang Y, et al. Automated delineation of nasopharynx gross tumor volume for nasopharyngeal carcinoma by plain CT combining contrast-enhanced CT using deep learning. J Radiat Res Appl Sci 2020; 13(1):568–77.

124. Men K, Chen X, Zhu J, et al. Continual improvement of nasopharyngeal carcinoma segmentation with less labeling effort. Phys Med 2020;80:347–51.

125. Liu K, Xia W, Qiang M, et al. Deep learning pathological microscopic features in endemic nasopharyngeal cancer: prognostic value and protentional role for individual induction chemotherapy. Cancer Med 2020;9(4):1298–306.

126. Guo F, Shi C, Li X, et al. Image segmentation of nasopharyngeal carcinoma using 3D CNN with long-range skip connection and multi-scale feature pyramid. Soft Comput 2020;24(16):12671–80.

127. Du D, Feng H, Lv W, et al. Machine learning methods for optimal radiomics-based differentiation between recurrence and inflammation: application to nasopharyngeal carcinoma post-therapy PET/CT images. Mol Imaging Biol 2020; 22(3):730–8.

128. Liu J, Mao Y, Li Z, et al. Use of texture analysis based on contrast enhanced MRI to predict treatment response to chemoradiotherapy in nasopharyngeal carcinoma. J Magn Reson Imaging 2016;44(2):445–55.

129. Zhang B, He X, Ouyang F, et al. Radiomic machine-learning classifiers for prognostic biomarkers of advanced nasopharyngeal carcinoma. Cancer Lett 2017; 403:21–7.

130. Zhang B, Tian J, Dong D, et al. Radiomics features of multiparametric MRI as novel prognostic factors in advanced nasopharyngeal carcinoma. Clin Cancer Res 2017;23(15):4259–69.

131. Cui C, Wang S, Zhou J, et al. Machine learning analysis of image data based on detailed MR image reports for nasopharyngeal carcinoma prognosis. BioMed Res Int 2020;2020:8068913.

132. Yang Q, Guo Y, Ou X, et al. Automatic T staging using weakly supervised deep learning for nasopharyngeal carcinoma on MR images. J Magn Reson Imag 2020;52(4):1074–82.

133. Xie C, Du R, Ho JWK, et al. Effect of machine learning re-sampling techniques for imbalanced datasets in 18F-FDG PET-based radiomics model on prognostication performance in cohorts of head and neck cancer patients. Eur J Nucl Med Mol Imaging 2020;47(12):2826–35.

134. Ke L, Deng Y, Xia W, et al. Development of a self-constrained 3D DenseNet model in automatic detection and segmentation of nasopharyngeal carcinoma using magnetic resonance images. Oral Oncol 2020;110:104862.

135. Jing B, Deng Y, Zhang T, et al. Deep learning for risk prediction in patients with nasopharyngeal carcinoma using multi-parametric MRIs. Comput Methods Programs Biomed 2020;197:105684.

136. Sher DJ, Avkshtol V, Moon D, et al. Recurrence and quality-of-life following involved node radiotherapy for head and neck squamous cell carcinoma: initial results from the phase II INRT-air trial. Int J Radiat Oncol Biol Phys 2021;111(3):e398.

137. Bur AM, Holcomb A, Goodwin S, et al. Machine learning to predict occult nodal metastasis in early oral squamous cell carcinoma. Oral Oncol 2019;92:20–5.

138. Kim K-Y, Cha I-H. A novel algorithm for lymph node status prediction of oral cancer before surgery. Oral Oncol 2011;47(11):1069–73.

139. Mermod M, Jourdan EF, Gupta R, et al. Development and validation of a multivariable prediction model for the identification of occult lymph node metastasis in oral squamous cell carcinoma. Head Neck 2020;42(8):1811–20.

140. Karadaghy OA, Shew M, New J, et al. Development and assessment of a machine learning model to help predict survival among patients with oral squamous cell carcinoma. JAMA Otolaryngol Neck Surg 2019;145:1115.

141. Lavanya L, Chandra J. Oral cancer analysis using machine learning techniques. Int J Eng Res Technol 2019;12:596–601.

142. Alabi RO, Elmusrati M, Sawazaki-Calone I, et al. Machine learning application for prediction of locoregional recurrences in early oral tongue cancer: a web-based prognostic tool. Virchows Arch 2019;475:489–97.

143. Tseng W-T, Chiang W-F, Liu S-Y, et al. The application of data mining techniques to oral cancer prognosis. J Med Syst 2015;39.

144. Chang S-W, Abdul-Kareem S, Merican AF, et al. Oral cancer prognosis based on clinicopathologic and genomic markers using a hybrid of feature selection and machine learning methods. BMC Bioinf 2013;14.

145. Chang S-W, Sameem A, Amir Feisal Merican AM, et al. A hybrid prognostic model for oral cancer based on clinicopathologic and genomic markers. Sains Malays 2014;43:567–73.

146. Ritthipravat P, Kumdee O, Bhongmakap T. Efficient missing data technique for prediction of nasopharyngeal carcinoma recurrence. Inf Technol J 2013;12:1125–33.

147. Jiang R, You R, Pei X-Q, et al. Development of a ten-signature classifier using a support vector machine integrated approach to subdivide the M1 stage into M1a and M1b stages of nasopharyngeal carcinoma with synchronous metastases to better predict patients' survival. Oncotarget 2016;7(3):3645–57.
148. Zhu W, Kan X, Calogero RA. Neural network cascade optimizes MicroRNA biomarker selection for nasopharyngeal cancer prognosis. PLoS One 2014; 9(10):e110537.
149. Narla A, Kuprel B, Sarin K, et al. Automated Classification of Skin Lesions: From Pixels to Practice. J Invest Dermatol 2018 Oct;138(10):2108–10.

Artificial Intelligence in Laryngology, Broncho-Esophagology, and Sleep Surgery

Obinna I. Nwosu, MD[a,b], Matthew R. Naunheim, MD, MBA[a,b,*]

KEYWORDS

- Otolaryngology • Laryngology • Sleep • Artificial intelligence • Machine learning
- Deep learning • Broncho-esophagology

KEY POINTS

- Advances in artificial intelligence (AI), especially machine learning and deep learning, are enhancing diagnosis and treatment in voice, swallowing, and sleep disorders.
- AI tools, notably in computer vision and voice and speech processing, are proving more accurate than traditional methods in identifying and analyzing laryngological pathologies.
- Effective AI integration in clinical practice requires addressing data quality, security, and ethical issues surrounding transparency and bias in AI systems.

INTRODUCTION

Laryngology, broncho-esophagology, and sleep surgery have experienced marked technological advancements in recent years, and with this has come an increasing amount of data for consideration in the workup and management of otolaryngologic disease. Artificial intelligence (AI) affords new and astonishing methods for digesting and interpreting the vast amounts of data that otolaryngologists are faced with. AI, a branch of computer science, enables machines to perform tasks that typically require human intelligence, such as problem-solving, pattern recognition, and decision-making. Within otolaryngology specifically, there has been a marked increase in the development of novel diagnostic and therapeutic approaches employing AI techniques, namely machine/deep learning and computer vision.[1] Machine learning (ML) utilizes patterns within data and algorithmic modeling to learn from data and perform tasks without specific task-oriented programming. Deep learning (DL), a subtype of ML, employs neural networks to tackle increasingly complex tasks through layers of processing. DL algorithms are commonly utilized in computer vision (CV)

[a] Department of Otolaryngology–Head & Neck Surgery, Massachusetts Eye & Ear, Boston, MA, USA; [b] Department of Otolaryngology–Head & Neck Surgery, Harvard Medical School, Boston, MA, USA
* Corresponding author. Department of Otolaryngology–Head & Neck Surgery, Massachusetts Eye & Ear, 243 Charles Street, Boston, MA 02114.
E-mail address: mnaunheim@mgb.org

Otolaryngol Clin N Am 57 (2024) 821–829
https://doi.org/10.1016/j.otc.2024.04.002
0030-6665/24/© 2024 Elsevier Inc. All rights reserved.

tasks, wherein programs are developed to extract information from visual data. CV models are often developed with a convolutional neural network (CNN), a multilayered system, which processes key features of visual data in grid-like manner. Neural networks are frequently employed in audio-processing tasks such as speech recognition or generation.[2]

In this study, we review recent applications of AI in laryngology, broncho-esophagology, and sleep surgery. As the majority of these AI applications have been diagnostic and preclinical in nature, our review focuses on AI innovations aimed at improved diagnosis. Still, we discuss tools for outcome prediction and personalized care. Finally, we note challenges and barriers to integration of AI-based solutions into common practice.

DISCUSSION
Artificial Intelligence in Laryngoscopy

The vast majority of diagnostic AI tools in laryngology focus on the analysis of endoscopic data. Indeed, many of the most notable AI-based innovations in laryngology have been CV models for image and video analysis of laryngoscopic data. These applications fall into 1 of 2 categories: classification and detection. To date, these have been applied to an array of clinical scenarios including pathology identification, localization, motion analysis, and quality assurance.

Classification, which typically involves categorization of laryngoscopic data, may be multiclass tasks (ie, normal vs polyp vs carcinoma, and so forth) or binary (normal vs pathologic). Ren and colleagues and Cho and colleagues developed multiclass models capable of categorizing endoscopic images as containing no pathology, nodules, polyps, or malignant lesions.[3,4] Both groups demonstrated superior accuracy in classifying images compared to clinician observers, highlighting the possibility for well-trained CV models to improve the diagnostic accuracy of clinicians. Classification approaches have even been applied to curation of endoscopic image datasets with the extraction of only high-quality, informative frames.[5,6] Endoscopic evaluation of the larynx is often hindered by blur, varying illumination, and glare and reflections of wet surfaces. In 2 separate studies, Moccia and colleagues and Yao and colleagues employed a classification DL approach to remove uninformative frames from laryngoscopic videos that often represent a high proportion of the entire video sample.[5,6]

Distinct from classification approaches are detection models that involve localization of laryngeal structures and pathologies. Azam and colleagues developed a model capable of localizing laryngeal malignancies in laryngoscopic frames achieving a Dice score of 81.4%.[7] Detection can be extended to segmentation where structures are localized and classified. Hamad and colleagues published their work creating segmentation models for delineation of the laryngeal framework and measurement of common intralaryngeal angles.[8] Adamian and colleagues extended this approach in their creation of a segmentation model for tracking vocal fold motion and calculating the anterior glottic angle (AGA). They used the model, capable of detecting vocal fold paralysis with 77% sensitivity and 92% specificity, to define the relationship between patient-reported voice outcomes and their AGA.[9,10] This study highlights the potential use of AI as a predictive tool for diagnosis, assessment of treatment response, monitoring, and patient-reported outcomes.

Artificial Intelligence in Automated Voice Processing

Automated voice processing is another area where AI has made a significant impact, with a growing number of publications describing AI techniques for voice analysis.[11]

Laryngologists and speech language pathologists routinely collect and utilize patient voice data for diagnostics and outcome monitoring. This acoustic and aerodynamic data can, in turn, be used to develop AI models capable of screening and potentially diagnosing a wide range of diseases. As the field of voice AI research grows, there is increasing effort to standardize and consolidate collection of voice data to develop robust, balanced voice datasets for training representative and generalizable models.[11] Even with disparate collection of voice data, the speech processing models published in recent literature have still demonstrated promise for the detection of primary laryngeal, psychiatric, as well as neurologic disorders. A variety of ML methods have been employed for the analysis of voice data including hidden Markov models, Gaussian mixture models, support vector machines, artificial neural networks (ANNs), decision trees, linear classifier, K-means clustering, and combined classifiers.

The application of ML voice tools is broad with some groups focused on the basic distinction between normal and abnormal voice as a screening tool. Compton and colleagues described an ANN that detected binary presence of laryngeal pathology with an F1 score of 98%.[12] They suggest this model may prove a useful screening tool in the primary care setting where otolaryngology equipment is unavailable. Similarly, Chen and colleagues developed a binary predictor for the presence of dysphonia. Interestingly, they trained the model with Chinese voice samples and tested it with German voice samples without a drop in the model's strong performance.[13] Bensoussan and colleagues developed a binary classification model for predicting gender on the basis of voice samples, a tool they intend to be used as an outcome measure for gender-affirming voice interventions.[14] Other approaches have focused on more complex predictions such as the works by Liu and colleagues and Hu and colleagues who both trained separate multiclass CNNs capable of differentiating voice pathologies such as adductor dysphonia, unilateral vocal paralysis, laryngitis, or presence of a vocal lesion. Both groups demonstrated the highest accuracy for detecting absence of pathology, though each model was capable at predicting class-specific pathology with similar performance to real clinicians.[15,16]

Automated voice and speech processing has also been pivotal in neurocognitive research domains. Liu and colleagues published on their ML approach for detecting Alzheimer's disease using voice data. In their cohort, they predicted the likelihood of Alzheimer's diagnosis with an accuracy of 84% using spectrograms automatically extracted from raw speech data.[17] Syed and colleagues incorporated an ensemble approach, combining multiple ML models into one predictor, to diagnose Alzheimer's disease with an accuracy of 95% from voice samples.[18] In a cohort of 115 patients, Suppa and colleagues utilized a vector machine ML approach to detect Parkinson's disease in affected patients using voice data processed into thousands of acoustic features.[19] While many of these models focused on diagnosis, the field of neurocognitive AI research continues to expand with a shift toward model development for patient-specific prognostication and disease monitoring as well as diagnosis.[20]

Several studies have demonstrated the feasibility of using voice and speech data for the diagnosis of psychiatric disorders such as depression and bipolar disorder.[21] Select acoustic features have been identified as key diagnostic indicators of psychiatric dysfunction.[22] These features can be automatically extracted from voice samples, converted into standard data elements such as spectrograms, or visual representations of speech, and used as input features in predictive models. Romero and colleagues utilized a CNN and ensemble method to develop a robust model for diagnosing depression using vocal spectrograms.[23] McGinnis and colleagues demonstrated that an ML approach could outperform parents in detecting their children's anxiety and depression based on speech samples.[24]

Finally, neuroimaging AI may also play an increasing role in the diagnosis of voice disorders. Spasmodic dysphonia, also known as laryngeal dystonia, causes a weak, strained, or breathy voice with irregular breaks or spasms. Although the exact pathophysiologic underpinning of spasmodic dysphonia is poorly understood, recent advances in neuroimaging enabled the identification of key brain regions involved in the disorder.[25] Capitalizing on this, Simonyan and colleagues employed a DL network to automatically identify these areas on structural brain imaging. Automated analysis of structural abnormalities in these areas permitted their model to predict the presence of dystonia with an accuracy of 98.8%.[25,26] Their model, capable of diagnosing a wide spectrum of focal dystonias (ie, blepharospasm, cervical dystonia, laryngeal dystonia) highlights the manner in which AI innovations in one domain can catalyze care in others.

Artificial Intelligence in Broncho-Esophagology

Apart from the larynx, other areas the upper aerodigestive tract have received less attention but have nonetheless seen significant advancement. One key area within the field that has benefited from advances in AI techniques is the management of dysphagia. Video fluoroscopic swallowing studies (VFSS) and fiberoptic endoscopic evaluation of swallowing (FEES) are the gold standard tests for evaluating patients with oropharyngeal dysphagia. These tests, however, are subject to interrater and intrarater variability as they are ultimately interpreted by an expert examiner.[27] Consequently, clinicians have incorporated manual techniques, such as quantitative temporal measurements of swallowing phases, to increase the objectivity of study evaluation. Unfortunately, this manual analysis can be time-consuming.

AI approaches offer an automated alternative. Lee and colleagues developed a DL model employing a CNN to detect the pharyngeal phase of swallow during VFSS, while Bandini and colleagues extended this functionality to track bolus location.[28,29] A DL model capable of detecting and measuring the duration of all phases was developed by Yun Jeong and colleagues and achieved an accuracy of 98.1%.[30] Aspiration detection has also been a target of DL analysis. Lee and colleagues developed a DL binary detection model that identified occurrence of aspiration in a VFSS.[29] Conversely, Weng and colleagues developed a more computational and graphically demanding model that segmented laryngeal anatomy during FEES to monitor for airway penetration/aspiration.[31] Both of these models provide an automated method for improving sensitivity of these tests.

As laryngoscopy is used in the diagnosis and management of bronchoesophagologic disease, some of the previously described approaches employed for automated pathology and motion analysis have been employed within the field. Laryngopharyngeal reflux is a common disorder and may be diagnosed on an endoscopic examination by the presence of characteristic laryngeal features. Witt and colleagues and Kuo and colleagues automatically detected the color and texture features of the vocal folds in laryngoscopic images. These features were in turn used to train a classification model capable of predicting the presence of laryngopharyngeal reflux.[32,33]

AI techniques have also been used in the workup of airway obstruction. Spirometry is a commonly employed noninvasive tool for evaluating airway pathology. Wang and colleagues used a CNN to differentiate causes of upper airway obstruction based on images of flow–volume curves.[34] Kim and colleagues tackled a similar problem in their development of a DL model for the detection of tracheostomy obstruction. Their model utilized airway sounds captured near the tracheostoma and was able to classify airway sounds as normal, sputum, or blood/crusts. They suggest that the use of this model in the immediate postoperative period may prevent adverse events in the early detection of tracheostomy obstruction.[35]

Artificial Intelligence in Sleep Surgery

Many of the techniques that are revolutionizing laryngology and broncho-esophagology are likewise transforming the landscape of sleep surgery. In a recent position statement, the American Academy of Sleep Medicine noted that AI is well-suited for the analysis of electrophysiologic sleep data and has the potential to stream-line care and improve patient outcomes.[36] Recent efforts to use AI for automated analysis of electrophysiologic data have yielded astounding results, particularly in the management of obstructive sleep apnea (OSA). OSA is one of the most common sleep disorders managed by sleep surgeons; it affects nearly 1 billion people worldwide and carries significant health risk.[37] Yet diagnosis remains challenging due to inefficient workflows and provider shortages.[38] The gold standard for OSA diagnosis is polysom-nography (PSG), a multiparameter test whose interpretation can be time-consuming, labor-intensive, and fraught with interrater and intrarater variability.[39]

There have been many recent applications of ML and DL methodologies to PSG interpretation with promising results. Levy and colleagues detailed a DL model for diagnosing OSA using only continuous oximetry from the PSG.[40] In addition to PSG data, researchers have utilized acoustic data, observing characteristic sounds related to upper airway obstruction, to screen for OSA. Nakano and colleagues employed a CNN within a DL architecture to predict the presence of OSA using tracheal sounds alone.[41] Pépin and colleagues describe the use of a wearable inertial monitoring unit, which measures mandibular movement to detect the presence of OSA. The mandibular movement data are transmitted to a smartphone app in real time and pro-cessed by an ML program capable of predicting the likelihood of underlying OSA.[42] These models use input data (oximetry, sound, and mandibular movement) that could be captured by a home sleep study device and may someday permit the development of a fully automated home test.

AI has also been employed in patient selection for surgical intervention and predict-ing outcome following treatment. A model for predicting which children with OSA were most likely to benefit from adenotonsillectomy was developed by Liu and colleagues. Their model utilized preoperative symptomatology and PSG results to predict improvement postoperatively with high accuracy.[43] They conclude that with the use of their model, children with mild symptoms preoperatively may be observed as opposed to undergoing a surgery with limited benefit. In adults, Lou and colleagues utilized an ML approach to identify patients likely to benefit from hypoglossal nerve stimulator placement by characterizing key patterns on preprocedural PSG.[44] Simi-larly, Kim and colleagues trained an ML model capable of predicting surgical success, as determined by the postoperative sleep study, based on preoperative information including demographics, physical examination features as well as preoperative PSG results.[45] These studies demonstrate the manner in which AI is enabling personalized treatment approaches in sleep care.

Ethical Considerations and Future Directions

Despite its promise, AI faces integration and ethical challenges. First, to develop high-performing ML/DL models, large amounts of high-quality data are required. Conse-quently, there has been a push for electronic health record (EHR) systems to streamline clinical data transmission into formats usable for model development. Novel EHR are being developed with built-in AI capabilities enabling clinicians to access and analyze patient data more efficiently.[46] This has particular importance in otolaryngology, where many models developed rely on protected health information in the form of images and acoustic data, as voice print is considered a biometric identifier.

Second, there are ethical considerations surrounding the oversight and maintenance of AI systems. AI models must be fair, transparent and interpretable in their functionality, and secure in their handling of patient data.[47] This is crucial not only in their development but also once used in real practice. As more AI-driven solutions are created for clinical problems in the fields of laryngology, broncho-esophagology, and sleep surgery, clinicians must partner with developers and regulators to ensure systems are safe, transparent, explainable, and unbiased.

SUMMARY

Herein we discuss the emerging role of AI in diagnosing and treating disorders related to the voice, swallowing, and sleep. AI, particularly ML and DL, is being utilized to efficiently process increasingly complex data stemming from technological advancement. The AI-based analyses of video, acoustic, and imaging data are revolutionizing diagnosis and enabling predictive modeling for personalized care. Though advancements in AI offer great potential in transforming otolaryngology, challenges in implementation and ethical considerations remain.

CLINICS CARE POINTS

- The fields of laryngology, broncho-esophagology, and sleep surgery have seen significant technological advancements, leading to a vast increase in clinical data available for decision-making.
- AI, particularly ML and DL, is increasingly used. These AI techniques help in problem-solving, pattern recognition, and decision-making, which are crucial for diagnosing and treating complex cases.
- The majority of AI applications in otolaryngology are focused on diagnostics. This includes the use of CV for analyzing endoscopic data and automated speech processing for voice analysis. These AI tools have shown higher accuracy in some cases compared to clinicians.
- AI is not only used for diagnostics but also for predicting treatment outcomes and personalizing patient care. This includes detecting laryngeal pathologies, managing dysphagia, and selecting appropriate treatments for sleep disorders like OSA.
- The integration of AI into clinical practice faces challenges, including the need for high-quality data, secure handling of patient information, and ensuring the transparency and fairness of AI systems. Ethical considerations are paramount to ensure that AI tools are used safely and effectively in patient care.

REFERENCES

1. Crowson MG, Ranisau J, Eskander A, et al. A contemporary review of machine learning in otolaryngology–head and neck surgery. Laryngoscope 2020;130(1):45–51.
2. Paderno A, Holsinger FC, Piazza C. Videomics: bringing deep learning to diagnostic endoscopy. Curr Opin Otolaryngol Head Neck Surg 2021;29(2):143–8.
3. Ren J, Jing X, Wang J, et al. Automatic recognition of laryngoscopic images using a deep-learning technique. Laryngoscope 2020;130(11):E686–93.
4. Cho WK, Lee YJ, Joo HA, et al. Diagnostic accuracies of laryngeal diseases using a convolutional neural network-based image classification system. Laryngoscope 2021;131(11):2558–66.

5. Moccia S, Vanone GO, Momi ED, et al. Learning-based classification of informative laryngoscopic frames. Comput Methods Progr Biomed 2018;158:21–30.

6. Yao P, Witte D, Gimonet H, et al. Automatic classification of informative laryngoscopic images using deep learning. Laryngoscope Investigative Otolaryngology 2022; Apr;7(2):460–6.

7. Azam MA, Sampieri C, Ioppi A, et al. Deep learning applied to white light and narrow band imaging videolaryngoscopy: toward real-time laryngeal cancer detection. Laryngoscope 2022;132(9):1798–806.

8. Hamad A, Haney M, Lever TE, et al. Automated segmentation of the vocal folds in laryngeal endoscopy videos using deep convolutional regression networks. In: Computer Vision Foundation, editor. 2019 IEEE/CVF Conference on computer vision and pattern recognition Workshops (CVPRW). Columbia, MO: IEEE; 2019. p. 140–8. https://doi.org/10.1109/CVPRW.2019.00023.

9. Adamian N, Naunheim MR, Jowett N. An open-source computer vision tool for automated vocal fold tracking from videoendoscopy. Laryngoscope 2021; 131(1):E219–25.

10. Wang TV, Adamian N, Song PC, et al. Application of a computer vision tool for automated glottic tracking to vocal fold paralysis patients. Otolaryngol Head Neck Surg 2021;165(4):556–62.

11. Evangelista E, Kale R, McCutcheon D, et al. Current practices in voice data collection and limitations to voice AI research: a national survey. Laryngoscope 2023. https://doi.org/10.1002/lary.31052.

12. Compton EC, Cruz T, Andreassen M, et al. Developing an artificial intelligence tool to predict vocal cord pathology in primary care settings. Laryngoscope 2023;133(8):1952–60.

13. Chen Z, Zhu P, Qiu W, et al. Deep learning in automatic detection of dysphonia: Comparing acoustic features and developing a generalizable framework. Int J Lang Commun Disord 2023;58(2):279–94.

14. Bensoussan Y, Pinto J, Crowson M, et al. Deep learning for voice gender identification: proof-of-concept for gender-affirming voice care. Laryngoscope 2021; 131(5):E1611–5.

15. Liu GS, Hodges JM, Yu J, et al. End-to-end deep learning classification of vocal pathology using stacked vowels. Laryngoscope Investig Otolaryngol 2023;8(5): 1312–8.

16. Hu HC, Chang SY, Wang CH, et al. Deep learning application for vocal fold disease prediction through voice recognition: preliminary development study. J Med Internet Res 2021;23(6):e25247.

17. Liu L, Zhao S, Chen H, et al. A new machine learning method for identifying Alzheimer's disease. Simulat Model Pract Theor 2020;99:102023.

18. Syed ZS, Syed MSS, Lech M, et al. Automated recognition of alzheimer's dementia using bag-of-deep-features and model ensembling. IEEE Access 2021;9: 88377–90.

19. Suppa A, Costantini G, Asci F, et al. Voice in Parkinson's Disease: A Machine Learning Study. Front Neurol 2022;13:831428.

20. Javeed A, Dallora AL, Berglund JS, et al. machine learning for dementia prediction: a systematic review and future research directions. J Med Syst 2023; 47(1):17.

21. Low DM, Bentley KH, Ghosh SS. Automated assessment of psychiatric disorders using speech: A systematic review. Laryngoscope Investig Otolaryngol 2020; 5(1):96–116.

22. Cohen AS, Ellevåg B. Automated computerized analysis of speech in psychiatric disorders. Curr Opin Psychiatr 2014;27(3):203–9.

23. Vázquez-Romero A, Gallardo-Antolín A. Automatic detection of depression in speech using ensemble convolutional neural networks. Entropy 2020;22(6):688.

24. McGinnis EW, Anderau SP, Hruschak J, et al. Giving voice to vulnerable children: machine learning analysis of speech detects anxiety and depression in early childhood. IEEE J Biomed Health Inform 2019;23(6):2294–301.

25. Valeriani D, Simonyan K. A microstructural neural network biomarker for dystonia diagnosis identified by a DystoniaNet deep learning platform. Proc Natl Acad Sci USA 2020;117(42):26398–405.

26. Yao D, O'Flynn LC, Simonyan K. DystoniaBoTXNet: novel neural network biomarker of botulinum toxin efficacy in isolated dystonia. Ann Neurol 2023; 93(3):460–71.

27. Baijens L, Barikroo A, Pilz W. Intrarater and interrater reliability for measurements in videofluoroscopy of swallowing. Eur J Radiol 2013;82(10):1683–95.

28. Bandini A, Smaoui S, Steele CM. Automated pharyngeal phase detection and bolus localization in videofluoroscopic swallowing study: Killing two birds with one stone? Comput Methods Progr Biomed 2022;225:107058.

29. Lee JT, Park E, Jung TD. Automatic detection of the pharyngeal phase in raw videos for the videofluoroscopic swallowing study using efficient data collection and 3d convolutional networks. Sensors 2019;19(18):3873.

30. Jeong SY, Kim JM, Park JE, et al. Application of deep learning technology for temporal analysis of videofluoroscopic swallowing studies. Sci Rep 2023;13(1): 17522.

31. Weng W, Imaizumi M, Murono S, et al. Expert-level aspiration and penetration detection during flexible endoscopic evaluation of swallowing with artificial intelligence-assisted diagnosis. Sci Rep 2022;12(1):21689.

32. Kuo CFJ, Kao CH, Dlamini S, et al. Laryngopharyngeal reflux image quantization and analysis of its severity. Sci Rep 2020;10(1):10975.

33. Witt DR, Chen H, Mielens JD, et al. detection of chronic laryngitis due to laryngopharyngeal reflux using color and texture analysis of laryngoscopic images. J Voice 2014;28(1):98–105.

34. Wang Y, Li Y, Chen W, et al. Deep learning for automatic upper airway obstruction detection by analysis of flow-volume curve. Respir Int Rev Thorac Dis 2022; 101(9):841–50.

35. Kim H, Koh D, Jung Y, et al. Breathing sounds analysis system for early detection of airway problems in patients with a tracheostomy tube. Sci Rep 2023;13(1): 21029.

36. Goldstein CA, Berry RB, Kent DT, et al. Artificial intelligence in sleep medicine: an American Academy of Sleep Medicine position statement. J Clin Sleep Med 2020;16(4):605–7.

37. Benjafield AV, Ayas NT, Eastwood PR, et al. Estimation of the global prevalence and burden of obstructive sleep apnoea: a literature-based analysis. Lancet Respir Med 2019;7(8):687–98.

38. Watson NF, Rosen IM, Chervin RD. The past is prologue: the future of sleep medicine. J Clin Sleep Med 2017;13(01):127–35.

39. Watson NF, Fernandez CR. Artificial intelligence and sleep: Advancing sleep medicine. Sleep Med Rev 2021;59:101512.

40. Levy J, Álvarez D, Del Campo F, et al. Deep learning for obstructive sleep apnea diagnosis based on single channel oximetry. Nat Commun 2023;14(1):4881.

41. Nakano H, Furukawa T, Tanigawa T. Tracheal sound analysis using a deep neural network to detect sleep apnea. J Clin Sleep Med 2019;15(8):1125–33.

42. Pépin JL, Letesson C, Le-Dong NN, et al. Assessment of mandibular movement monitoring with machine learning analysis for the diagnosis of obstructive sleep apnea. JAMA Netw Open 2020;3(1):e1919657.

43. Liu X, Pamula Y, Immanuel S, et al. Utilisation of machine learning to predict surgical candidates for the treatment of childhood upper airway obstruction. Sleep Breath Schlaf Atm 2022;26(2):649–61.

44. Lou B, Rusk S, Nygate YN, et al. Association of hypoglossal nerve stimulator response with machine learning identified negative effort dependence patterns. Sleep Breath Schlaf Atm 2023;27(2):519–25.

45. Kim JY, Kong HJ, Kim SH, et al. Machine learning-based preoperative datamining can predict the therapeutic outcome of sleep surgery in OSA subjects. Sci Rep 2021;11(1):14911.

46. Yang X, Chen A, PourNejatian N, et al. A large language model for electronic health records. Npj Digit Med 2022;5(1):1–9.

47. Nwosu OI, Crowson MG, Rameau A. Artificial intelligence governance and otolaryngology-head and neck surgery. Laryngoscope 2023;133(11):2868–70.

Artificial Intelligence in Rhinology

Noel F. Ayoub, MD, MBA*, Jordan T. Glicksman, MD, MPH

KEYWORDS

- Rhinology • Allergy • Skull base surgery • Artificial intelligence • Machine learning
- Deep learning • Natural language processing

KEY POINTS

- There is considerable interest in employing artificial intelligence (AI) applications across the fields of rhinology, allergy, and skull base surgery.
- The numerous data sources in rhinology, including endoscopic images and videos from clinic and operating room, radiography, pathology, and quality of life metrics provide ample datapoints to train large language models.
- Existing applications of AI within rhinology largely concentrate on inflammatory disease, sinonasal and skull base tumors, imaging, and preoperative planning. The overwhelming majority of published studies reflect in silico evaluations.
- Improved data quality and integrity, validation of existing models, and additional testing are important challenges and next steps.

INTRODUCTION

Rhinologic conditions remain some of the most prevalent of all disorders. Over 12% of the US population is diagnosed with sinusitis each year,[1] and up to 60% of the world's population is affected by rhinitis.[2] These disorders can also have significant negative impact on patient quality of life (QOL).[3,4] Other rhinologic conditions, while less common, can be life-threatening, such as certain sinonasal malignancies and skull base tumors.[5] Because of the prevalence of rhinologic conditions, and the potential impact on QOL and patient survival, rhinology often employs revolutionary solutions to improve patient outcomes.

Since its inception, rhinology has been a leading force in technological innovation, from image-guided intraoperative navigation to minimally invasive approaches to the skull base.[6] Repeated breakthroughs in technology, surgical expertise, and pharmaceutic discoveries have expanded the capability of rhinologists to diagnose and

Department of Otolaryngology–Head & Neck Surgery, Mass Eye and Ear/Harvard Medical School, Boston, MA, USA
* Corresponding author. Division of Rhinology and Skull Base Surgery, Department of Otolaryngology–Head & Neck Surgery, Mass Eye and Ear/Harvard Medical School, 243 Charles Street, Boston, MA 02114.
E-mail address: fayoub@meei.harvard.edu

Otolaryngol Clin N Am 57 (2024) 831–842
https://doi.org/10.1016/j.otc.2024.04.010
0030-6665/24/© 2024 Elsevier Inc. All rights reserved.

oto.theclinics.com

manage sinonasal conditions. As a subspecialty that employs state-of-the-art technology daily, rhinology has also been a pioneer in health care applications of artificial intelligence (AI). Perhaps because of the ubiquity of rhinologic disorders, there has been considerable interest in employing AI across rhinology, and numerous studies have been published demonstrating the potential of AI-enabled solutions.[7–10] Rhinology represents a particularly unique field in that the majority of the clinic and operating room evaluations and procedures are performed with an endoscope, highlighting the extensive image and video data that can be collected from these patients. The endoscopic images, in addition to the radiographic and pathologic data, provide researchers with tremendous amounts of variables to study. This review briefly reviews definitions of AI, then highlights a selection of the existing and potential applications of AI within rhinology.

BRIEF DEFINITIONS

AI is an overarching term that contains many subcategories, each of which is applicable to rhinologic use cases. AI broadly describes the creation of machines that can think or act like humans. Machine learning (ML) is a subset of AI that uses complex algorithms to learn from data and improve its own performance continually.[11] Even further, deep learning (DL) is a specific method of ML that utilizes artificial neural networks (ANN), modeled after neuronal connections in the human brain, to perform more complex tasks independently and without human input.

Within ML and DL, *supervised learning* describes a form of training that requires more human input. An application that utilizes supervised learning requires "labeled" datasets. "Labeled" implies that the raw data have descriptions (eg, name) that provide context or meaning to the value. Unsupervised learning, in contrast, does not require labeled data. Unsupervised models are fed unlabeled data and autonomously discover patterns, then categorize the data itself. For example, in a model developed to diagnose malignancy on computed tomography (CT) or magnetic resonance imaging (MRI), a supervised learning model would be trained using images with clearly labeled tumors. In an unsupervised version, the model would be given many images at once without being told which scans show a malignancy. The model would then find patterns among images and independently sort them into "malignancy" or "no malignancy" groups. This model can then use these learned patterns to categorize all future images it sees. Unsupervised learning techniques thus reduce some of the obstacles seen with supervised data, including the cost and time necessary to label data, and the potential for poorly labeled data.

INFLAMMATORY SINONASAL DISEASE

Chronic rhinosinusitis (CRS) is an appropriate focus of attention for AI applications. As clinicians learn more about biological pathways and immune dysregulation involved in CRS, our understanding of the heterogeneity of the disease process continues to increase.[12] For example, the traditional classification of CRS as having (CRSwNP) or lacking (CRSsNP) polyps has evolved into more specific categories, such as endotypes, specific inflammatory mediators, and polyp location.[12] The various genetic, environmental, anatomic, and iatrogenic contributions to the condition illustrate the difficulty of utilizing precision medicine to diagnose and manage the condition appropriately.[12,13]

The increased complexity of CRS classification necessitates precision medicine with individualized diagnostic and treatment approaches for each person. The more widespread use of expensive monoclonal antibody therapy to treat CRS, and the variable patient responses, additionally invites more personalized treatment plans.[14] A better understanding of who may respond to various treatments could help guide clinical decision-making and reduce the cost of care. While it may be difficult, time-consuming, and expensive for humans to deliver personalized care, these AI-enabled solutions could help advance precision approaches for inflammatory sinonasal disease.

Rhinology utilizes multiple modalities to assess patients with sinonasal symptoms, including the patient history, physical examination, nasal endoscopy, radiography, pathology, and genetics.[10] Researchers can utilize these numerous datapoints to build models that aid clinicians in diagnosing and classifying patients with CRS. An increasing number of researchers have focused their attention to grouping CRS patients into clusters. Clustering is a type of unsupervised learning that can identify groups of patients with similar features.[15] Clustering can thus analyze unlabeled datasets to group, or cluster, patients according to common characteristics, such as the location of opacification on a CT scan. While these commonalities may go unnoticed by the human eye, this grouping may permit better diagnostic or treatment approaches.

Many of these data-centric clustering techniques correlate CRS symptomatology and outcomes with multi-omics (genomic, epigenomic, transcriptomic, proteomic, and metabolomic) datasets. Soler and colleagues analyzed preoperative clinical data to group patients into phenotypic clusters, which in turn could be used to predict medication usage.[16] Additional cluster analyses have been performed to identify patterns of olfactory dysfunction,[17] CRS endotypes,[18] and surgical outcomes based on endotype and phenotype.[19] For example, Morse and colleagues found that elevated Th2 cytokines interleukin IL-5 and IL-13 are strongly associated with reduced olfaction.[17] Qi and colleagues used a variety of clinical variables to help explain the heterogeneity of patient responses to antibiotic treatment.[20] Kim and colleagues showed that subepithelial neutrophilic infiltration can predict refractory CRSwNP.[21]

Because CRS significantly affects QOL, additional research has focused on the prediction of preoperative and postoperative QOL outcomes from medical and surgical interventions. Many of these studies utilize established patient-reported outcome measures (PROMs). Divekar and colleagues clustered patients based on preoperative Sino-Nasal Outcome Test (SNOT-22) scores using unsupervised learning.[22] Chowdury and colleagues model demonstrated that mucus cytokines can help predict postoperative changes in SNOT-22 scores.[23] For example, IL-5 was associated with greater improvement in SNOT-22 scores while IL-2 showed the inverse. Preoperative SNOT scores have also been used to predict postoperative endoscopic sinus surgery (ESS) outcomes,[10] and Szaleniec and colleagues utilized neural networks to anticipate persistent postoperative facial pain.[24] These findings can be used as additional data points to help guide clinical decision-making and provide patients with more informed preoperative counseling.

The interest in using AI to help predict outcomes for inflammatory conditions extends beyond rhinology. For example, models have been built to assist clinicians in diagnosing allergic rhinitis.[25,26] Kim and colleagues similarly identified asthmatic and non-asthmatic clusters within a cohort of patients with CRSwNP.[27] Molecular studies have been utilized to cluster patients with asthma and predict asthma exacerbations, an anticipatory approach that could be useful in rhinology and allergy.[28] The potential to identify patients who are at higher risk of experiencing an asthma exacerbation and preemptively manage this has correlates with CRS. The ability to predict which CRS patients will have an exacerbation and when may reduce the time to treatment. Additionally, as the access to remote patient monitoring devices increases, the availability of continuous patient data will expand.[29,30] For example, the greater availability of relatively inexpensive and mobile personal at-home endoscopes can increase endoscopic data at different timepoints during a patient's care cycle, including at the onset of CRS exacerbations. This continuous data can be used to build more robust models across all aspects of rhinology.

BENIGN AND MALIGNANT SINONASAL AND NASOPHARYNGEAL TUMORS

Sinonasal malignancies represent less than 5% of head and neck cancers.[31,32] However, prognosis can be poor, and treatment can have a detrimental impact on QOL. As endoscopic techniques have advanced, so has the ability of surgeons to endoscopically endonasally resect, and subsequently reconstruct, benign and malignant sinonasal and nasopharyngeal tumors.[33] Neoadjuvant and adjuvant chemotherapy and/ or radiation, and targeted therapy, are also employed. Because of the impact on patient survival and QOL, the multiple treatment modalities, and the diverse pathology, there has been substantial interest in employing AI to improve the diagnosis and management of these conditions.

Radiography, endoscopy, and histology are 3 main tools used to aid in the diagnosis of these neoplasms. Researchers have used both endoscopic and radiographic data to generate predictive models to improve the diagnostic techniques and prognosis estimates of tumors. For example, existing applications have helped differentiate between squamous cell carcinoma (SCC) and inverted papilloma (IP),[34] tumors that have progressed from IP to SCC,[35] and treatment outcomes of sinonasal SCC.[36] Fujima and colleagues developed algorithms that had high sensitivity, specificity, positive predictive value, and negative predictive value when using MRI to predict local control and failure for sinonasal SCC.[36] Li X and colleagues analyzed CT scans to differentiate between IP and inflammatory nasal polyps.[37] Similarly, Girdler and colleagues used endoscopic images to differentiate between IP and nasal polyps,[10] and more recently, Guo and colleagues's models showed greater than 90% area under the curve (AUC) score performance in similarly differentiating between IP and inflammatory polyps.[38]

Numerous studies have been published for the evaluation and management of patients with nasopharyngeal masses, including detection of nasopharyngeal carcinoma (NPC),[39] NPC recurrence,[40] NPC segmentation,[41,42] treatment failure, and progression-free survival.[43] Li C and colleagues's study notably demonstrated greater accuracy in the model's detection of NPC from endoscopic images when compared to the oncologist.[39] Wong and colleagues's convolutional neural network (CNN) had accuracy greater than 90% in detecting early-stage NPC using MRI.[44] DL applications of Raman spectroscopy have also shown high sensitivity in NPC staging.[45]

SKULL BASE SURGERY

Since the 1990s, endoscopic techniques have advanced significantly, and the definition of what is considered endoscopically resectable has continued to expand. These more extensive surgical opportunities warrant more accurate and precise risk stratification models, and there has been growing interest in utilizing AI for endonasal skull base surgery.[7,9] Additionally, the heterogeneity of skull base tumors, variable tumor characteristics, and differing prognoses make pre-treatment predictions more difficult. Improved preoperative predictive analytics could potentially help guide decision making, informed consent discussions, medical and surgical management, and long-term care.

Researchers have built various ML models based on radiomic, clinical, and pathologic data to provide surgeons with greater insight into a variety of surgical and non-surgical outcomes. One area of focus involves preoperative radiographic evaluation of the features of skull base tumors, such as tumor size, location, and radiographic features.[7] Published studies have analyzed preoperative images to predict tumor histology,[46–48] consistency,[49–51] Ki labeling,[52,53] and aggressiveness.[6,10,54] One study developed models to predict the care cycle costs of patients who were diagnosed with pituitary adenomas.[55] Another major area of focus has analyzed clinicopathological data to predict intraoperative or postoperative complications, including cerebrospinal fluid leak,[56–58] hypopituitarism,[59] hyponatremia,[60] and unplanned readmission.[61] Additional studies have sought to predict rates of gross total resection, recurrence, remission, improvement in vision, and normalization of hormone levels.[62–66] In one study, Zhang and colleagues used preoperative MRI scans to predict postoperative visual field recovery after endoscopic endonasal resection of pituitary lesions.[64] Such knowledge can be instrumental for clinical decision-making and preoperative patient counseling.

IMAGING AND SURGICAL PLANNING

Radiographic modalities, including CT and MRI, are often used to diagnose sinonasal disorders. Because radiography is so vital to the field of rhinology, this is a considerable area of interest for AI applications, including for diagnosis, prognosis, and surgical planning.

Segmentation involves dividing an image (eg, CT scan slice) into several smaller parts based on specific characteristics of the different structures in the image. Automated segmentation can rapidly process images, label structures, and potentially detect abnormalities. Various automated segmentation programs have been developed for rhinologic applications. From the surgical planning approach, these models can provide surgeons with more preoperative data, including identification of various normal anatomic structures, such as the anterior ethmoid artery,[67] inferior turbinate,[68] and sphenoid sinus.[69] These innovations have the potential to help trainees, radiologists, and rhinologists read and analyze radiography. Other models have been developed to recognize anatomic variations, such as concha bullosa,[70] maxillary defects,[71] and olfactory fossa depth.[72] Diagnostically, segmentation has been used to detect mucosal thickening and mucosal retention cysts,[10] fungus balls,[73] and a volume-based modified Lund-Mackay score.[10] These methods can also analyze nasal computational fluid dynamics[10] and identify specific pathology, such as maxillary sinus lesions, more rapidly than manual techniques.[74]

Segmentation of skull base anatomy can also be used to improve intraoperative three-dimensional navigation.[75] In one study, automated segmentation was used to identify and segment skull base structures, such as the internal carotid artery, optic nerve, and superior turbinate.[75]

Natural language processing has also been utilized to predict future operative steps, with goals of improving surgical training and reducing surgical errors.[76] From the administrative perspective generative AI programs have been tested to generate operative reports[77] and clinical practice guidelines,[78] both of which represent opportunities to reducing the administrative burden of physicians.

POTENTIAL RISKS AND LIMITATIONS

The existing and potential future, applications of AI within rhinology highlight the extensive opportunity to advance the field and positively impact patients and clinicians alike. Despite the tremendous advancements within rhinology's nascent AI programs, there are limitations. The data and algorithms in the studies are often heterogeneous, making comparisons across models difficult. The use of endoscopic and radiographic data, while useful, necessitates standardization of images. Most existing studies lack external validation, as they have not been tested in different clinical settings. These models have also not yet demonstrated consistent, widespread improvements in clinical outcomes, cost effectiveness, or value-based care. The cost of developing and implementing these applications, the rigidity of these models and impractical use within clinical medicine, and limited translation thus far to the bedside are just a few examples of the existing hurdles of health care-focused AI.

The heterogeneity of the disease processes in rhinology highlights that large datasets are necessary to provide meaningful clinical impact. The ability to gather large datasets, develop accurate and precise algorithms, evaluate external validity, and ensure equity and transparency are challenges that must be overcome to unlock AI's true potential in this field. Because larger datasets are needed, some health systems have collaborated to pool patient data. This, however, introduces risks associated with data sharing. Federated learning is one area of interest wherein patient data itself is not shared among institutions.[79] Instead, patient data is kept within each institution in a decentralized format, but the data from each site can still be used to develop the AI model. The model parameters are shared from each institution to train and validate the model.

These technological innovations likewise are not without risk. Similar to the stringent regulations that dictate the use of medical devices and the Institutional Review Board requirements that oversee unproven medical interventions, AI applications in rhinology should undergo thorough scrutiny, testing, and evaluation prior to implementation in the real world. Efforts must be taken to ensure that untested or unproven software does not negatively impact patient care. The ability to oversee software is more difficult than medical devices, especially with the greater access to generative AI programs. The widespread dissemination of generative AI and other forms of large language models has further broadened the potential of how AI can change the field. Guidelines and regulation for developing and reporting AI-based models in rhinology are vital.

The lack of transparency, especially with generative AI applications, introduces risks of bias, as the clinician is unable to determine how the model came to a specific answer.[80] Explainable AI (XAI) stresses the need for AI to be explainable, transparent, and interpretable.[81] Rhinology applications of AI should strive to maximize transparency and reduce the risk of faulty models. Continued monitoring of these programs is also necessary to ensure accuracy.

NEXT STEPS

AI has the potential to provide useful data to patients and surgeons for a variety of rhinologic and skull base conditions. This remains a rapidly evolving field with numerous challenges and opportunities ahead. Despite, and because of, these concerns, rhinologists should strive to ensure that the establishment of AI within health care occurs safely, responsibly, and collaboratively. First and foremost, rhinologists must learn more about this technology and better understand how it can affect the quality of care provided and the impact it will have on patient, provider, and staff experiences. Clinicians must continue to advocate for patients and can develop best practice benchmarks, create and enforce quality assurance and improvement programs, and appropriately define and measure AI-related outcomes. Every effort should be made to evaluate the cost effectiveness of building, employing, and maintaining these within health systems.

SUMMARY

The integration of AI into rhinology represents a major paradigm shift with immense potential. Numerous models have already been developed for rhinology, allergy, skull base surgery, imaging, and surgical planning. Additional extensive research and testing is necessary prior to widespread implementation of AI in direct clinical practice within rhinology. Furthermore, extensive research is necessary to understand these models' impact on clinical outcomes.

CLINICS CARE POINTS

- There is immense potential for artificial intelligence applications within rhinology, allergy, and skull base surgery.
- Machine learning algorithms have the ability to augment diagnostics and aid in the analysis of endoscopic, imaging, and histologic data.
- Improved diagnostics, predictive analytics, and risk stratification can enhance patient-centered, personalized treatment plans.
- AI applications within healthcare require careful review and rigorous scrutiny.

DISCLOSURE

None of the authors have any financial disclosures or conflicts of interest relevant to this article.

REFERENCES

1. Albu S. Chronic Rhinosinusitis-An Update on Epidemiology, Pathogenesis and Management. J Clin Med 2020;9(7). https://doi.org/10.3390/jcm9072285.
2. Savoure M, Bousquet J, Jaakkola JJK, et al. Worldwide prevalence of rhinitis in adults: A review of definitions and temporal evolution. Clin Transl Allergy 2022; 12(3):e12130.
3. Rudmik L, Smith TL. Quality of life in patients with chronic rhinosinusitis. Curr Allergy Asthma Rep 2011;11(3):247–52.
4. Segboer CL, Terreehorst I, Gevorgyan A, et al. Quality of life is significantly impaired in nonallergic rhinitis patients. Allergy 2018;73(5):1094–100.
5. Hafstrom A, Sjovall J, Persson SS, et al. Outcome for sinonasal malignancies: a population-based survey. Eur Arch Oto-Rhino-Laryngol 2022;279(5): 2611–22.
6. Fang Y, Wang H, Feng M, et al. Application of Convolutional Neural Network in the Diagnosis of Cavernous Sinus Invasion in Pituitary Adenoma. Front Oncol 2022; 12:835047.
7. Maroufi SF, Dogruel Y, Pour-Rashidi A, et al. Current status of artificial intelligence technologies in pituitary adenoma surgery: a scoping review. Pituitary 2024. https://doi.org/10.1007/s11102-023-01369-6.
8. Osie G, Darbari Kaul R, Alvarado R, et al. A Scoping Review of Artificial Intelligence Research in Rhinology. Am J Rhinol Allergy 2023;37(4):438–48.
9. Yang DB, Smith AD, Smith EJ, et al. The State of Machine Learning in Outcomes Prediction of Transsphenoidal Surgery: A Systematic Review. J Neurol Surg B Skull Base 2023;84(6):548–59.

10. Niu J, Zhang S, Ma S, et al. Preoperative prediction of cavernous sinus invasion by pituitary adenomas using a radiomics method based on magnetic resonance images. Eur Radiol 2019;29(3):1625–34.

11. Bzdok D, Krzywinski M, Altman N. Points of Significance: Machine learning: a primer. Nat Methods 2017;14(12):1119–20.

12. Grayson JW, Hopkins C, Mori E, et al. Contemporary Classification of Chronic Rhinosinusitis Beyond Polyps vs No Polyps: A Review. JAMA Otolaryngol Head Neck Surg 2020;146(9):831–8.

13. Luu VP, Fiorini M, Combes S, et al. Challenges of artificial intelligence in precision oncology: public-private partnerships including national health agencies as an asset to make it happen. Ann Oncol 2024;35(2):154–8.

14. Godse NR, Keswani A, Lane AP, et al. Biologics for Nasal Polyps: Synthesizing Current Recommendations into a Practical Clinical Algorithm. Am J Rhinol Allergy 2023;37(2):207–13.

15. Altman N, Krzywinski M. Clustering. Nat Methods 2017;14:545–6.

16. Soler ZM, Hyer JM, Ramakrishnan V, et al. Identification of chronic rhinosinusitis phenotypes using cluster analysis. Int Forum Allergy Rhinol 2015;5(5):399–407.

17. Morse JC, Shilts MH, Ely KA, et al. Patterns of olfactory dysfunction in chronic rhinosinusitis identified by hierarchical cluster analysis and machine learning algorithms. Int Forum Allergy Rhinol 2019;9(3):255–64.

18. Lal D, Hopkins C, Divekar RD. SNOT-22-based clusters in chronic rhinosinusitis without nasal polyposis exhibit distinct endotypic and prognostic differences. Int Forum Allergy Rhinol 2018;8(7):797–805.

19. Adnane C, Adouly T, Khallouk A, et al. Using preoperative unsupervised cluster analysis of chronic rhinosinusitis to inform patient decision and endoscopic sinus surgery outcome. Eur Arch Oto-Rhino-Laryngol 2017;274(2):879–85.

20. Qi W, Abu-Hanna A, van Esch TEM, et al. Explaining heterogeneity of individual treatment causal effects by subgroup discovery: An observational case study in antibiotics treatment of acute rhino-sinusitis. Artif Intell Med 2021;116:102080.

21. Kim DK, Lim HS, Eun KM, et al. Subepithelial neutrophil infiltration as a predictor of the surgical outcome of chronic rhinosinusitis with nasal polyps. Rhinology 2021;59(2):173–80.

22. Divekar R, Patel N, Jin J, et al. Symptom-Based Clustering in Chronic Rhinosinusitis Relates to History of Aspirin Sensitivity and Postsurgical Outcomes. J Allergy Clin Immunol Pract 2015;3(6):934–940 e3.

23. Chowdhury NI, Li P, Chandra RK, et al. Baseline mucus cytokines predict 22-item Sino-Nasal Outcome Test results after endoscopic sinus surgery. Int Forum Allergy Rhinol 2020;10(1):15–22.

24. Szaleniec JSM, Stre̜k P. A stepwise protocol for neural network modeling of persistent postoperative facial pain in chronic rhinosinusitis. Bio Algorithm Med Syst 2016;12(2):81–8.

25. Caimmi D, Baiz N, Sanyal S, et al. Discriminating severe seasonal allergic rhinitis. Results from a large nation-wide database. PLoS One 2018;13(11):e0207290.

26. Jabez Christopher J, Khanna Nehemiah H, Kannan A. A clinical decision support system for diagnosis of Allergic Rhinitis based on intradermal skin tests. Comput Biol Med 2015;65:76–84.

27. Kim JW, Huh G, Rhee CS, et al. Unsupervised cluster analysis of chronic rhinosinusitis with nasal polyp using routinely available clinical markers and its implication in treatment outcomes. Int Forum Allergy Rhinol 2019;9(1):79–86.

28. Ray A, Das J, Wenzel SE. Determining asthma endotypes and outcomes: Complementing existing clinical practice with modern machine learning. Cell Rep Med 2022;3(12):100857.
29. Manning LA, Gillespie CM. E-Health and Telemedicine in Otolaryngology: Risks and Rewards. Otolaryngol Clin North Am 2022;55(1):145–51.
30. Somani SN, Yu KM, Chiu AG, et al. Consumer Wearables for Patient Monitoring in Otolaryngology: A State of the Art Review. Otolaryngol Head Neck Surg 2022; 167(4):620–31.
31. Dutta R, Dubal PM, Svider PF, et al. Sinonasal malignancies: A population-based analysis of site-specific incidence and survival. Laryngoscope 2015;125(11): 2491–7.
32. Turner JH, Reh DD. Incidence and survival in patients with sinonasal cancer: a historical analysis of population-based data. Head Neck 2012;34(6):877–85.
33. Thawani R, Kim MS, Arastu A, et al. The contemporary management of cancers of the sinonasal tract in adults. CA Cancer J Clin 2023;73(1):72–112.
34. Ramkumar S, Ranjbar S, Ning S, et al. MRI-Based Texture Analysis to Differentiate Sinonasal Squamous Cell Carcinoma from Inverted Papilloma. AJNR Am J Neuroradiol 2017;38(5):1019–25.
35. Liu GS, Yang A, Kim D, et al. Deep learning classification of inverted papilloma malignant transformation using 3D convolutional neural networks and magnetic resonance imaging. Int Forum Allergy Rhinol 2022;12(8):1025–33.
36. Fujima N, Shimizu Y, Yoshida D, et al. Machine-Learning-Based Prediction of Treatment Outcomes Using MR Imaging-Derived Quantitative Tumor Information in Patients with Sinonasal Squamous Cell Carcinomas: A Preliminary Study. Cancers 2019;11(6). https://doi.org/10.3390/cancers11060800.
37. Li X, Zhao H, Ren T, et al. Inverted papilloma and nasal polyp classification using a deep convolutional network integrated with an attention mechanism. Comput Biol Med 2022;149:105976.
38. Guo M, Zang X, Fu W, et al. Classification of nasal polyps and inverted papillomas using CT-based radiomics. Insights Imaging 2023;14(1):188.
39. Li C, Jing B, Ke L, et al. Development and validation of an endoscopic images-based deep learning model for detection with nasopharyngeal malignancies. Cancer Commun 2018;38(1):59.
40. Kumdee OBT, Ritthipravat P. Prediction of nasopharyngeal carcinoma recurrence by neuro-fuzzy techniques. Fuzzy Set Syst 2012;203:95–111.
41. Zeng Y, Zeng P, Shen S, et al. DCTR U-Net: automatic segmentation algorithm for medical images of nasopharyngeal cancer in the context of deep learning. Front Oncol 2023;13:1190075.
42. Qi Y, Li J, Chen H, et al. Computer-aided diagnosis and regional segmentation of nasopharyngeal carcinoma based on multi-modality medical images. Int J Comput Assist Radiol Surg 2021;16(6):871–82.
43. Farhidzadeh HKJ, Scott JG, Goldgof DB, et al. Classification of progression free survival with nasopharyngeal carcinoma tumors. Proceedings of SPIE 9785, Medical Imaging: Computer-Aided Diagnosis 2016;87851I.
44. Wong LM, King AD, Ai QYH, et al. Convolutional neural network for discriminating nasopharyngeal carcinoma and benign hyperplasia on MRI. Eur Radiol 2021; 31(6):3856–63.
45. Shu C, Zheng W, Lin K, et al. Real-time in vivo cancer staging of nasopharyngeal carcinoma patients with rapid fiberoptic Raman endoscopy. Talanta 2023;259: 124561.

46. Peng A, Dai H, Duan H, et al. A machine learning model to precisely immunohistochemically classify pituitary adenoma subtypes with radiomics based on preoperative magnetic resonance imaging. Eur J Radiol 2020;125:108892.

47. Li H, Zhao Q, Zhang Y, et al. Image-driven classification of functioning and nonfunctioning pituitary adenoma by deep convolutional neural networks. Comput Struct Biotechnol J 2021;19:3077–86.

48. Baysal B, Eser MB, Dogan MB, et al. Multivariable Diagnostic Prediction Model to Detect Hormone Secretion Profile From T2W MRI Radiomics with Artificial Neural Networks in Pituitary Adenomas. Medeni Med J 2022;37(1):36–43.

49. Zeynalova A, Kocak B, Durmaz ES, et al. Preoperative evaluation of tumour consistency in pituitary macroadenomas: a machine learning-based histogram analysis on conventional T2-weighted MRI. Neuroradiology 2019;61(7):767–74.

50. Cuocolo R, Ugga L, Solari D, et al. Prediction of pituitary adenoma surgical consistency: radiomic data mining and machine learning on T2-weighted MRI. Neuroradiology 2020;62(12):1649–56.

51. Wan T, Wu C, Meng M, et al. Radiomic Features on Multiparametric MRI for Preoperative Evaluation of Pituitary Macroadenomas Consistency: Preliminary Findings. J Magn Reson Imaging 2022;55(5):1491–503.

52. Ugga L, Cuocolo R, Solari D, et al. Prediction of high proliferative index in pituitary macroadenomas using MRI-based radiomics and machine learning. Neuroradiology 2019;61(12):1365–73.

53. Shu XJ, Chang H, Wang Q, et al. Deep Learning model-based approach for preoperative prediction of Ki67 labeling index status in a noninvasive way using magnetic resonance images: A single-center study. Clin Neurol Neurosurg 2022;219: 107301.

54. Feng T, Fang Y, Pei Z, et al. A Convolutional Neural Network Model for Detecting Sellar Floor Destruction of Pituitary Adenoma on Magnetic Resonance Imaging Scans. Front Neurosci 2022;16:900519.

55. Muhlestein WE, Akagi DS, McManus AR, et al. Machine learning ensemble models predict total charges and drivers of cost for transsphenoidal surgery for pituitary tumor. J Neurosurg 2018;131(2):507–16.

56. Zanier O, Zoli M, Staartjes VE, et al. Machine learning-based clinical outcome prediction in surgery for acromegaly. Endocrine 2022;75(2):508–15.

57. Mattogno PP, Caccavella VM, Giordano M, et al. Interpretable Machine Learning-Based Prediction of Intraoperative Cerebrospinal Fluid Leakage in Endoscopic Transsphenoidal Pituitary Surgery: A Pilot Study. J Neurol Surg B Skull Base 2022;83(5):485–95.

58. Villalonga JF, Solari D, Cuocolo R, et al. Clinical application of the "sellar barrier's concept" for predicting intraoperative CSF leak in endoscopic endonasal surgery for pituitary adenomas with a machine learning analysis. Front Surg 2022;9: 934721.

59. Fang Y, Wang H, Feng M, et al. Machine-Learning Prediction of Postoperative Pituitary Hormonal Outcomes in Nonfunctioning Pituitary Adenomas: A Multicenter Study. Front Endocrinol 2021;12:748725.

60. Voglis S, van Niftrik CHB, Staartjes VE, et al. Feasibility of machine learning based predictive modelling of postoperative hyponatremia after pituitary surgery. Pituitary 2020;23(5):543–51.

61. Crabb BT, Hamrick F, Campbell JM, et al. Machine Learning-Based Analysis and Prediction of Unplanned 30-Day Readmissions After Pituitary Adenoma Resection: A Multi-Institutional Retrospective Study With External Validation. Neurosurgery 2022;91(2):263–71.

62. Chen YJ, Hsieh HP, Hung KC, et al. Deep Learning for Prediction of Progression and Recurrence in Nonfunctioning Pituitary Macroadenomas: Combination of Clinical and MRI Features. Front Oncol 2022;12:813806.
63. Staartjes VE, Serra C, Muscas G, et al. Utility of deep neural networks in predicting gross-total resection after transsphenoidal surgery for pituitary adenoma: a pilot study. Neurosurg Focus 2018;45(5):E12.
64. Zhang Y, Chen C, Huang W, et al. Machine Learning-Based Radiomics of the Optic Chiasm Predict Visual Outcome Following Pituitary Adenoma Surgery. J Pers Med 2021;11(10). https://doi.org/10.3390/jpm11100991.
65. Huber M, Luedi MM, Schubert GA, et al. Machine Learning for Outcome Prediction in First-Line Surgery of Prolactinomas. Front Endocrinol 2022;13:810219.
66. Qiao N, Shen M, He W, et al. Machine learning in predicting early remission in patients after surgical treatment of acromegaly: a multicenter study. Pituitary 2021; 24(1):53–61.
67. Huang J, Habib AR, Mendis D, et al. An artificial intelligence algorithm that differentiates anterior ethmoidal artery location on sinus computed tomography scans. J Laryngol Otol 2020;134(1):52–5.
68. Kuo CFJLY, Hu DJ, Huang CC, et al. Application of intelligent automatic segmentation and 3D reconstruction of inferior turbinate and maxillary sinus from computed tomography and analyze the relationship between volume and nasal lesion. Biomed Signal Process Contro 2020;57:101660.
69. Gibelli D, Cellina M, Gibelli S, et al. Volumetric assessment of sphenoid sinuses through segmentation on CT scan. Surg Radiol Anat 2018;40(2):193–8.
70. Parmar P, Habib AR, Mendis D, et al. An artificial intelligence algorithm that identifies middle turbinate pneumatisation (concha bullosa) on sinus computed tomography scans. J Laryngol Otol 2020;134(4):328–31.
71. Wang X, Pastewait M, Wu TH, et al. 3D morphometric quantification of maxillae and defects for patients with unilateral cleft palate via deep learning-based CBCT image auto-segmentation. Orthod Craniofac Res 2021;24(Suppl 2):108–16.
72. Almushayti ZA, Almutairi AN, Almushayti MA, et al. Evaluation of the Keros Classification of Olfactory Fossa by CT Scan in Qassim Region. Cureus 2022;14(2): e22378.
73. Kim KS, Kim BK, Chung MJ, et al. Detection of maxillary sinus fungal ball via 3-D CNN-based artificial intelligence: Fully automated system and clinical validation. PLoS One 2022;17(2):e0263125.
74. Jung SK, Lim HK, Lee S, et al. Deep Active Learning for Automatic Segmentation of Maxillary Sinus Lesions Using a Convolutional Neural Network. Diagnostics 2021;11(4). https://doi.org/10.3390/diagnostics11040688.
75. Neves CA, Tran ED, Blevins NH, et al. Deep learning automated segmentation of middle skull-base structures for enhanced navigation. Int Forum Allergy Rhinol 2021;11(12):1694–7.
76. Bieck R, Heuermann K, Pirlich M, et al. Language-based translation and prediction of surgical navigation steps for endoscopic wayfinding assistance in minimally invasive surgery. Int J Comput Assist Radiol Surg 2020;15(12):2089–100.
77. Wildfeuer VKV, Bieck R, Sorge M, et al. Clinical evaluation of keyword-based, computer-generated reports of sinus operations. Laryngo-Rhino-Otol 2021; 100:S32.
78. Maniaci A, Saibene AM, Calvo-Henriquez C, et al. Is generative pre-trained transformer artificial intelligence (Chat-GPT) a reliable tool for guidelines synthesis? A preliminary evaluation for biologic CRSwNP therapy. Eur Arch Oto-Rhino-Laryngol 2024. https://doi.org/10.1007/s00405-024-08464-9.

79. Rahman A, Hossain MS, Muhammad G, et al. Federated learning-based AI approaches in smart healthcare: concepts, taxonomies, challenges and open issues. Cluster Comput 2022;1–41.

80. Zakka C, Shad R, Chaurasia A, et al. Almanac - Retrieval-Augmented Language Models for Clinical Medicine. NEJM 2024;1(2). https://doi.org/10.1056/aioa2300068.

81. DARPA's explainable AI (XAI) program: A retrospective. Applied AI Letters 2021; 2:e61.

Artificial Intelligence in Facial Plastics and Reconstructive Surgery

Ki Wan Park, MD, Mohamed Diop, MD, Sierra Hewett Willens, BS,
Jon-Paul Pepper, MD*

KEYWORDS

- Artificial intelligence • Deep learning • Machine learning
- Facial plastic and reconstructive surgery

KEY POINTS

- Artificial intelligence (AI), particularly convolutional neural networks and computer vision, is poised to revolutionize facial plastic and reconstructive surgery (FPRS) by improving diagnostic accuracy, refining surgical planning, and enhancing post-operative evaluation.
- Innovative, active applications of AI in FPRS include objective grading of facial nerve palsy, advanced preoperative counseling for procedures such as rhinoplasty and facelift, and improved objectivity in post-operative outcome assessments.
- AI will impact FPRS by enabling real-time image analysis and voice input capabilities, thereby facilitating patient education and streamlining clinical workflows.
- Despite its transformative potential, integrating AI in FPRS faces challenges such as algorithmic bias, ethical concerns, and the need for accurate and explainable AI systems.

INTRODUCTION

Artificial intelligence (AI) is poised to bring significant changes to health care. Several landmark studies have already demonstrated AI's ability to streamline medical diagnosis and treatment, including skin cancer detection and tumor detection on radiographs using deep learning.[1,2] In Otolaryngology—Head & Neck Surgery, early AI tools have been used for tumor margin identification, diagnosis, surgical training, and hearing loss management.[3–5] However, the formal adoption of AI in daily clinical practice has yet to be fully realized.

In facial plastic and reconstructive surgery (FPRS), as final aesthetic outcomes rely heavily on subjective visual diagnosis and prediction, AI can enhance objectivity and standardization. Several AI tools have already been developed to standardize

Department of Otolaryngology–Head and Neck Surgery, Stanford University School of Medicine, 801 Welch Road, Palo Alto, CA 94305, USA
* Corresponding author.
E-mail address: jpepper@stanford.edu

Otolaryngol Clin N Am 57 (2024) 843–852
https://doi.org/10.1016/j.otc.2024.05.002
0030-6665/24/© 2024 Elsevier Inc. All rights reserved, including those for text and data mining, AI training, and similar technologies.

measurements before and after surgery, with initial efforts to model post-operative outcomes with generative AI.[6-9] Additionally, AI applications have been utilized in FPRS to improve physician workflow in the clinic and enhance patient adherence to discharge instructions.[10-15] This review focuses on current and emerging AI technologies in FPRS for the clinic setting. Separately, the authors discuss the limitations and concerns of this technology. The authors place special emphasis on deep learning and foundation models given their prevalence and level of access for consumers.

ARTIFICIAL INTELLIGENCE APPLICATIONS IN FACIAL PLASTIC AND RECONSTRUCTIVE SURGERY

Applications in AI for FPRS are numerous, including medical diagnosis, pre-operative modeling, risk stratification, objective post-operative assessments, and increasing clinic efficiency (**Fig. 1**). The authors discuss the current state of AI technologies for the FPRS clinic setting in this review.

Medical Diagnosis

Facial palsy assessment
Automated evaluation of patients in FPRS with computer vision remains promising given the significant advancements over the past decade. In particular, deep learning-driven systems with convolutional neural networks (CNNs) have dominated computer vision since Krizhevsky *and colleagues* demonstrated significantly lower

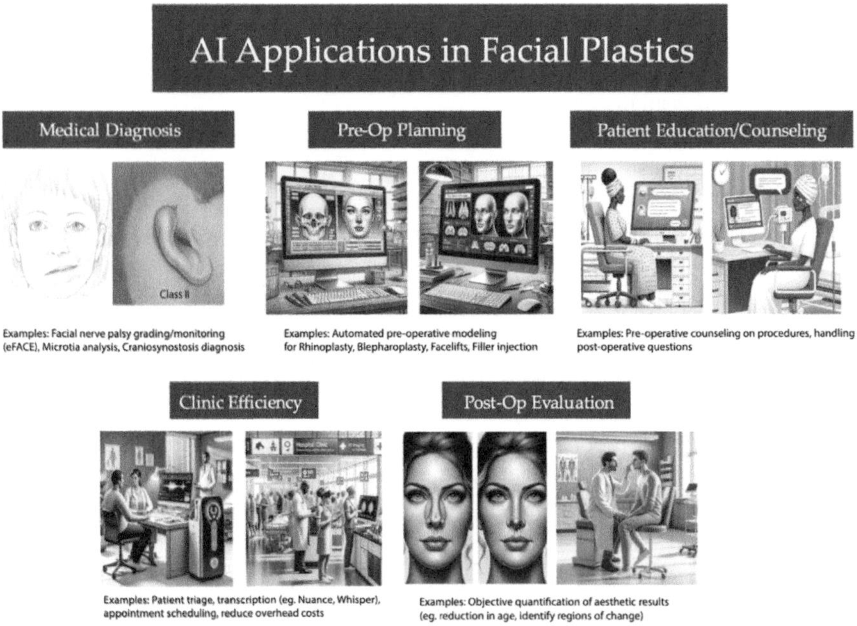

Fig. 1. Artificial intelligence (AI) applications in facial plastic and reconstructive surgery. Applications of AI include medical diagnosis, pre-operative planning/modeling, objective post-operative assessments, patient education, and increasing clinic efficiency. (All images with exception of medical diagnosis were generated using artificial intelligence with DALL-E from OpenAI.)

error rates in image classification compared to existing mainstream techniques in 2012.[16] As facial plastic surgery is a visual field, it is inherently subject to bias and interpretation by the provider. While bias may be present in AI models, computer vision methods may help provide objective measures and allow comparability across providers.

One emerging utilization of computer vision is for the assessment of facial palsy. Traditional grading mechanisms for facial palsy, such as the House-Brackmann Grading System (HBGS), have faced challenges with observer subjectivity and an inherent weakness in grading synkinesis and variable facial weakness.[17] To overcome these limitations, more sophisticated schemas such as the electronic clinician-graded facial function scale (eFACE) were developed. The eFACE utilizes a visual analog scale of 15 items[18] and has the advantage of maintaining high inter-reliability and intra-reliability between users[19] while expanding on prior scales in evaluating synkinesis and both static and dynamic domains. However, it remains reliant on clinician experience, time-consuming data collection, and confers subjectivity bias.

Recent strategies and advances in deep learning offer advantages with automatic computation of facial measurements and facial landmark assessment. One such model, Emotrics, utilizes 2-dimensional (2D) front-facing photographs to automate several facial measurements by scaling pixel width to mean iris diameter.[20] Furthermore, a recent addition has added nasolabial fold as a parameter to Emotrics, which would allow evaluation of a total of 13 parameters of the eFACE.[21] Subsequently, an auto-eFACE machine learning software was developed from Emotrics to produce an automatic mini eFACE score.[22] Compared to clinician scoring, the auto-eFACE predicted more asymmetry in patients without facial palsy and less asymmetry in patients with synkinesis/flaccid palsy.[22]

A limitation of the auto-eFACE is its reliance on static photographs for analysis compared to standardized video. This reliance is a notable drawback because static images are unable to capture the dynamic temporal movements that are crucial for clinical assessment with the eFACE. This limitation not only reduces the effectiveness of the auto-eFACE in fully replicating the eFACE assessment, but also introduces potential bias in image selection for analysis. Additionally, as only severe cases of facial palsy (flaccid paralysis and severe synkinesis) were used in the analysis, more data analysis would be needed when analyzing patients with mild or moderate facial palsy, and there is likely to be greater interrater variability for these cases. Future directions should explore video-based approaches to assessing facial palsy to provide real-time feedback and measurements in a streamlined fashion. Other objective ML algorithms have also been explored but there has been limited adoption due to the complexity of setup, hardware, and data processing required. One example is the use of Kinect v2 hardware and accompanying SDK 2.0 software to assess facial animation units.[23] However, a key limitation is the absence of validated measures of facial palsy with facial animation units in the existing literature. Another limitation is limited access to large-scale databases of patient videos due to privacy protections that may forbid access for computational model training.[24]

Other conditions relevant to facial plastic and reconstructive surgery

Deep learning algorithms have already been applied to external ear malformations. Hallac *and colleagues* developed a CNN model with near-perfect accuracy in classifying normal and abnormal ears from 2D photographs.[25] Similarly, Wang and colleagues, demonstrated the use of deep CNNs in grading microtia severity with high accuracy and providing an objective, automated assessment.[26] These models have been extended to other craniofacial conditions, such as grading the severity of unilateral cleft lip[27] and diagnosing craniosynostosis, which is challenging even for experienced craniofacial surgeons.[28,29] These novel applications of AI show its promise in grading disease severity using a targeted, visual prompt. ML techniques have been utilized to analyze computed tomography (CT) images, yielding accuracy comparable to experienced radiologists.[30,31] These diagnostic tools are particularly beneficial for communities with limited resources, as they could not only significantly accelerate the diagnosis process but also expand access to care in geographically isolated or underserved areas. Furthermore, AI's enhancement in efficiency and its improved capacity for diagnosing rare diseases can substantially elevate patient care accessibility.

Pre-operative Assessment

Recent studies have assessed the ability of AI tools to provide standardized measurements in pre-operative states and offer personalized recommendations to patients. In the field of facial rejuvenation, Alrabiah *and colleagues* developed a CNN model to determine whether forehead filler injections are needed based on the detection of wrinkles, achieving a wrinkle detection rate of 85.3%.[6] Alternatively, Shah *and colleagues* developed models based on deep learning and regression models to predict the 3-dimensional (3D) post-operative facial rejuvenation outcome after intervention, with accuracy rates up to 89.5% with real-world data, and even higher accuracy rates of up to 90.1% with synthetic data.[32] Li *and colleagues* piloted a customized precision facial assessment tool to quantify facial microexpressions.[33] The tool detected decreases in negative facial expressions 1 and 3 months after treatment in a small sample of 3 patients. However, further studies are needed to validate the system's efficacy.

For rhinoplasty, several studies have assessed automated pre-operative planning for nasal contour design. In a study, a deep neural network was trained using 3D facial images from 209 patients to perform automatic aesthetic design specifically for Asian faces.[7] The model achieved results closely mirroring manual designs, with a minimal deviation of just 0.8 mm. Similarly, Chinski *and colleagues* developed an AI model based on surgeon criteria to generate simulated post-operative images of rhinoplasty.[9] Evaluators had total or partial agreement 68.4% of the time with AI-generated post-operative images. Other models such as "RhinoNet" utilized a training set of 22,686 images from publicly available sources and achieved a prediction accuracy of 85% for rhinoplasty status on test images.[8] While the iOS application for RhinoNet is not currently active on the Apple app store, source code for RhinoNet is currently publicly available on github.

AI has been instrumental in identifying critical anatomic landmarks imperative for surgical planning, including the determination of skeletal profiles, midfacial plane, and location of perforator vessels.[34] Furthermore, several models have made advancements in risk stratification for plastic surgery, such as forecasting surgical reconstruction needs, along with anticipating clinical and technical outcomes—such as blood loss, the incidence of surgical site infections after free flap reconstruction, failure of surgical flaps, and overall patient survival.[34–36]

Post-Operative Assessment

AI has the potential to provide a more unbiased and objective approach through computational modeling, making aesthetic assessment more objective. In a study, FaceReader, a commercially available facial expression recognition software, was used to objectively measure changes in facial expression following a browlift.[37] There was a statistically significant decrease in emotions of sadness along with an increase in happiness. A study by Gibstein *and colleagues* assessed a CNN to quantify reduction in apparent age following facelift procedures.[38] More involved procedures (fat grafting, superficial musculoaponeurotic system [SMAS]-involved procedures) expectedly had a greater objective reduction in age. This allowed for quantitative measurements of post-operative outcomes and was correlated with patient satisfaction.

Other CNN models have also assessed objective changes in age following rhinoplasty. The extent of objective age reduction was strongly correlated with patient satisfaction. In a study by Dorfman *and colleagues,* rhinoplasty patients were assessed using Microsoft Azure Face API, a cloud-based algorithm for facial detection, and found to be, on average, 3 years younger post-operatively.[39] There was a strong correlation coefficient ($r = 0.91$) between the actual age and the predicted age after the operation. Ultimately, AI can provide a more unbiased and objective approach through computational modeling and provide surgeons a method to measure success of a procedure. It also highlights the transformative impact of AI in surgical planning and signals a shift toward more objective post-operative evaluations.

Patient Education and Counseling

Large language models (eg, ChatGPT) have an immense potential to excel in patient education. AI can, in theory, rapidly translate complex medical information into understandable terms for patients. As a result, it has begun to be employed in FPRS, supported by multiple studies demonstrating ChatGPT's abilities to counsel patients on blepharoplasty, rhinoplasty, and other aesthetic procedures.[10–12]

The literature supports ChatGPT's potential in efficiently generating patient educational handouts for head and neck microvascular reconstruction procedures and complex wound reconstruction.[40,41] The generated FAQ sheets have been deemed highly accurate (95.6%) but somewhat nonspecific (67.8%) suggesting that ChatGPT can be used to streamline clinical work-flow, albeit with limitations.[40,41] In a study by Durairaj *and colleagues*, researchers studying ChatGPT's ability to preoperatively counsel patients prior to rhinoplasty collected 2 sets of responses for questions: one from the expert surgeon and the other from ChatGPT 3.5.[13] Responses were independently assessed by an expert rhinoplasty surgeon and ChatGPT 3.5 outperformed the expert rhinoplasty surgeon in pre-operative consultations. ChatGPT excelled in all areas except empathy, although this category was not statistically significant. This indicates that ChatGPT can effectively counsel and educate patients with accurate and comprehensive responses to preoperative inquiries. Nonetheless, it is important to note that the value of human connection and empathy in clinical interactions, which AI cannot fully replace.

Research

AI applications extend to being a key player in advancing FPRS research, a crucial aspect of advancing the field via the discovery of new medical knowledge, refining surgical techniques, and improving patient outcomes. Gupta *and colleagues* utilized ChatGPT to generate 240 novel systemic review questions in plastic surgery, of which 132 questions were deemed novel after review.[42] Another study assessed the ability of ChatGPT to identify high-frequency keywords in plastic surgery over a 5-year period, demonstrating the ability to identify trends in "research hotspots."[43] Nonetheless, there are concerns regarding inaccuracies and plagiarism with the use of AI chatbots, with a case study showing ChatGPT was only able to offer shallow answers to esoteric questions with fabricated references.[44] Concerningly, in a study evaluating the quality of references generated by ChatGPT, 47% of references were found to be fabricated and 46% were authentic but inaccurate.[45] AI chatbots are also increasingly utilized for scientific writing with similar legal and ethical concerns regarding inaccuracies, bias, and possible plagiarism.[46]

LIMITATIONS

The implementation of AI in medical settings has shown immense potential in enhancing diagnostic accuracy, predicting patient outcomes, and personalizing treatment plans. However, despite its significant potential, limitations inherent to AI models have prevented its widespread use and raised ethical and security concerns.[47,48] A significant limitation of AI models, especially those based on deep learning, is their reliance on large datasets for training. Small datasets unfortunately predispose deep learning models to overfitting, in which the machine memorizes the training set and fails on new data. As such, large, diverse datasets are crucial for the models to learn patterns, identify correlations, and make accurate predictions. In the medical field, acquiring such extensive datasets can be challenging due to privacy concerns, data variability, and the rarity of certain conditions.

Privacy protections of sensitive medical data restrict the sharing and public distribution of health-related information, making publicly available datasets scarce. Specifically, regarding facial images, HIPA (Health Insurance Portability and Accountability Act) privacy rules require deidentification of full-face photographs or comparable images. Common deidentification techniques such as blurring, however, cannot fully evade AI facial recognition technologies as they continue to evolve.[49,50] There have been efforts to develop digital masking algorithms to separate biometric identifiers while maintaining relevant medical information but will require further validation studies.[49] Additionally, the limited availability of diverse, large-scale datasets poses a considerable challenge in training robust and generalizable AI models. Furthermore, the variability in how medical data, particularly imaging data, are captured across different health care centers compounds these challenges. Imaging techniques and protocols can vary significantly from one institution to another, influenced by factors like equipment type, imaging settings, and operator expertise. This variability introduces inconsistencies in the data, making it difficult not only to train an AI model, but also to ensure its performance is universally applicable.

As a result, concerns are appropriately raised about an AI model's validity, reliability, and robustness when deployed in different clinical environments, especially in underserved communities with limited resources. Therefore, ensuring the standardization of data collection methods and broadening access to high-quality, diverse datasets are crucial steps toward the successful integration of AI in health care.

Furthermore, many published studies use training data sets that are retrospective rather than prospective, which may affect real-world performance.[51] Comparability between AI algorithms in published studies also is an issue, due to a lack of standardization of measured metrics and algorithm techniques.[51] Ultimately, randomized controlled studies will need to be conducted with standardized metrics prior to widespread implementation in the clinical setting.

Beyond the lack of public datasets, rare diseases pose a unique challenge due to their low prevalence and smaller datasets that are insufficient for traditional AI model training. This limitation can lead to underrepresentation of rare diseases in AI research and development, potentially skewing predictions, and creating poorer tools for these conditions. For aesthetic surgery, the concept of beauty is subjective and changes depending on cultural influences. As AI applies an objective measure to these parameters, it may perpetuate and apply a generalized aesthetic to every patient. Patients of color have traditionally been underrepresented in aesthetic surgery, which will further limit robust training datasets for AI algorithms.[52]

Deep learning and machine-based approaches are often criticized for the black box paradigm, in which an AI system produces a solution without understanding the decision- making process.[53] This can lead to mistrust among physicians and a barrier for adoption given conventional decision-making in medicine is evidence based. To mitigate the "black box" nature of AI, the development and integration of visualization models that elucidate where and how the AI is deriving its conclusions are gaining traction. In diagnostic imaging, this approach, often referred to as "heat mapping," visually indicates the regions of an image most influential in the AI's decision-making process.[54] Nonetheless, creation of interpretable AI algorithms will be critical for implementation of AI in the clinical setting.

Nonetheless, AI tools are poised to significantly change the field facial plastic surgery. Surgeons may someday use generative AI tools to create and evaluate potential surgical outcomes. This aids in refining procedures and establishing realistic expectations for future patients. Reviewing AI-simulated images empowers surgeons and patients to strive for optimal results. AI optimization in administrative tasks, such as documentation and appointment coordination, improves practice efficiency and reduces costs.

SUMMARY

AI application in FPRS spans various domains, including automated evaluation of facial palsy, preoperative planning using predictive models, and objective assessment of post-operative outcomes. Notably, AI tools have improved the objectivity in facial assessments, contributing to more precise surgical planning and better patient outcomes. In clinical practice, AI is enhancing efficiency by streamlining administrative tasks like documentation and appointment scheduling, thereby improving overall health care delivery. Prior to widespread integration in the clinical setting, issues such as algorithmic bias, ethical considerations, and need for validation must be addressed.

CLINICS CARE POINTS

- AI, particularly CNNs and computer vision, is poised to revolutionize facial plastic and reconstructive surgery by improving diagnostic accuracy, refining surgical planning, and enhancing post-operative evaluation.

- Innovative applications of AI in FPRS include objective grading of facial palsy, advanced preoperative counseling for procedures such as rhinoplasty and facelift, and improved objectivity in post-operative outcome assessments.

- Generative AI has allowed post-operative outcome modeling for procedures in rhinoplasty and facelifts, but will require further validation and consideration of gender, socioeconomic, and cultural biases.

- AI has significantly impacted FPRS by enabling real-time image analysis and voice input capabilities, thereby facilitating patient education and streamlining clinical workflows.

- Despite its transformative potential, integrating AI in FPRS faces challenges such as algorithmic bias, ethical concerns, and the need for accurate and explainable AI systems.

- Looking forward, AI tools hold promise for revolutionizing preoperative planning in FPRS, offering the potential for creating and evaluating simulated surgical outcomes. This will aid the physician in setting realistic expectations and improving surgical results.

REFERENCES

1. Zhang C, Sun X, Dang K, et al. Toward an expert level of lung cancer detection and classification using a deep convolutional neural network. Oncol 2019;24(9):1159–65.
2. Esteva A, Kuprel B, Novoa RA, et al. Dermatologist-level classification of skin cancer with deep neural networks. Nature 2017;542(7639):115–8.
3. Pertzborn D, Nguyen HN, Huttmann K, et al. Intraoperative Assessment of Tumor Margins in Tissue Sections with Hyperspectral Imaging and Machine Learning. Cancers 2022;15(1).
4. Varas J, Coronel BV, Villagran I, et al. Innovations in surgical training: exploring the role of artificial intelligence and large language models (LLM). Rev Col Bras Cir 2023;50:e20233605.
5. Zeng J, Kang W, Chen S, et al. A Deep Learning Approach to Predict Conductive Hearing Loss in Patients With Otitis Media With Effusion Using Otoscopic Images. JAMA Otolaryngol Head Neck Surg 2022;148(7):612–20.
6. Alrabiah A, Alduailij Mai, Crane Martin. Computer-based approach to detect wrinkles and suggest facial fillers. Int J Adv Comput Sci Appl 2019;10(9).
7. Li R, Shu F, Zhen Y, et al. Artificial Intelligence for Rhinoplasty Design in Asian Patients. Aesthetic Plast Surg 2023. https://doi.org/10.1007/s00266-023-03534-5.
8. Borsting E, DeSimone R, Ascha M, et al. Applied Deep Learning in Plastic Surgery: Classifying Rhinoplasty With a Mobile App. J Craniofac Surg Jan/2020;31(1):102–6.
9. Chinski H, Lerch R, Tournour D, et al. An Artificial Intelligence Tool for Image Simulation in Rhinoplasty. Facial Plast Surg 2022;38(2):201–6.
10. Liu HY, Alessandri-Bonetti M, Arellano JA, et al. Can ChatGPT be the plastic surgeon's new digital assistant? a bibliometric analysis and scoping review of ChatGPT in plastic surgery literature. Aesthetic Plast Surg 2023. https://doi.org/10.1007/s00266-023-03709-0.
11. Seth I, Cox A, Xie Y, et al. Evaluating chatbot efficacy for answering frequently asked questions in plastic surgery: a chatgpt case study focused on breast augmentation. Aesthetic Surg J 2023;43(10):1126–35.
12. Kang Y, Xia Z, Zhu L. When ChatGPT meets plastic surgeons. Aesthetic Plast Surg 2023;47(5):2190–3.
13. Durairaj KK, Baker O, Bertossi D, et al. Artificial intelligence versus expert plastic surgeon: comparative study shows ChatGPT "wins" rhinoplasty consultations: should we be worried? Facial Plast Surg Aesthet Med 2023. https://doi.org/10.1089/fpsam.2023.0224.
14. Abramoff MD, Whitestone N, Patnaik JL, et al. Autonomous artificial intelligence increases real-world specialist clinic productivity in a cluster-randomized trial. NPJ Digit Med 2023;6(1):184.
15. Jindal A, Sumodhee D, Brandao-de-Resende C, et al. Usability of an artificially intelligence-powered triage platform for adult ophthalmic emergencies: a mixed methods study. Sci Rep 2023;13(1):22490.
16. Krizhevsky A, Sutskever Ilya, Hinton Geoffrey E. ImageNet classification with deep convolutional neural networks. Adv Neural Inf Process Syst 2012;25:1097–105.
17. Reitzen SD, Babb JS, Lalwani AK. Significance and reliability of the House-Brackmann grading system for regional facial nerve function. Otolaryngol Head Neck Surg 2009;140(2):154–8.

18. Banks CA, Bhama PK, Park J, et al. Clinician-graded electronic facial paralysis assessment: the eFACE. Plast Reconstr Surg 2015;136(2):223e–30e.

19. Banks CA, Jowett N, Hadlock TA. Test-retest reliability and agreement between in-person and video assessment of facial mimetic function using the eFACE facial grading system. JAMA Facial Plast Surg 2017;19(3):206–11.

20. Guarin DL, Dusseldorp J, Hadlock TA, et al. A machine learning approach for automated facial measurements in facial palsy. JAMA Facial Plast Surg 2018; 20(4):335–7.

21. Ein L, Trzcinski L, Perry L, et al. Embellishing emotrics for a more complete emotion analysis: addition of the nasolabial fold. Facial Plast Surg Aesthet Med Sep-Oct 2023;25(5):409–14.

22. Miller MQ, Hadlock TA, Fortier E, et al. The Auto-eFACE: machine learning-enhanced program yields automated facial palsy assessment tool. Plast Reconstr Surg 2021;147(2):467–74.

23. Gaber A, Taher MF, Abdel Wahed M, et al. Comprehensive assessment of facial paralysis based on facial animation units. PLoS One 2022;17(12):e0277297.

24. Boochoon K, Mottaghi A, Aziz A, et al. Deep learning for the assessment of facial nerve palsy: opportunities and challenges. Facial Plast Surg 2023;39(5):508–11.

25. Hallac RR, Jackson SA, Grant J, et al. Assessing outcomes of ear molding therapy by health care providers and convolutional neural network. Sci Rep 2021;11(1): 17875.

26. Wang D, Chen X, Wu Y, et al. Artificial intelligence for assessing the severity of microtia via deep convolutional neural networks. Front Surg 2022;9:929110.

27. Miranda F, Choudhari V, Barone S, et al. Interpretable artificial intelligence for classification of alveolar bone defect in patients with cleft lip and palate. Sci Rep 2023;13(1):15861.

28. Paro M, Lambert WA, Leclair NK, et al. Machine Learning-Driven Clinical Image Analysis to Identify Craniosynostosis: A Pilot Study of Telemedicine and Clinic Patients. Neurosurgery 2022;90(5):613–8.

29. Anderson MG, Jungbauer D, Leclair NK, et al. Incorporation of a biparietal narrowing metric to improve the ability of machine learning models to detect sagittal craniosynostosis with 2D photographs. Neurosurg Focus 2023;54(6):E9.

30. Harmon SA, Sanford TH, Xu S, et al. Artificial intelligence for the detection of COVID-19 pneumonia on chest CT using multinational datasets. Nat Commun 2020;11(1):4080.

31. Yan C, Wang L, Lin J, et al. A fully automatic artificial intelligence-based CT image analysis system for accurate detection, diagnosis, and quantitative severity evaluation of pulmonary tuberculosis. Eur Radiol 2022;32(4):2188–99.

32. Shah SAA, Bennamoun Mohammed, Molton Michael K. Machine learning approaches for prediction of facial rejuvenation using real and synthetic data. IEEE 2019;7:23779–87.

33. Li CW, Wang CC, Chou CY, et al. Customized precision facial assessment: an ai-assisted analysis of facial microexpressions for advanced aesthetic treatment. Plast Reconstr Surg Glob Open 2020;8(3):e2688.

34. Spoer DL, Kiene JM, Dekker PK, et al. A systematic review of artificial intelligence applications in plastic surgery: looking to the future. Plast Reconstr Surg Glob Open 2022;10(12):e4608.

35. O'Neill AC, Yang D, Roy M, et al. Development and evaluation of a machine learning prediction model for flap failure in microvascular breast reconstruction. Ann Surg Oncol 2020;27(9):3466–75.

36. Kuo PJ, Wu SC, Chien PC, et al. Artificial neural network approach to predict surgical site infection after free-flap reconstruction in patients receiving surgery for head and neck cancer. Oncotarget 2018;9(17):13768–82.
37. Boonipat T, Lin J, Bite U. Detection of baseline emotion in brow lift patients using artificial intelligence. Aesthetic Plast Surg 2021;45(6):2742–8.
38. Gibstein AR, Chen K, Nakfoor B, et al. Facelift surgery turns back the clock: artificial intelligence and patient satisfaction quantitate value of procedure type and specific techniques. Aesthetic Surg J 2021;41(9):987–99.
39. Dorfman R, Chang I, Saadat S, et al. Making the subjective objective: machine learning and rhinoplasty. Aesthetic Surg J 2020;40(5):493–8.
40. Tian WM, Sergesketter AR, Hollenbeck ST. The role of ChatGPT in microsurgery: assessing content quality and potential applications. J Reconstr Microsurg 2023. https://doi.org/10.1055/a-2098-6509.
41. Lanzano G. Harnessing the potential of ChatGPT in breast reconstruction: a revolution in patient communication and education. Aesthetic Plast Surg 2023;47(5): 2215–6.
42. Gupta R, Park JB, Bisht C, et al. Expanding cosmetic plastic surgery research with ChatGPT. Aesthetic Surg J 2023;43(8):930–7.
43. Zhou J, Jia Y, Qiu Y, et al. The potential of applying ChatGPT to extract keywords of medical literature in plastic surgery. Aesthetic Surg J 2023;43(9):NP720–3.
44. Xie Y, Seth I, Rozen WM, et al. Evaluation of the artificial intelligence Chatbot on breast reconstruction and its efficacy in surgical research: a case study. Aesthetic Plast Surg 2023. https://doi.org/10.1007/s00266-023-03443-7.
45. Bhattacharyya M, Miller VM, Bhattacharyya D, et al. High rates of fabricated and inaccurate references in ChatGPT-generated medical content. Cureus 2023; 15(5):e39238.
46. Salvagno M, Taccone FS, Gerli AG. Can artificial intelligence help for scientific writing? Crit Care 2023;27(1):75.
47. Kavian JA, Wilkey HL, Patel PA, et al. Harvesting the power of artificial intelligence for surgery: uses, implications, and ethical considerations. Am Surg 2023. https://doi.org/10.1177/00031348231175454. 31348231175454.
48. Bassiri-Tehrani B, Cress PE. Unleashing the power of ChatGPT: revolutionizing plastic surgery and beyond. Aesthetic Surg J 2023;43(11):1395–9.
49. Yang Y, Lyu J, Wang R, et al. A digital mask to safeguard patient privacy. Nat Med 2022;28(9):1883–92.
50. Thornton SM, Attaluri PK, Wirth PJ, et al. Picture perfect: standardizing and safekeeping clinical photography in plastic surgery. Aesthet Surg J Open Forum 2024;6:ojae012.
51. Kelly CJ, Karthikesalingam A, Suleyman M, et al. Key challenges for delivering clinical impact with artificial intelligence. BMC Med 2019;17(1):195.
52. Tirrell AR, Bekeny JC, Baker SB, et al. Patient representation and diversity in plastic surgery social media. Aesthetic Surg J 2021;41(9):1094–101.
53. Poon AIF, Sung JJY. Opening the black box of AI-Medicine. J Gastroenterol Hepatol 2021;36(3):581–4.
54. Lysdahlgaard S. Utilizing heat maps as explainable artificial intelligence for detecting abnormalities on wrist and elbow radiographs. Radiography 2023;29(6): 1132–8.

Artificial Intelligence and Pediatric Otolaryngology

Alice E. Huang, MD, Tulio A. Valdez, MD, MSc*

KEYWORDS

- Artificial intelligence • Machine learning • Neural network • ChatBot
- Education technology • Patient education • Pediatric otolaryngology

KEY POINTS

- Artificial intelligence has exciting potential to enhance the efficiency, safety, and efficacy of otolaryngologic surgery.
- Automated machine learning tools may have the capacity to engage in diagnosis and triaging of common pediatric otolaryngologic conditions, such as acute otitis media and middle ear effusions.
- The use of artificial intelligence within robotic-assisted surgery and computer-aided planning is an evolving field of study.
- Preliminary studies show widely variable accuracy of chatBot-generated health information and capacity for reliable patient education.

INTRODUCTION

Artificial intelligence (AI) studies show how to program computers to simulate human intelligence and perform data interpretation, learning, and adaptive decision-making. Large language models (LLMs) are trained on massive datasets from the Internet to generate human-like responses to inquiries. Advances in AI can fundamentally change the practice of medicine by automating image acquisition and data analysis, providing patient education and clinical decision support, and prognosticating disease and treatment decisions. Otolaryngology as a field lends itself well to machine learning models due to the wide assortment of image-based technologies in otolaryngologic practice, such as endoscopy, otoscopy, and rhinoscopy, and cross-sectional-based surgical planning. Pediatric otolaryngology comprises a vast spectrum of diseases, from the most common childhood infections, such as acute otitis media (AOM), to exceedingly rare congenital conditions requiring highly subspecialized management. Given this breadth, AI and open access LLM models may play an exponentially

Department of Otolaryngology–Head & Neck Surgery, Stanford University School of Medicine, Stanford, CA, USA
* Corresponding author. Department of Otolaryngology–Head & Neck Surgery, Stanford Hospital and Clinics, 801 Welch Road, Stanford, CA 94304.
E-mail address: tvaldez1@stanford.edu

Otolaryngol Clin N Am 57 (2024) 853–862
https://doi.org/10.1016/j.otc.2024.04.011
0030-6665/24/© 2024 Elsevier Inc. All rights reserved.

growing role in patient education, trainee education, telemedicine, and surgical planning and the execution of surgical procedures. The current review highlights advancements in AI and pediatric otolaryngology.

ARTIFICIAL INTELLIGENCE AND DIAGNOSTICS
Acute Otitis Media

Perhaps one of the most studied applications of AI in pediatric otolaryngology is in the diagnosis of AOM. With technological advances in otoscope and endoscopes and enhanced capacity to digitize acquired images, the role of AI for reliable diagnostic workups continues to expand.[1] Given the high incidence of AOM and the burden of untreated infections, various studies have investigated the feasibility of deep learning algorithms and image recognition software to facilitate the diagnosis of middle ear effusions and AOM. Ngombu and colleagues performed a state-of-the-art review of advances in AI for the diagnosis of otitis media in which many of the following studies are highlighted.[2] In a recent large retrospective cohort study, Crowson and colleagues developed a neural network model trained on a set of 639 images representing normal tympanic membranes (TM), otitis media with effusion (OME), and AOM.[3] Their model outperformed human clinicians with a mean diagnostic accuracy of 80.8% versus 60.5%. A proprietary commercial image classifier offered within the Google Cloud Platform outperformed both models with a diagnostic accuracy of 85.4%. The same author group performed a congruent study in the intraoperative setting for patients undergoing myringotomy with possible tympanostomy tube placement and demonstrated an 83.8% prediction accuracy of the neural network model with an area under the receiver operating characteristic curve of 0.93.[4] Other groups are using similar approaches for automated detection of other structures, such as the presence of tympanostomy tubes.[5]

A group led by Hoberman described and developed a smartphone-based technique using an attached endoscope to acquire images and applying an algorithm to distinguish OME from AOM.[6] Using a different smartphone-based approach, Chan and colleagues employed a machine learning algorithm to assess TM mobility using data from built-in phone speakers and microphones and achieved 85% sensitivity and 82% specificity in the detection of OME, comparable to detection rates with tympanometry and pneumatic otoscopy.[7] Optical coherence tomography is a noninvasive cross-sectional imaging technique that can assess for changes in TM thickness or the presence of middle ear biofilms and has recently been shown to be a robust method for in vivo real-time human imaging with accurate diagnosis of OME and AOM.[8,9]

AI technology has important implications for telemedicine and in settings of limited health care access. Habib and colleagues utilized a deep learning method to develop an image classification algorithm for triaging otoscopic images from a teleotology ear health screening of rural and remote aboriginal children in Australia.[10] The AI model achieved 99.3% accuracy for AOM, 96.3% for chronic otitis media, 77.8% for OME, and 98.2% for identifying cerumen-impacted or obstructed canal. Kashani and colleagues developed an otoscope capable of visualizing and capturing middle ear structures and fluid using short-wave infrared light and a subsequent machine-learning approach to automate the analysis of these images (**Fig. 1**). Their device and method diagnosed middle ear effusions with a sensitivity and specificity of 90%.[11] Notably, machine learning applications for these image-based processes rely on large diverse image databases and remain in development and testing stages. Nonetheless, improving the point-of-care diagnostic accuracy of otitis media with AI and machine learning technology has far-reaching benefits across multiple provider specialties.

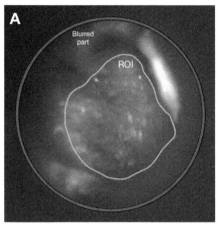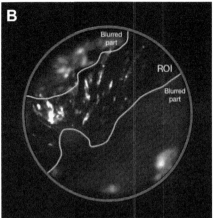

Fig. 1. Examples of manual image review, where each frame of the shortwave infrared oto-scopy video was annotated to label artifacts such as cerumen, hair, and nonfocused regions. (*A*) Portion of tympanic membrane is nonfocused, bounded between the red and yellow lines. (*B*) Another example of annotations performed to exclude nonfocused regions of the tympanic membrane. (*From* Kashani RG, Młyńczak MC, Zarabanda D, Solis-Pazmino P, Huland DM, Ahmad IN, Singh SP, Valdez TA. Shortwave infrared otoscopy for diagnosis of middle ear effusions: a machine-learning-based approach. Sci Rep. 2021 Jun 15;11(1):12509; with permission.)

Pediatric Obstructive Sleep Apnea

Yet another common pediatric otolaryngologic condition being met with advances in AI is obstructive sleep apnea (OSA). Though lateral cephalograms are not routinely obtained during workups for suspected adenoid hypertrophy, children often undergo plain radiographic studies as part of routine dental care or when presenting to a dental or oral maxillofacial specialist with many of the craniofacial changes from chronic mouth breathing. Using a convolutional neural network trained on 581 lateral cephalograms, Zhao and colleagues developed an AI model capable of assessing adenoid hypertrophy with a sensitivity of 90.6% and specificity of 93.8%, offering a potential alternative to the often challenging nasal endoscopic examination in the pediatric population.[12]

Beyond diagnostics, AI has begun to play a role in the perioperative management of pediatric OSA as well. In contrast to adults, pediatric patients with suspected OSA may not undergo polysomnography (PSG) due to challenges with administration, resource allocation, and clinical practice guidelines suggestive of low diagnostic yield when presenting symptoms and examination findings are strongly concordant with OSA or sleep-disordered breathing. However, PSG can be useful in quantifying OSA severity and determining postoperative care and monitoring. Using machine learning, Bertoni and colleagues published a study in *Nature Pediatric Research* utilizing a machine learning approach to analyze oximetry and actigraphy data—both potentially obtained from wearable or portable devices—to categorize the severity of OSA in 190 children and demonstrated a 95% to 96% predictive accuracy for identifying patients with an apnea-hypopnea index of greater than 10 (ie, severe OSA).[13] Liu and colleagues enrolled 323 children from the Child Adenotonsillectomy Trial and used multidomain analysis of PSG markers in conjunction with machine learning to generate a more comprehensive picture of OSA syndrome and predict whether each patient would benefit from surgical intervention.[14]

Pediatric Dysphagia and Aspiration

Up to one-third of pediatric patients with feeding disorders demonstrate oropharyngeal aspiration and frequently undergo serial examinations, including nasolaryngoscopy, functional endoscopic evaluation of swallow, and video fluoroscopic swallow studies (VFSS). Each technique has limitations and downsides, including but not limited to ease of administration and radiation exposure. These constraints have prompted the investigation of alternative modalities, most notably machine learning-based methods, for noninvasive diagnosis of swallow dysfunction. Frakking and colleagues describe the use of an automated speech recognition approach to analyze sounds obtained with digital cervical auscultation and demonstrated a 98% overall accuracy in the diagnosis of oropharyngeal aspiration when compared to the gold standard of VFSS.[15] A group in Belgium similarly utilized an artificial neural network to model and quantify the severity of swallow dysfunction and aspiration sequelae using pharyngeal pressure-flow analysis.[16] Though the latter study was conducted in an adult sample, use of machine learning to detect aspiration in children is an evolving and important field.

Diagnosis of Craniofacial Anomalies and Congenital Syndromes

Any otolaryngologist will recall the plethora of congenital syndromes involving craniofacial or head and neck anomalies with which we are required to be familiar. Diagnosis of these often multisystem, multiorgan syndromes, many of which are highly variable in presentation, can be challenging and heavily reliant on multidisciplinary vigilance and collaboration. As aptly stated by Hennocq and colleagues, "Two to three thousand syndromes modify facial features: their screening requires the eye of an expert in dysmorphology."[17] With the increasing digitization of patient care documentation and expanding database of facial images, multiple studies have examined the use of AI and automated diagnosis of rare or congenital diseases with characteristic craniofacial features. Hennocq developed a pipeline to create automated annotation models adapted to faces with congenital anomalies and facilitate diagnosis of common conditions such as Treacher Collins syndrome. The same medical group developed a model based on external ear dysmorphology to differentiate nonsyndromic control ears from ears of patients with Treacher Collins syndrome, CHARGE syndrome, and Nager syndrome, the main differential diagnoses among others with mandibulofacial dysostosis.[18] While AI remains in its infancy, its potential in facial analysis and diagnosis of genetic conditions will only expand and with ameliorated accuracy as larger and more diverse datasets become available and widely studied.[19]

ARTIFICIAL INTELLIGENCE IN SURGICAL PLANNING AND PERFORMANCE

With the capacity for precise and refined movements in confined spaces, excellent 3 dimensional (3D) depth perception, and untiring action, robotic technology and robotic-assisted surgery has ushered in a new era of minimally invasive surgery, particularly in the realm of transoral head and neck surgery. Use of AI with robotic technology, such as live intraoperative analysis of oncologic margins or automated adjustment of surgical technique, is being studied in the adult population.[20,21] Within pediatric otolaryngology, robotic surgery has been explored since 2007 with especially poignant potential benefits given their smaller anatomy.[22] However, its utilization has been limited to large institutions, and adoption is limited by a sparsity of controlled trials and feasibility studies.[23] Konuthula and colleagues published a comprehensive narrative review of uses of robotics in pediatric otolaryngology and advanced surgical planning.[23] In our review, we highlight specific uses of AI within robotic and robotic-assisted surgery.

Robotic Ear Surgery

The complexity of cochlear implantation (CI) offers various opportunities for optimization with machine learning and AI. In a structured narrative review by Crowson and colleagues, machine learning applications in CI surgery involved speech and signal processing optimization, automated evoked potential measurement, prediction of postoperative performance and efficacy, and aiding in or prediction of surgical anatomy.[24] With the goal of a minimally invasive approach to the cochlea, innovations in robotic technology are being developed and studied.[25–28] Bell and colleagues aimed to replace a standard mastoidectomy with a small diameter tunnel from the lateral temporal bone surface directly to the cochlea for electrode array insertion and developed an image-based robotic system to automatically calculate the distance from the drill tunnel to the round window with impressive accuracy.[26] In another study by Pile and colleagues, the authors developed a robotic system to automatically detect electrode tip fold-over intraoperatively, a complication that is usually detected on postoperative imaging or CI performance assessments when revision would require a return to the operating room.[25] With pediatric CI, Bom Braga and colleagues demonstrated the feasibility of planning and performing implantation in phantom models of pediatric subjects.[29] Robotic-assisted surgical planning and navigation also have the potential to improve outcomes in complex clinical scenarios such as CI in cases of postmeningitic labyrinthitis ossificans.[30] Beyond utilization for CI, robotic assistance for the optimization of transcanal and endoscopic approaches to the middle ear—for example, for congenital cholesteatoma resection—holds promise but remains in very early stages.[31]

Computer-Aided Planning for Craniofacial Surgery

Virtual surgical planning and 3D printing have become essential components in craniofacial and orthognathic surgery.[32,33] Multiple studies establish the value of computed tomography-based virtual reality systems in facilitating surgical planning and improving functional outcomes in pediatric patients with Pierre Robin sequence or mandibular hypoplasia who undergo mandibular distraction.[34–36] More recently, the development of specialized, intelligent, planning-based navigation systems has exciting prospects for broad applications, including craniofacial surgery such as mandibular distraction osteogenesis (MDO). MDO is a main component of the treatment algorithm for hemifacial microsomia, one of the most common craniofacial congenital anomalies. Postoperative outcome and patient function are highly dependent on the precision of bony, soft tissue, and neurovascular lengthening, complicated by the narrow exposure offered by a standard intraoral incision.[37] Zhang and colleagues investigated the efficacy and safety of an AI-based surgical navigation system for MDO for hemifacial microsomia in an early phase single-arm clinical study including 4 patients. Using computed tomography image data and considering the mandibular deformity, occlusal plane, and inferior alveolar nerve position, the system compiled a preoperative design plan including "the position of the osteotomy plane and the distractor, the direction, and the expected length of distraction."[38] The series produced high postoperative patient satisfaction and no adverse events.

PATIENT EDUCATION IN PEDIATRIC OTOLARYNGOLOGY

Development of open access LLM platforms, such as the Chat Generative Pre-trained Transformer (ChatGPT) launched by OpenAI in November 2022, has the potential to fundamentally change the landscape of patient education and health care-seeking behavior. As the fastest-growing consumer application to date, ChatGPT has been undergoing vigorous study in various fields and subspecialties with regards to its ability to provide accurate medical information and coherent answers to patient questions. Few such studies have been performed within pediatric otolaryngology. To come full circle in this review, **Table 1** shows the output from ChatGPT when we queried the chatBot about potential uses of AI in pediatric otolaryngology.

Table 1
Artificial intelligence applications in pediatric otolaryngology according to ChatGPT

Domain	Examples
Diagnosis and imaging	• AI-assisted interpretation of imaging (MRI, CT, radiographs) for ear, nose, and throat (ENT) conditions in children • Detection of abnormalities or anomalies in pediatric head and neck images
Speech and language development	• AI-based tools for assessing and monitoring speech and language development in pediatric patients • Speech recognition technology to aid in speech therapy exercises for children with communication disorders
Hearing loss screening	• AI algorithms for automated hearing loss screening in newborns and young children • Analysis of audiometric data to identify hearing impairments at an early stage
Treatment planning	• AI-driven decision support systems to assist in developing personalized treatment plans for pediatric ENT conditions • Integration of patient data, medical history, and clinical guidelines to optimize treatment strategies
Virtual consultations	• AI-powered virtual assistants for initial consultations, providing basic information, and guidance to parents before scheduling an in-person visit • Telemedicine applications using AI to facilitate remote consultations for routine ENT concerns
Education and training	• Virtual reality and augmented reality applications for simulating pediatric ENT procedures, allowing training for medical professionals in a risk-free environment • AI-enhanced educational platforms for residents and health care providers in pediatric otolaryngology
Patient monitoring and follow-up	• Remote monitoring of pediatric patients after surgery or during treatment using wearable devices with AI capabilities • Automated follow-up reminders and guidance for parents to ensure proper postoperative care
Data analysis for research	• AI tools for analyzing large datasets of pediatric otolaryngology cases, identifying patterns, and contributing to research on trends and outcomes • Mining electronic health records for valuable insights into the prevalence and management of specific conditions in children
Assistive devices for communication	• Development of AI-powered assistive devices to aid children with communication disorders, including voice synthesizers and language translation tools • Customized communication devices based on AI algorithms that adapt to the specific needs of the child
Predictive analytics for complications	• AI models predicting potential complications or adverse events in pediatric otolaryngology procedures, helping health care providers take preventive measures • Early identification of risk factors and proactive intervention strategies based on historical data

Moise and colleagues compared ChatGPT-generated responses to parent questions regarding tympanostomy tube placement, the most common pediatric otolaryngologic procedure, with recommendations based on the most recent clinical practice guidelines from the American Academy of Otolaryngology–Head and Neck Surgery Foundation (AAO-HNSF). A total of 23 ChatGPT responses were generated, of which 22 (95.7%) were deemed by 2 independent otolaryngologists to be highly reliable and accurate.[39] For the single question to which the chatBot's response exhibited a slight discrepancy from AAO-HNSF guidelines, there was deemed to be no risk should the parents have followed ChatGPT's recommendation. This point is particularly important to recognize in medicine and health care given the high stakes of misinformation.

In general otolaryngology, 2 studies have found impressive results with the same chatBot's performance. Zalzal and colleagues inputted 30 patient-generated otolaryngology questions to ChatGPT, such as "Is tonsil removal dangerous?" and "Will ear tubes make me lose my hearing?" Interestingly, they found otolaryngologists rated the responses higher (98.3% were rated as accurate) than laypeople, who appeared to have lower confidence or trust in the ChatGPT's responses.[40] Moreover, in a follow-up study evaluating the concordance of ChatGPT responses with expert otolaryngologists, when posed with more high-level questions, they demonstrated a much lower ability to provide accurate responses to sophisticated otolaryngologic questions reliably.[41] In a parallel vein of study, Qu and colleagues queried the most updated ChatGPT version with 20 physician-written clinical vignettes in otolaryngology and demonstrated a high level of agreement between physician and chatBot responses regarding differential diagnoses and recommendations for management.[42] Given the importance of emergent AI applications for patient care and education, further studies will be paramount to understand the accuracy and reliability of open access AI tools in provision of medical information, especially in response to unstructured or nuanced questions and in highly subspecialized fields such as pediatric otolaryngology.

SUMMARY

AI and automated machine learning have exciting potential to enhance the efficiency, safety, and efficacy of otolaryngologic surgery. Within pediatric otolaryngology, there is a growing body of evidence for the role of AI in diagnosis and triaging of AOM and middle ear effusion, pediatric sleep disorders, and syndromic craniofacial anomalies. The use of automated machine learning with robotic devices intraoperatively is an evolving field of study, particularly in the realms of pediatric otologic surgery and computer-aided planning for maxillofacial reconstruction, and we will likely continue seeing novel applications of machine learning in otolaryngologic surgery. With preliminary studies showing widely variable accuracy of chatBot-generated health information, perhaps the most critical area of need for future study is the impact and role of machine learning platforms on patient education and provider–patient interaction as open access tools become increasingly ubiquitous.

DISCLOSURE

None.

REFERENCES

1. Ezzibdeh R, Munjal T, Ahmad I, et al. Artificial intelligence and tele-otoscopy: A window into the future of pediatric otology. Int J Pediatr Otorhinolaryngol 2022;160.

2. Ngombu S, Binol H, Gurcan MN, et al. Advances in artificial intelligence to diagnose otitis media: state of the art review. Otolaryngol Head Neck Surg 2023; 168(4):635–42.
3. Crowson MG, Bates DW, Suresh K, et al. "Human vs machine" validation of a deep learning algorithm for pediatric middle ear infection diagnosis. Otolaryngol Head Neck Surg 2023;169(1):41–6.
4. Crowson MG, Hartnick CJ, Diercks GR, et al. Machine learning for accurate intraoperative pediatric middle ear effusion diagnosis. Pediatrics 2021;147(4).
5. Wang X, Valdez TA, Bi J. Detecting tympanostomy tubes from otoscopic images via offline and online training. Comput Biol Med 2015;61:107–18.
6. Kuruvilla A, Shaikh N, Hoberman A, et al. Automated diagnosis of otitis media: vocabulary and grammar. Int J Biomed Imag 2013;2013. https://doi.org/10.1155/2013/327515.
7. Chan J, Raju S, Nandakumar R, et al. Detecting middle ear fluid using smartphones. Sci Transl Med 2019;11(492).
8. Pichichero ME. Can machine learning and AI replace otoscopy for diagnosis of otitis media? Pediatrics 2021;147(4).
9. Hubler Z, Shemonski ND, Shelton RL, et al. Real-time automated thickness measurement of the in vivo human tympanic membrane using optical coherence tomography. Quant Imag Med Surg 2015;5(1):69.
10. Habib AR, Crossland G, Patel H, et al. An artificial intelligence computer-vision algorithm to triage otoscopic images from australian aboriginal and torres strait islander children. Otol Neurotol 2022;43(4):481–8.
11. Kashani RG, Młyńczak MC, Zarabanda D, et al. Shortwave infrared otoscopy for diagnosis of middle ear effusions: a machine-learning-based approach. Sci Rep 2021;11(1):12509.
12. Zhao T, Zhou J, Yan J, et al. Automated adenoid hypertrophy assessment with lateral cephalometry in children based on artificial intelligence. Diagnostics 2021;11(8).
13. Bertoni D, Sterni LM, Pereira KD, et al. Predicting polysomnographic severity thresholds in children using machine learning. Pediatr Res 2020;88(3):404–11.
14. Liu X, Pamula Y, Immanuel S, et al. Utilisation of machine learning to predict surgical candidates for the treatment of childhood upper airway obstruction. Sleep Breath 2022;26(2):649–61.
15. Frakking TT, Chang AB, Carty C, et al. Using an automated speech recognition approach to differentiate between normal and aspirating swallowing sounds recorded from digital cervical auscultation in children. Dysphagia 2022;37(6):1482–92.
16. Kritas S, Dejaeger E, Tack J, et al. Objective prediction of pharyngeal swallow dysfunction in dysphagia through artificial neural network modeling. Neuro Gastroenterol Motil 2016;28(3):336–44.
17. Hennocq Q, Bongibault T, Bizière M, et al. An automatic facial landmarking for children with rare diseases. Am J Med Genet 2023;191(5):1210–21.
18. Hennocq Q, Bongibault T, Marlin S, et al. AI-based diagnosis in mandibulofacial dysostosis with microcephaly using external ear shapes. Front Pediatr 2023;11:1171277.
19. Kruszka P, Tekendo-Ngongang C. Application of facial analysis Technology in Clinical Genetics: Considerations for diverse populations. Am J Med Genet C Semin Med Genet 2023;193(3).
20. Loperfido A, Celebrini A, Marzetti A, et al. Current role of artificial intelligence in head and neck cancer surgery: a systematic review of literature. Explor Target Antitumor Ther 2023;4(5):933–40.

21. Costantino A, Sampieri C, Pirola F, et al. Development of machine learning models for the prediction of positive surgical margins in transoral robotic surgery (TORS). Head Neck 2023;45(3):675–84.

22. Rahbar R, Ferrari LR, Borer JG, et al. Robotic surgery in the pediatric airway: application and safety. Arch Otolaryngol Head Neck Surg 2007;133(1):46–50.

23. Konuthula N, Parikh SR, Bly RA. Robotics in pediatric otolaryngology-head and neck surgery and advanced surgical planning. Otolaryngol Clin North Am 2020;53(6):1005–16.

24. Crowson MG, Lin V, Chen JM, et al. Machine learning and cochlear implantation - a structured review of opportunities and challenges. Otol Neurotol 2020;41(1): E36–45.

25. Pile J, Wanna GB, Simaan N. Robot-assisted perception augmentation for online detection of insertion failure during cochlear implant surgery. Robotica 2017; 35(7):1598–615.

26. Bell B, Williamson T, Gerber N, et al. An image-guided robot system for direct cochlear access. Cochlear Implants Int 2014;15(Suppl 1).

27. Danilchenko A, Balachandran R, Toennies JL, et al. Robotic mastoidectomy. Otol Neurotol 2011;32(1):11–6.

28. Labadie RF, Chodhury P, Cetinkaya E, et al. Minimally invasive, image-guided, facial-recess approach to the middle ear: demonstration of the concept of percutaneous cochlear access in vitro. Otol Neurotol 2005;26(4):557–62.

29. Bom Braga GOT, Schneider D, Muller F, et al. Feasibility of pediatric robotic cochlear implantation in phantoms. Otol Neurotol 2020;41(2):e192–200.

30. Al Saadi M, Heuninck E, De Raeve L, et al. Robotic cochlear implantation in post-meningitis ossified cochlea. American Journal of Otolaryngology - Head and Neck Medicine and Surgery 2023;44(1).

31. Simon F, Nguyen Y, Loundon N, et al. Robot-assisted transcanal endoscopic ear surgery for congenital cholesteatoma. J Vis Exp 2023;2023(202).

32. Gray R, Gougoutas A, Nguyen V, et al. Use of three-dimensional, CAD/CAM-assisted, virtual surgical simulation and planning in the pediatric craniofacial population. Int J Pediatr Otorhinolaryngol 2017;97:163–9.

33. Weitz J, Wolff KD, Kesting MR, et al. Development of a novel resection and cutting guide for mandibular reconstruction using free fibula flap. J Cranio-Maxillofacial Surg 2018;46(11):1975–8.

34. Zanaty O, El Metainy S, Abo Alia D, et al. Improvement in the airway after mandibular distraction osteogenesis surgery in children with temporomandibular joint ankylosis and mandibular hypoplasia. Paediatr Anaesth 2016;26(4):399–404.

35. Vanesa V, Irene MP, Marta AS, et al. Accuracy of virtually planned mandibular distraction in a pediatric case series. J Cranio-Maxillofacial Surg 2021;49(2): 154–65.

36. Resnick CM. Precise osteotomies for mandibular distraction in infants with Robin sequence using virtual surgical planning. Int J Oral Maxillofac Surg 2018;47(1): 35–43.

37. Al-Mahdi AH, Al-Hasnawi SN, Al-Jumaily HA. Changes in soft tissue measurements after mandibular distraction osteogenesis. J Craniofac Surg 2016;27(7):e702–7.

38. Zhang Z, Zhao Z, Han W, et al. Accuracy and safety of robotic navigation-assisted distraction osteogenesis for hemifacial microsomia. Front Pediatr 2023;11:1158078.

39. Moise A, Centomo-Bozzo A, Orishchak O, et al. Can ChatGPT guide parents on tympanostomy tube insertion? Children 2023;10(10).

40. Zalzal HG, Abraham A, Cheng J, et al. Can ChatGPT help patients answer their otolaryngology questions? Laryngoscope Investig Otolaryngol 2023. https://doi.org/10.1002/lio2.1193.
41. Zalzal HG, Cheng J, Shah RK. Evaluating the current ability of chatgpt to assist in professional otolaryngology education. OTO Open 2023;7(4):e94.
42. Qu RW, Qureshi U, Petersen G, et al. Diagnostic and management applications of ChatGPT in structured otolaryngology clinical scenarios. OTO Open 2023;7(3):e67.

GOVERNANCE AND IMPLEMENTATION

Artificial Intelligence in Otolaryngology
Topics in Epistemology & Ethics

Katie Tai, MD[a], Robin Zhao, BS[b], Anaïs Rameau, MD, MS, MPhil[b],*

KEYWORDS

- Artificial intelligence ethics • Artificial intelligence governance
- Artificial intelligence epistemology • Explainability • Bias

KEY POINTS

- Artificial intelligence (AI)/machine learning/large language models have unique epistemic limitations that pose ethical dilemma in the clinical setting of otolaryngology.
- Issues around opacity, reproducibility, and risk of bias of AI systems can harm the patients, and the authors have a fiduciary responsibility to understand and mitigate these risks.
- Numerous solutions exist, including specific efforts toward explainability and transparency, reproducibly and replicability, and risk of bias alleviation.

INTRODUCTION

The past years have witnessed rapid acceleration of artificial intelligence (AI) development, specifically in machine learning (ML) and large language models (LLMs). AI is the study and development of computer systems that mimic human intelligence in the performance of varied tasks. ML is the subfield of AI in which algorithms are developed to learn from data without being explicitly programmed to make precise predictions based on new data.[1] LLMs are natural language processing models based on transformer architecture that can predict the next word in a sequence and to measure

Funding: 1. Developing an App-Based Voice Clinical Decision Support Tool to Augment the Sensitivity of the Bedside Swallow Evaluation in Older Adults K76- AG079040 RAMEAU, ANAIS. 2. Bridge2AI: Voice as a Biomarker of Health - Building an ethically sourced, bioacoustic database to understand disease like never before OT2-OD032720 RAMEAU, ANAIS.

[a] New York Presbyterian Hospital, 1300 York Avenue, New York, NY 10065, USA; [b] Department of Otolaryngology–Head & Neck Surgery, Sean Parker Institute for the Voice, Weill Cornell Medical College, 240 East 59th Street, New York, NY 10022, USA

* Corresponding author. Department of Otolaryngology–Head & Neck Surgery, Sean Parker Institute for the Voice, Weill Cornell Medical College, 240 East 59th Street, New York, NY, 10022.

E-mail address: anr2783@med.cornell.edu

Otolaryngol Clin N Am 57 (2024) 863–870
https://doi.org/10.1016/j.otc.2024.04.008
oto.theclinics.com

attention or calculate the context of words.[2] There is currently enormous interest in applications of ML and LLM in medicine, from supporting precision care, to multiplying innovations in medicine and reducing "pajama time" or the time required for documentation in the electronic health record outside work hours, contributing to provider burnout.

Despite the hype around AI in health care, concerns surrounding governance have been multiplying and caution around deployment has been urged. In October 2022, the White House established a Blueprint for an AI Bill of Rights outlining best practices on AI use and development, emphasizing equity and access.[3] This was followed the next year with the United States' first AI Executive Order, requiring several federal agencies including the Department of Health and Human Services to launch an Artificial Intelligence Task Force to drive regulatory frameworks and guide policy.[4] In the Europe Union, the AI Act aims to regulate AI with a risk-based approach, including bans on intrusive and discriminatory uses of AI systems, such as those that "exploit vulnerabilities and social scoring."[5]

Among the most pressing governance challenges of AI in health care are the management of potential risks of AI, including risk of bias and ensuing harm, privacy and security infringement, and opacity and associated distrust. *Bias* may occur when AI training data is implicitly biased or does not represent diverse populations, leading to algorithmic output incorporating these biases or with unequal predictive capabilities in different populations, potentially exacerbating health care disparities. *Privacy and security* concerns arise when the anonymity of health data are jeopardized and with cybersecurity threats. The *opacity* problem refers to AI/ML algorithms as "black-box" tools with limited human insights on how they function. Opacity compounded by the potential of bias and privacy breaches may lead to mistrust in AI and potential damage to the patient-physician relationship.

Because AI is designed to mimic human intelligence and is currently being applied in expert fields of human knowledge, at the basis of these ethical concerns are also questions regarding truth and knowledge. These include questions like how can one ensure that the answers provided by AI are accurate? How is knowledge generated by AI/ML different from that created by human researchers or health care providers? The authors turn to epistemology, the theoretic field of human knowledge and understanding to address these questions. Here, the authors will discuss several key epistemic issues tightly associated with the ethical conundrums of AI applications in health care broadly and otolaryngology specifically, including explainability & transparency, reproducibility & replicability, and risk of bias.

EXPLAINABILITY & TRANSPARENCY

Though understanding, interpretability, and explainability have been used interchangeably in the medical literature, these terms represent different concepts. In health care applications of AI, *understanding* is defined as functional knowledge of algorithmic processes.[6,7] This would be akin to the epistemic relationship between AI coders and the algorithmic "black box". *Interpretability* relates to how well an AI system map abstract concepts, such as image pixels, into knowledge domains humans understand. Interpretability is in turn distinct from *explainability*, or the ability to describe a collection of interpretable features that have contributed to a result or decision.[8]

As AI systems become increasingly more advanced in predicting phenomena in the real world, they also become increasingly complex and opaque.[9] Otherwise known as the "black-box" problem, the lack of transparency of AI models limits users' and even coders' understanding of algorithmic functioning.[10,11] This lack of explainability creates epistemic concerns regarding the validity and reliability of AI systems in health care. This can lead to mistrust, particularly among patient groups who are already skeptical of the medical enterprise, such as underrepresented groups in medicine. Several studies, including in otolaryngology, have demonstrated that increased explainability could improve providers' trust and willingness to use AI/ML/LLM. Chen and colleagues found that otolaryngologists were more likely to follow the diagnostic suggestion of an AI clinical decision support tool in stroboscopy assessment when presented with a specific explanation of its logic,[12] as opposed to a general or no explanation.

While human providers are not always called upon to describe their exact thought processes and decision making, accountability for these decisions and ability to reason and defend them is foundational for building trust in a provider-patient relationship. Lack of equivalent transparency and explainability in AI/ML/LLM may challenge trust and fracture the provider-patient relationship. This could be particularly challenging during the informed consent process if the clinician is unable to explain how AI functions and may impact surgical decision-making, for instance.

To address explainability, 2 possible solutions have been posited.[9] First, the posthoc analysis may provide explanations for specific AI decision recommendations or predictions with a partial explanation of the system as a whole. For example, a post hoc explanation for an automated laryngoscopy diagnosis could be a supplemental image with an overlying heat map highlighting a suspicious lesion. This allows clinicians to apply their independent reasoning to assess the result. Second, a human-in-the-loop approach can promote "glass-box" AI, as a counterpoint to the "black-box". Expert input on the design of the AI system at every step, allowing high-quality automation with continuous human feedback and increasing transparency on the hidden knowledge in the data, could improve transparency.[9,13]

Governance framework in AI applied to health increasingly calls for transparency and explainability. For instance, the Agency for Healthcare Research and Quality and the National Institute for Minority Health and Health Disparities conceptual framework for governance across an algorithm's life cycle require that algorithms are transparent and explainable.[14] Guidelines such as this put the onus on all groups involved with AI/ML/LLM in medicine to make algorithms transparent, from computer scientists to health care institutions, fostering a culture of collaboration and responsibility in achieving explainable AI.

REPRODUCIBILITY & REPLICABILITY

Some researchers are alarmed by a possible reproducibility crisis with the advent of AI/ML/LLM in medical research.[15–17] *Reproducibility* is defined as the ability of independent investigators to draw the same conclusions from an experiment by following the documentation shared by the original investigators.[18] Of concern, one study found that only 63.5% of 255 papers using AI methods could be reproduced as reported.[19] Ultimately, AI systems in clinical care should not be designed to function in highly controlled experimental conditions but rather to function in diverse real-world situations. AI/ML/LLM output should, thus, ideally be replicable (obtaining consistent results with the same methodology but with new data) and repeatable in real-world situations. This can only be tested with external validation or prospective studies. Lack of reproducibility and replicability is both an epistemological and ethical dilemma. A poorly reliable AI-based diagnostic tool may cause harm. Yet, non-maleficence is one of the pillars of medical ethics. Flooding the literature with poor quality research of limited real-world value for clinical practice obscures impactful research and may indirectly harm patients.

The potential causes for reproducibility and replicability issues in AI/ML/LLM applications to health care are multifaceted. ML classification of visual objects, such as radiology or pathology images, may not reproducible and replicable in large part because of methodologic flaws and biased image data sets.[16,17] Medical datasets used for ML training are often limited in size and diversity, and may not reflect the complexities of the real world, adequately. It is unfortunately not rare for AI application in health care to demonstrate poor generalizability and replicability. Many algorithms may suffer from overfitting, that is, they perform well with their training datasets, but their performance drops with new data.[20] For instance, a study found that 62 published ML models for coronavirus disease 2019 diagnosis based on chest radiographs or computed tomography (CT) scans could have performed better in real-world clinical scenarios.[21] "Data leakage" describes a situation where data from the training dataset are also used to test an ML algorithm, a widespread issue in AI/ML.[15] Overfitting because of data leakage create over-optimistic results, lacking in external validity.

To support reproducibility and replicability studies, the biomedical scientific community has been calling for transparency in the form of the actual computer code used to train a model and arrive at its final set of parameters.[22] For instance, this can be easily done by sharing the code on GitHub. In addition, there have been calls for openly sharing medical data used to train ML. However, medical data contain personal health information that are protected by Health Insurance Portability and Accountability Act, and openly sharing sensitive health data raise significant concerns regarding privacy and security. Despite these challenges, there is a growing trend of sharing raw data in the biomedical sciences for transparency and reproducibility purposes, from under 1% in the early 2000s to 20% today.[23] A growing number of journals, such as PLoS ONE, are requiring authors to make all data underlying the finding described fully available without restriction, with rare exceptions.[24] Other recommendations include detailed description of data acquisition protocols and data processing before training ML algorithms, which can easily be demonstrated on small artificial datasets or public datasets[22] if there is reluctance to share training data. The National Institute of Health (NIH) now requires a data sharing plan and associated budget for grant submitted after January 2023.

Despite these concerns about the reproducibility of AI in health care, some researchers believe these challenges represent a temporary hindrance.[16] From that perspective, poor quality data are necessary growing pain in this nascent and rapidly growing field that will over time be offset by more impactful studies. Over time, they predict that AI/ML systems will converge and with improved datasets and algorithms, their performance will organically continue to improve.

RISK OF BIAS

Another prominent ethical concern regarding AI applications in health care that is tightly linked to epistemology is the risk of AI catalyzing bias perpetuation in medicine, ultimately exacerbating existing health disparities and systemic discrimination. Beyond risk of harm because of erroneous AI output, perseveration of biased patterns leads to mistrust among underrepresented patients who are inclined to avoid the health care system.

AI/ML/LLM depends on their training data's sizes, robustness, and accuracy. Biased training data lead to biased algorithms. Currently, clinical research biorepositories predominantly comprise Caucasian subjects, relying heavily on data from large hospitals with limited diversity in their patient populations.[25–27] Such dataset biases can cause unexpected and pervasive biases. In a pertinent study for otolaryngology, Koenecke and colleagues found that commercial automated speech recognition (ASR) systems exhibited substantial racial disparities because of limited black speech training data, with a significantly lower word error rate in white speakers compared with black speakers.[28] The authors propose that the "phonological, phonetic, or prosodic characteristics of African American Vernacular English rather than the grammatical or lexical characteristics" are what drive the gap in performance of the acoustic models.[28]

Bias is also prevalent in clinical applications of AI/ML because of inherent bias in the training datasets reflecting providers' implicit judgements. For example, AI algorithms are less likely to identify pathology on chest radiographs among underserved populations like African-Americans, Hispanics, and patients with Medicaid.[29] Another salient example studying multiple publicly utilized training datasets for interpreting chest radiograph imaging, demonstrated extensive bias against women. Despite a relatively balanced gender ratio in the datasets, the woman sample was more likely to be misdiagnosed likely because of inherent bias in the datasets.[30]

Another more subtle, yet powerful source of bias in AI/ML/LLM, is the rise of "algorithmic monoculture." Jain and colleagues investigated the overreliance on identical or similar foundation models, as a source of uniformity, institutionalizing standardized errors and limiting pluralism in AI-driven decision supporting tools.[25] As the authors argue, the focus on fairness, equal opportunity, and equal outcomes for different subgroups may limit the opportunity structure. Instead, algorithmic pluralism, as a state of affairs in which decision-making algorithms that structure opportunity are meaningfully pluralistic, allow for a plurality of paths to different outcomes, and reflecting different values and preferences. Such pluralism would be important in end-of-life decisions in head and neck cancer, for instance, as patients may have different preference reflecting their personal and community values or in the field of facial plastics, as not every patient will desire the same outcome.

Efforts are multiplying to address bias in AI/ML. Even in the cases of established AI/ML use, that is, not for research purposes, regular vigilance and lifecycle algorithmic auditing may be necessary to ensure quality and accuracy of results for different people as the algorithms are trained on additional data. Following their findings on bias in commercial ASR, Koenecke and colleagues advocate for more robust incorporation of voice samples from black people in speech training data as a solution.[28] Augmented datasheets in speech data for ASR offer a pragmatic intervention to ensure diversity in datasets.[31] Such datasheets include standardized information such as hours of speech, numbers of speakers, word counts, information on linguistic subpopulations and their relative contributions, non-speech mediums, and semantics.

To promote algorithmic pluralism, a diversity of perspective via a diverse workforce is needed in the design of AI/ML/LLM algorithm. A great example of effort in this direction includes the partnership between the "All of Us Research Program" led by the Common Fund and the NIH "Artificial Intelligence/Machine Learning Consortium to Advance Health Equity and Researcher Diversity" (AIM-AHEAD) and their myriad training programs aiming to build a diverse workforce of researchers skilled in the utilization of AI/ML through their application to the All of Us dataset.[32] Such programs aim to promote the incorporation of diverse perspectives not only at the level of the data, but also at the stage of algorithmic development and inception of research ideas. AIM-AHEAD Ethics and Equity Workgroup complements this work with continuous evaluation, critique, and guidance of ethical and equity issues in health care AI/ML.[33] Efforts have also been made to empower patients as equal stakeholders and address bias at all levels of algorithmic creation and implementation.

SUMMARY

The promise of AI/ML/LLM in medicine and otolaryngology is immense. To fully advance AI potential in clinical practice, it is essential that researchers understand its epistemic limitations, which are tightly linked to ethical dilemmas requiring careful consideration. As the authors reviewed, AI tools are fundamentally opaque systems, though there are methods to increase explainability and transparency. Reproducibility and replicability limitations can be overcomed with sharing computing code, raw data, and data processing methodology. Bias is a well-known risk of AI/ML/LLM, however, its insidiousness is complex and difficult to overcome. Algorithmic auditing, augmented datasheets with demographic information, and advocating for diverse workforce in AI can promote fair outcomes and algorithmic pluralism that best reflects our populations diversity of values and preferences.

DISCLOSURE

A. Rameau owns equity of Perceptron Health Inc. A. Rameau is a medical advisor for Sound Health Systems, Inc.

FUNDING

Anaïs Rameau was supported by a Paul A. Beeson Emerging Leaders Career Development Award in Aging (K76 AG079040) from the National Institute on Aging and by the Bridge2AI award (OT2 OD032720) from the NIH Common Fund.

REFERENCES

1. Michalski RS, Carbonell JG. In: Mitchell TM, editor. Machine learning: An artificial intelligence approach. Springer Science & Business Media; 2013.
2. Vaswani A, Shazeer N, Parmar N, et al. Attention is all you need. Adv Neural Inf Process Syst 2017;30.
3. Whitehouse.gov. Blueprint for an AI Bill of Rights. Whitehousegov. 2021. Available at: https://www.whitehouse.gov/ostp/ai-bill-of-rights/. Accessed March 14, 2024.
4. Whitehouse.gov, FACT SHEET: President Biden Issues Executive Order on Safe, Secure, and Trustworthy Artificial Intelligence 2023, Available at: https://www.whitehouse.gov/briefing-room/statements-releases/2023/10/30/fact-sheet-president-biden-issues-executive-order-on-safe-secure-and-trustworthy-artificial-intelligence/. Accessed March 14, 2024.
5. Europa.eu, AI Act: a step closer to the first rules on Artificial Intelligence 2023, Available at: https://www.europarl.europa.eu/news/en/press-room/20230505IPR84904/ai-act-a-step-closer-to-the-first-rules-on-artificial-intelligence. Accessed March 14, 2024.
6. Doran D, Schulz S, Besold T. What does explainable AI really mean? A new conceptualization of perspectives 2017.
7. Lipton Z. The Mythos of Model Interpretability. Commun ACM 2016;61.
8. Montavon G, Samek W, Müller K-R. Methods for interpreting and understanding deep neural networks. Digit Signal Process 2018;73:1–15.
9. Holzinger A, Langs G, Denk H, et al. Causability and explainability of artificial intelligence in medicine. Wiley Interdiscip Rev Data Min Knowl Discov 2019;9(4):e1312.
10. Topol EJ. High-performance medicine: the convergence of human and artificial intelligence. Nat Med 2019;25(1):44–56.

11. Wischmeyer. Artificial Intelligence and Transparency: Opening the Black Box. Regulating Artificial Intelligence 2020;75.

12. Chen H, Ma X, Rives H, et al. Trust in machine learning driven clinical decision support tools among otolaryngologists. Laryngoscope 2024.

13. Guillaume S. Designing fuzzy inference systems from data: An interpretability-oriented review. IEEE Trans Fuzzy Syst 2001;9(3):426–43.

14. Chin MH, Afsar-Manesh N, Bierman AS, et al. Guiding principles to address the impact of algorithm bias on racial and ethnic disparities in health and health care. JAMA Netw Open 2023;6(12):e2345050–.

15. Kapoor S, Narayanan A. Leakage and the reproducibility crisis in machine-learning-based science. Patterns 2023;4:100804.

16. Ball P. Is AI leading to a reproducibility crisis in science? Nature 2023;624(7990):22–5.

17. Dhar S, Shamir L. Evaluation of the benchmark datasets for testing the efficacy of deep convolutional neural networks. Visual Informatics 2021;5(3):92–101.

18. Erik GO. The fundamental principles of reproducibility. Philos Trans A Math Phys Eng Sci 2021;379(2197):20200210.

19. Raff E. A step toward quantifying independently reproducible machine learning research. Advances in Neural Information Processing Systems 2019;32.

20. Srivastava N, Hinton G, Krizhevsky A, et al. Dropout: a simple way to prevent neural networks from overfitting. J Mach Learn Res 2014;15(1):1929–58.

21. Roberts M, Driggs D, Thorpe M, et al. Common pitfalls and recommendations for using machine learning to detect and prognosticate for COVID-19 using chest radiographs and CT scans. Nat Mach Intell 2021;3(3):199–217.

22. Haibe-Kains B, Adam GA, Hosny A, et al. Transparency and reproducibility in artificial intelligence. Nature 2020 Oct 15;586(7829):E14–6.

23. Wallach JD, Boyack KW, Ioannidis JP. Reproducible research practices, transparency, and open access data in the biomedical literature, 2015–2017. PLoS Biol 2018;16(11):e2006930.

24. PLoS ONE, Data Availability, Available at: http://journals.plos.org/plosone/s/data-availability. Accessed March 14, 2024.

25. Jain SV,S, Creel K, Wilson A. Algorithmic pluralism: a structural approach to equal opportunity. arXiv preprint 2023.

26. Lee SS, Cho MK, Kraft SA, et al. "I don't want to be Henrietta Lacks": diverse patient perspectives on donating biospecimens for precision medicine research. Genet Med 2019;21(1):107–13.

27. Muñoz DC, Sant, C., Becedas, R.R., et al . Dangers of gender bias in CRVS and cause of death data: the path to health inequality. 2022:1–24.

28. Koenecke A, Nam A, Lake E, et al. Racial disparities in automated speech recognition. Proc Natl Acad Sci USA 2020;117(14):7684–9.

29. Seyyed-Kalantari L, Zhang H, McDermott MBA, et al. Underdiagnosis bias of artificial intelligence algorithms applied to chest radiographs in under-served patient populations. Nat Med 2021;27(12):2176–82.

30. Hein AE, Vrijens B, Hiligsmann M. A digital innovation for the personalized management of adherence: analysis of strengths, weaknesses, opportunities, and threats. Frontiers in medical technology 2020;2.

31. Papakyriakopoulos O, Choi ASG, Thong W, et al. Augmented datasheets for speech datasets and ethical decision-making. Proceedings of the 2023 ACM conference on fairness, accountability, and transparency. Chicago, IL: Association for Computing Machinery; 2023. p. 881–904.

32. AIM-AHEAD.net, AIM-AHEAD: All of Us Training Program, Available at: https://www.aim-ahead.net/data-science-tralniny-core/aim ahead-all-of-us-training-program/, 2023. Accessed March 14, 2024.

33. Hendricks-Sturrup R, Simmons M, Anders S, et al. Developing Ethics and equity principles, terms, and engagement tools to advance health equity and researcher diversity in artificial intelligence/machine learning: a modified delphi approach (preprint)2. JMIR AI; 2023.

Regulatory and Implementation Considerations for Artificial Intelligence

Si Chen, MD*, Brian C. Lobo, MD[1]

KEYWORDS

- Artificial intelligence in health • AI regulation • AI implementation • AI education

KEY POINTS

- Central to implementation of artificial intelligence (AI) in otolaryngology is fostering a culture of safe and responsible AI use, achieved through regulatory guidelines, proper standards, and educational programs.
- Regulatory frameworks are continually evolving to navigate the unique challenges of AI applications in health. Otolaryngologists need to understand AI application regulation and governance to determine the safe and effective use in their own practice.
- Professional societies have an opportunity to standardize data and establish benchmarks to facilitate the development and implementation of AI tools in otolaryngology.
- Otolaryngologists can support AI implementation in clinical practice through participation in strategic institutional initiatives, focusing on infrastructure, data security, and governance.
- To overcome barriers to AI implementation, clinicians require deliberate, organized, multidomain AI education tailored to the needs of otolaryngology practice.

INTRODUCTION

Recent decades have seen fluctuating interest and investment in artificial intelligence (AI), with a current surge driven by the popularization of self-driving cars, large language models like Chat Generative Pre-Trained Transformer (ChatGPT), and tremendous advances in computing power and data storage.[1] AI's potential to enhance health care has been realized in applications like diabetic retinopathy screening,[2] skin cancer diagnosis,[3] and polyp detection during colonoscopies,[4] showcasing its capability to match or exceed human diagnostic skills. As health care faces a proliferation of AI-powered

Department of Otolaryngology – Head and Neck Surgery, University of Florida College of Medicine, 1345 Center Drive, PO Box 100264, Gainesville, FL 32610, USA
[1] Present address. 2320 Northwest 38th Drive, Gainesville, FL 32605, USA.
* Corresponding author. 739 Southwest 125th Terrace, Newberry, FL 32669.
E-mail address: si.chen@ent.ufl.edu

Otolaryngol Clin N Am 57 (2024) 871–886
https://doi.org/10.1016/j.otc.2024.04.007
0030-6665/24/Published by Elsevier Inc.

oto.theclinics.com

software and medical devices emerging into the market, integration of AI into clinical practice is fraught with challenges, notably concerns regarding its safety, efficacy, and reliability.

To achieve broad implementation of AI in health care, it is crucial to foster a culture of safe and responsible AI use, a key element in garnering trust from both clinicians and patients.[1,2] This trust, often lacking outside of health care, is needed to prevent the kind of public dissatisfaction and loss of credibility witnessed in industries such as social media. Balanced regulatory guidelines, transparent performance metrics, and comprehensive AI education can build trust by clearly defining AI's role in clinical decisions, promote ongoing evaluation of AI outcomes, and delineate responsibility for their outcomes.[1] Ethical and technical challenges associated with AI applications are discussed in separate articles. This review focuses on the importance of regulation, standardization, and education in navigating the practical challenges of AI in otolaryngology.

REGULATORY CHALLENGES

The successful integration of AI in health care relies on establishing clear standards to evaluate AI products' safety and efficacy.[5] The regulation of AI can be facilitated by an AI governance model, such as the one proposed by Nwosu and colleagues for otolaryngology, emphasizing fairness, transparency, interpretability, privacy, security, and lifecycle oversight.[6] Regulations and oversight mechanisms boost confidence in AI technologies among doctors and patients.[7] Given the complexities of AI development, clinicians and patients often depend on regulatory approvals to gauge safety. Otolaryngologists need to understand the nuances of AI regulation, distinct from traditional medical devices, to make informed choices about their application in clinical settings.

AI tools present unique regulatory challenges summarized in **Table 1**; please refer to Reddy and colleagues, and Larson and colleagues for an in-depth discussion on AI regulations.[8,9] Machine learning (ML), a subset of AI, is notable for its ability to make predictions or decisions, improve with use, identify new patterns, and evolve without explicit reprogramming.[10] Consequently, algorithms can undergo unpredictable and unexplainable changes in decision-making, acquiring new features beyond their initial intended use.[8] This dynamic nature requires adaptive policies to monitor AI systems' performance and alert them to deviations affecting patient care.

The growth of AI tools has been substantial, outpacing the formalization of standards and accreditation systems to assess their safety and impact.[8] Regulatory standards are evolving across multiple levels. Entities like the US Food and Drug Administration (FDA) and the European Medicines Agency (EMA) are actively reforming and revising their regulatory frameworks[11,12]. Additionally, professional medical societies and academic institutions are pivotal in formulating policies and guidelines that specifically tackle challenges within subspecialty practices and patient populations. The next section examines the present regulatory landscape at these various levels for AI applications in otolaryngology.

FEDERAL REGULATION CHANGES

The FDA has tailored regulations for AI-based tools, differentiating them from conventional medical devices. FDA distinguishes Software in Medical Devices (SiMD) from Software as a Medical Device (SaMD).[13] SiMD is integrated into the hardware or drives the function of a medical device, such as software in an insulin pump or nerve monitor. On the other hand, SaMD refers to software that operates independently of any hardware, functioning as a medical device itself, such as stroke-detecting analysis software

Table 1	
Regulatory challenges for artificial intelligence /machine learning medical devices	
Continuous Learning and Adaption	Artificial intelligence/machine learning devices can evolve after learning from real-world data use, making it difficult to monitor its performance and safety.
Standardization and validation	Performance of artificial intelligence/machine learning (AI/ML) systems must be verified after training, and measured against ground truth or pre-determined standards, and validated for local, new and changing data.
Data quality and bias	AI models can perpetuate or amplify biases present in training data set, leading to unfair treatment or outcomes. Regulators must ensure AI applications are unbiased and equitable across different patient demographics.
Transparency	Many AI models, especially deep learning systems, are often described as "black boxes" due to their opaque decision-making processes. Regulators are challenged with ensuring that AI tools can be interpreted by clinical users, and explainable to users and patients.
Data Privacy and Security	Patient disclosure for data use, appropriate deidentification process must comply with laws like HIPAA (Health Insurance Portability and Accountability Act) in the United States, GDPR (General Data Protection Regulation) in Europe, and other regional regulations.
Patient autonomy	Patient's consent for data collection and usage, ability to request for removal of data
Accountability	Determining liability in cases where AI recommendations contribute to patient harm is complicated. Clarifying accountability between AI developers, health care providers, and institutions is essential for legal and ethical reasons.
Interoperability	Can the algorithms run on different equipment in different health systems

for MRIs. Recent updates in 2019[11] and 2021[13] have focused on SaMDs, indicating rapid growth and a projected 30% increase in AI-enabled SaMDs by 2023,[14] illustrated in **Fig. 1**. Radiology and cardiovascular applications dominate the current FDA-approved SaMDs,[14] seen in **Fig. 2**. There were 2 approved applications specific to otolaryngology: ENT EM by Brainlab AG (image-guided planning and navigation system) and VISIONAIR by PacificMD Biotech LLC (rhinoanemometer designed for measuring nasal decongestion).[14] Following sections will delve into the FDA's AI/ML SaMD review process, emphasizing the importance for otolaryngologists to stay informed on regulatory changes and critically assess AI tools' safety and efficacy.

Risk Stratification

The FDA approval process for SaMD involves the fundamental steps of risk designation and the review of clinical evidence to establish safety and efficacy. However, for SaMD, there are ongoing efforts to develop practices that regulate the algorithms' adaptability and potential for change.

Risk categorization, guided by the International Medical Device Regulators Forum, ranges from low-risk devices that inform clinical decisions to high-risk devices that diagnose or treat diseases.[15] This stratification influences the review intensity and necessary controls. FDA risk classes **Fig. 3**, from I (lowest risk) to III (highest risk), are

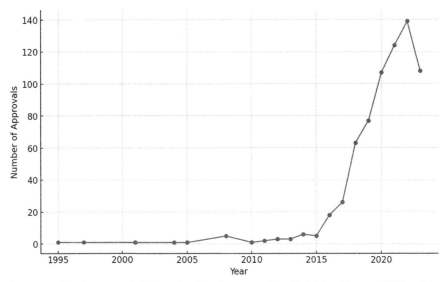

Fig. 1. Food and Drug Administration (FDA)-approved artificial intelligence (AI)/machine learning (ML) Software as a Medical Device (SaMD) per year.

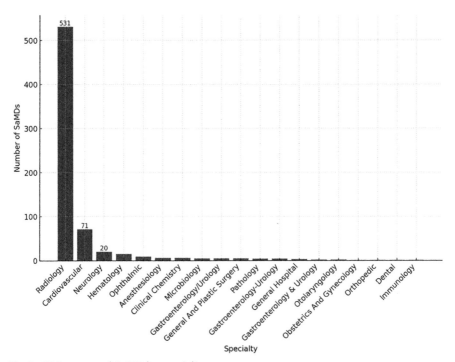

Fig. 2. FDA-approved SaMD by specialty.

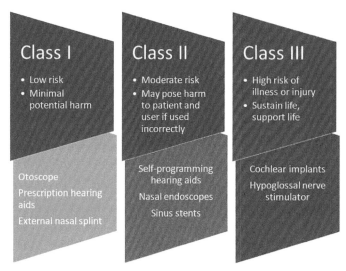

Fig. 3. FDA risk classifications and examples.

determined based on the device's use and potential impact on patient care.[16] For instance, in otolaryngology, Class I includes basic devices like prescription hearing aids, while most SaMDs, including FDA-cleared ENT EM and VISIONAIR, are in Class II. High-risk devices, such as implantable devices, fall into Class III, requiring special controls for assurance of safety and efficacy.

Risk categories guide the FDA approval route, as depicted in **Fig. 4**. SaMDs, like other devices, may be approved through exemption, 510(k) clearance, de novo classification for novel devices, or premarket approval, with the latter being most stringent.[11] The de novo route is for new Class I or II devices lacking a predicate, while 510(k) clearance relies on substantial equivalence to an existing device. Notably, over 90% of SaMDs cleared by the FDA followed the 510(k) process; often trace an average 1.5 previous generations of devices to non-AI/ML medical devices.[17,18] Experts raised concerns

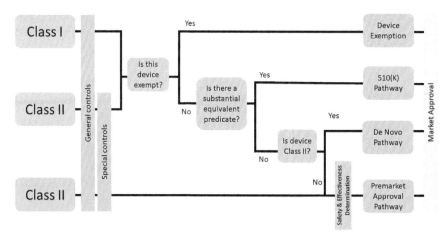

Fig. 4. FDA approval pathways.

of "predicate creep," that is, the AI/ML technology has changed in intended use different from the network of previously approved technologies.[18] Specialties such as radiology and ophthalmology also expressed concerns that the approval of most SaMDs has relied on retrospective data, urging the need for more prospective clinical trials in the SaMD approval process.[10,19,20]

Certain health care software applications may be exempt from FDA scrutiny if they meet the criteria listed in **Box 1**.[21] Notably, select AI radiology applications that simplify visualization, annotation, and interaction with medical images without modifying the original image qualified for FDA exemption. For otolaryngologists contemplating using these exempt AI tools, it is important to recognize that exemption from FDA review does not eliminate the need to assess bias, patient privacy, and data security.[22]

Capacity for Change

The FDA distinguishes "locked" algorithms from "adaptive" ML algorithms.[13] A "locked" algorithm consistently delivers the same result for identical inputs and does not change over time.[13] For instance, IDX-DR is a "locked" algorithm utilized for diabetic retinopathy screening.[2] It has been thoroughly trained on a substantial dataset and reliably identifies retinopathy from the same retinal scan taken at different times.[20] If developers wish to improve the SaMD's accuracy or enable it to suggest new treatment plans based on updated data, they need to retrain the SaMD with new data, perform testing, and lock the algorithm once more before submitting it for FDA review.[20] On the other hand, "adaptive" algorithms are defined by the FDA as those that "change their behavior through a defined learning process."[13] This means their outputs might vary for the same input if the algorithm has adapted from real-world usage.[1] To date, the FDA has only approved locked algorithms, but newer FDA regulations address adaptive SaMDs.[13]

As adaptive SaMDs learn from real-world data, they undergo notable changes, such as input modification, algorithm alteration, or new feature additions that redefine their use.[13] Typically, these significant changes would require FDA review through a de novo process or a full premarket approval for each iteration.[13] Because of their inherently frequent and unpredictable nature, it is felt that if subject to the traditional approval process, could stifle innovation. To circumvent these issues, the FDA has implemented a total product lifecycle regulatory approach for adaptive SaMDs,[11] which is detailed in **Fig. 5**. This approach is designed to comprehensively assess SaMDs before and after they enter the market, focusing on continuous monitoring, risk management, and detailed change documentation to ensure ongoing safety and efficacy.[11]

Box 1
Food and Drug Administration exemptions for medical software

1. Administrative support: Software designed for administrative purposes, such as scheduling or inventory management.

2. Health Lifestyle Maintenance: Applications aimed at promoting and maintaining a healthy lifestyle, such as mobile apps that monitor exercise routines.

3. Electronic Patient Records: Software that serves as electronic patient records, allowing patients to input and share their health information with health care providers.

4. Data Handling: Applications focused on transferring, storing, converting, or displaying data without making any alterations to the data itself.

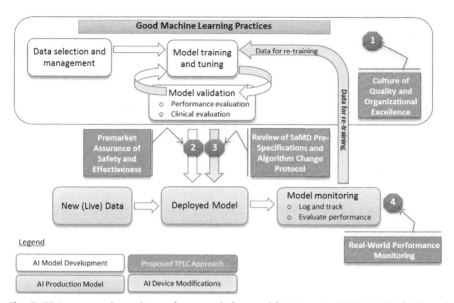

Fig. 5. FDA proposed regulatory framework for modifications to AI/ML SaMD. (*Adapted from* U.S. Food and Drug Administration. Artificial Intelligence and Machine Learning in Software as a Medical Device Action Plan. Published 2021. Accessed January 4, 2024. https://www.fda.gov/medical-devices/software-medical-device-samd/artificial-intelligence-and-machine-learning-software-medical-device.)

The FDA encourages AI developers to establish a "Predetermined Control Plan Protocol" to manage and document expected changes in SaMDs.[11] The FDA's Pre-Cert Pilot Program assesses developers on "good machine learning practices," emphasizing collaboration, transparency, and long-term oversight.[11] Companies like Apple and Fitbit have achieved precertification, streamlining the FDA review process with exemptions for low-risk SaMDs or expedited review for higher risk applications.[23] Senators Elizabeth Warren, Patty Murray, and Tina Smith have raised concerns that companies would be in charge of their own evaluation processes and may lead to a conflict of interest and potentially lower the bar for safety and efficacy standards.[24] These senators questioned the organization of the program as well as the fee structure for participants.[24] The financial aspect could influence how companies participate and could have implications for market dynamics.[24] Otolaryngologists are advised to seek clear information on product testing, performance, and certification criteria before adopting SaMDs.

CONSIDERATIONS FOR PROFESSIONAL SOCIETIES

Professional societies are crucial in collating data and establishing performance benchmarks to advance AI in otolaryngology. Data requirements for AI development are discussed in a different article. Still, insights can be gained from how organizations in radiology, cardiology, and ophthalmology have promoted standardized data aggregation and warehousing to facilitate AI implementation.

AI algorithms in clinical practice rely on measuring AI predictions against ground truths—the real, accurate clinical inputs and outputs that AI models seek to classify or predict. These models are evaluated using benchmarks or performance metrics like accuracy, sensitivity, harmonic means (F-Score), and the area under the receiver operating characteristic curve, depending on extensive sets of real clinical data. For instance, an AI algorithm that differentiates sinusitis from healthy sinuses requires training and verification in a vast collection of standardized CT images, with both normal and abnormal sinuses. There is an increased data requirement in rare diseases to minimize false positives.[10] Unfortunately, the lack of extensive and varied public datasets often hampers an AI tool's ability to perform consistently across different patient populations and health care environments.[25] This challenge can be overcome by specialty-wide efforts to gather and standardize data, ensuring AI evaluations are based on solid and representative benchmarks.

Radiology exemplifies the benefits of data standardization. Currently, over 80% of AI/ML devices approved by the FDA fall within the radiology sector.[14] The American College of Radiology (ACR) undertook a large survey of their members and found that 30% of radiologists are currently using AI apps in their practice.[26] Among the many factors that contributed to the rapid advancement of AI in radiology, data standardization was pivotal. In the 1980s ACR and National Electrical Manufacturers Association collaborated to develop the Digital Imaging and Communications in Medicine (DICOM), a universal format for storing, retrieving, sharing, and displaying medical images.[27] DICOM made it easier to transfer imaging data across various operating systems and image viewing software, ensuring interoperability for integration of AI algorithms.[10] Building on this, the ACR's Data Science Institute's AI-LAB now offers an expansive, well-annotated dataset repository that empowers radiologists to develop, test, and share AI models.[28] Additionally, the Radiological Society of North America (RSNA)'s International COVID-19 Open Annotated Radiology Database initiative has curated a large-scale open dataset for coronavirus disease 2019 (COVID-19) chest x-rays, enhancing AI diagnostic tools for diagnosis of COVID-19.[29] Radiologists have come together in a multi-society statement to recommend using society-developed resource to develop solutions that target true clinical needs rather than develop algorithms from existing technology simply because a dataset happens to be available.[10]

Ophthalmology is also making strides by standardizing data for AI tools to enhance the screening and management of retinal diseases.[2] In 2021, American Academy of Ophthalmology advocated that manufactures of ophthalmic devices standardize the format of digital images developed by American Academy of Ophthalmology.[20] Similarly, for elements of electronic health records that are challenging to standardize, the American College of Cardiology (ACC) and the American Heart Association (AHA) have jointly developed the ACC/AHA Clinical Data Standards.[30] These standards aim to unify the terminology and data elements in cardiovascular care.[30]

Mirroring these initiatives, American Academy of Otolaryngology—Head and Neck Surgery created the otolaryngology-specific Reg-ent Clinical Data Registry,[31] which collects and standardizes clinical data across practices for quality improvement and research. Future undertakings by professional otolaryngology societies can promote broader data utilization and innovation by encouraging the development of more datasets, foster collaborations between institutions, advocating for interoperability, and supporting open access initiatives.

STRATEGIC INITIATIVES AT INSTITUTIONS

At the institutional level, the challenge of implementing AI in health care involves not only the infrastructure and data concerns, but also establishing proper governance to manage AI performance in the local context. It is important to customize AI implementation strategies to match each institution's specific needs and resources.[10,32]

Health care institutions must recognize their own unique challenges, assess the alignment of AI solutions with these challenges, and establish clear, measurable objectives for AI performance to guarantee thorough monitoring, alerting, and evaluation tailored to individual cases.[10,32] Before deploying an AI model into patient care, health systems need to conduct prospective validation within their local demographic, allowing clinicians to confirm the model's efficacy for their population and troubleshoot any irregularities in the model, ensuring its outputs remain relevant and adaptable to the practice's patient demographics and clinical guidelines.[1]

Several institutions have outlined strategic initiatives and established specialized groups to build infrastructure to support AI in clinical practice through research, innovation, and education. Examples include the Mayo Clinic Platform, Stanford's Center for Artificial Intelligence In Medicine and Imaging, University of California Health's Center for Data-Driven Insights and Innovation, and University of Florida's Quality and Patient Safety Initiative. These institution-wide initiatives have created system-level data assets, such as Partners HealthCare's i2b2, University of Florida's GatorTron, and University of California's Observational Medical Outcomes Partnership . Such focused efforts are essential for accurately validating and monitoring the performance of AI algorithms as they are introduced to real clinical practice.

Due to significant data processing and storage needs, most institutions will likely adopt cloud-based AI tools, requiring careful legal review to safeguard patients, staff, and the institution.[33] Data use agreements must specify terms for using, sharing, and storing PHIand non-PHI data.[33] Understanding data usage and ownership, especially in scenarios like company changes, is essential for AI deployments. Additionally, standards and commercial tools for de-identifying PHI from electronic health records are available to ensure privacy. De-identified system-wide data assets like i2b2 and GatorTron further facilitate research and AI implementation, benefiting not only the originating institution but also others through collaboration.

Local AI governance bodies have been proposed to manage the transition of AI tools from development to clinical use, as discrepancies in performance may arise between premarket training and real clinical application.[10] Differences in equipment, protocols, and patient demographics may diminish performance in real-world settings.[10] Health care institutions must pay special attention to their specific population and monitor any significant changes that may affect an AI model's effectiveness.[10] Implementing regularly updated benchmarking datasets and local standards is recommended to preserve model accuracy, akin to the clinical laboratory validations conducted for blood-based biomarkers.[5] The criteria and timing for re-assessing AI models should consider factors such as disease specifics and patient risk.[32] Consequently, clinical experts, especially subspecialists such as otolaryngologists, at each institution must collaborate with their local AI governance group to ensure ongoing monitoring and guidance for AI implementations.

Otolaryngologists interested in AI implementation should work with institutional AI programs and governance bodies to customize and confirm the efficacy of AI models within their specific clinical settings before integration. Otolaryngologists must participate in collaborative AI projects, enabling them to tackle distinct clinical issues and cater to the specialized requirements of their field, considering the disease patterns and patient populations pertinent to otolaryngology.

INDIVIDUAL CHALLENGES TO ARTIFICIAL INTELLIGENCE IMPLEMENTATION

For individual clinicians, the barriers to implementing AI in everyday medical practice often stem from a need for more awareness and knowledge. Many clinicians and patients are unfamiliar with AI, harboring concerns about the absence of human oversight and the potential for mistakes that could affect patient care.[34,35] Babu and colleagues illustrated this through a scenario where AI misjudged the cancer risk in a patient, leading to a decision against biopsy due to the patient's inability to undergo anesthesia.[36] The lesion later grew, demonstrating the consequences of relying on AI without adequate understanding. The authors argue that although it is not necessary for otolaryngologists to completely explain the algorithms before using the AI tool, there is a need to understand AI's capabilities and limitations to build trust and confidence in AI-assisted clinical decision.[36]

AI literacy and education have been demonstrated to mitigate fear of AI and manage more realistic expectations of AI.[37] The subsequent section explores initial efforts in AI education aimed at fostering understanding and trust, which will require more work to achieve wide acceptance AI implementation.[35] It highlights strategies for educational initiatives and how individual physicians can prepare for AI integration in clinical practice. By adopting an intentional, structured, specialty-specific, multi-domain approach to AI education, it is possible to decrease fear and instill trust at every phase of AI implementation: conceptualization, design, application, assessment, and ongoing oversight.[35]

AI education varies widely in its content and aim; however, the curriculum can be effectively designed to emphasize patient safety and care quality.[35] Clinicians can learn to form a robust approach to mitigating *biases*, identifying real clinical needs, setting *performance standards*, and discussing *accountability* in AI clinical decision making.[10] To achieve AI implementation after algorithm development, the clinical users need to have a basic understanding of the tool's algorithm and output (*interpretability*) and explain the medical decision- making to patients and colleagues (*explainability*).[10] Clinicians need to learn how to assess and maintain transparency in AI-human teams. *Transparency* involves clear communication about the AI system's purpose, operational conditions, and accuracy expectations. It also includes informing patients about the use of their data in AI development or when AI influences their care.[10] Modern clinicians must understand how to balance *interpretability* and *explainability* with potential trade-offs in *performance*, *privacy*, and proprietary information *security*.[10] AI governance principles should be emphasized and woven into education across all levels.

Innovative AI curriculum (**Table 2**) encompasses multiple domains: cognitive, psychomotor, and affective.[38] This approach emphasizes the importance of affective skills such as communicating empathy and compassion in patient interactions with AI diagnostics.[39] Additional psychomotor skills are important for clinicians to navigate and maximize their functions in human-machine teams, such as automation bias (the increasing reliance on algorithms that could overshadow human judgment) and confirmation bias (clinicians might trust AI outputs that confirm their pre-existing beliefs or hypotheses, while disregarding outputs that contradict them).[5] Moreover, the growing role of AI in clinical decision-making could alter the physician's sense of personal accountability.[5] Clinicians must become adept at identifying and managing the uncertainties present in human-machine interactions. Developing these affective and psychomotor skills is essential for establishing trust between doctors and patients, a fundamental component for effectively integrating AI technologies into health care.[35,39]

The AI curriculum has expanded to cover implementation science and change management. Implementation science explores the effective incorporation of evidence-based research into clinical practice, providing strategies for facilitating adoption of innovation.[40] An otolaryngology relevant example is Studts's application for hearing

Table 2
Education curriculum/competencies for artificial intelligence implementation

	Cognitive	Psychomotor	Affective
Introduction to artificial intelligence (AI) in health care	History, definitions, types of AI	—	Discussion on the impact of AI on patient care and health care delivery to foster a positive attitude toward technology advancement.
Data science basics	Data types, data collection, data preprocessing techniques, data governance	Hands-on exercises in data handling and analysis using health care datasets.	Ethical considerations in AI, including patient privacy, data security, addressing bias in AI algorithms, and ensuring fairness across patient populations.
Machine learning and deep learning	Supervised vs non-supervised learning, reinforcement learning	Practical sessions on building basic machine learning models using health care data, such as patient outcome prediction.	—
Clinical applications of AI	Understanding decision science and probabilities from AI diagnostic and therapeutic algorithms to then meaningfully apply them in clinical decision-making	Interactive case studies exploring the use of AI tools in clinical settings	Practice clinical translation and interpretation of model outputs with transparency to build patient trust
Bias and fairness	Guidelines and best practices for ethical AI use in health care.	Experience examples of various such as sample bias, label bias, algorithm automation bias, confirmation bias	Understand pitfalls and errors, unintended consequences of perpetuating bias
Regulatory and policy	Understanding regulatory frameworks governing AI in health care, Food and Drug Administration (FDA) approval processes for AI tools, and international standards.	Trace an example of adaptive algorithm change that warrant new FDA approval	Building a culture of responsible AI use in product development

(continued on next page)

Table 2
(continued)

	Cognitive	Psychomotor	Affective
Implementation science and change management	Strategies for implementing AI in health care settings, including integration with existing health IT systems.	Simulation exercises on deploying AI tools and managing change in health care organizations.	Building resilience and adaptability to technological changes among health care teams.
Communication and patient engagement	Learning to use data visualization to present and describe outputs from AI tools	Mastering how to communicate results with patients in a personalized and meaningful way and discuss the use of AI in the medical decision-making process	Cultivating and expressing empathy and compassion when communicating with patients
Ethics issues	Understanding and building awareness of ethics, equity, inclusion, patient rights, and confidentiality when using AI tools	Discuss cases of ethical dilemmas and conflicts of interest in AI deployment	—

health.[40] Change management deals with managing the human aspects of organizational change, emphasizing the need for leadership and communication skills to engage stakeholders and guide them toward new technology or methodology.[41] While not directly related to AI algorithm development, training in these areas aligns health care teams with new directions, relevant for introducing technology to different groups who might not be fully understanding or receptive.

Various models for AI education are in early development, most recognize the need to organize vast amount of information and skills throughout different educational phases.[35,38] Undergraduate and medical students learn the basics and AI capabilities, while advanced skills like validation and clinical limitations are taught at the graduate level.[38] Ethical considerations and psychomotor/affective competencies are woven into the curriculum at all levels. This groundwork sets the stage for deeper exploration of AI's regulatory, economic, and societal implications in continued medical education for practicing clinicians to take on leadership roles.[38]

Initiatives to introduce AI fundamentals into the medical curriculum at both the undergraduate and post-graduate levels are gaining momentum. These fundamentals cover AI terminology, machine learning algorithms, bioinformatics, and data science. Tools to gauge the AI readiness of medical students and faculty focus on their grasp of AI concepts and attitudes toward its application.[42–44] Radiologists, as early AI adopters in the medical field, have introduced AI education in residency,[44] and considered AI literacy as a core competency for residents.[44,45] Similarly, otolaryngology trainees and educators are encouraged to familiarize themselves with AI/ML basics, the power of big data, and AI's potential in their specialty.

For most clinicians already in practice, accessing AI education is a challenge due to time and financial constraints.[35,38] Less than 5% of AI-related medical education articles focus on continuing medical education (CME) courses, highlighting a gap in ongoing professional development in AI.[38] Recent years have seen the introduction of online courses and certificate programs to bridge this gap, offering self-paced "AI for Healthcare" programs. However, these programs are often too generalized. Specialized AI curricula tailored to individual medical specialties are needed. In radiology, organizations like the ACR and RSNA have already started offering specialty-specific AI courses.[46–48] Looking ahead, otolaryngology professional societies are encouraged to develop targeted AI education programs to meet the unique needs of our field.

Overall, the evolution of AI education in health care is moving toward a comprehensive approach that balances technical knowledge with communication and leadership skills, aiming to prepare clinicians evaluate the AI tools on the market, comprehend the underlying algorithms, and articulate how these tools impact patient care decisions, and lead a team to monitor its safety and effectiveness.[38]

SUMMARY

This review delves into the complexities of AI implementation, emphasizing the pivotal role of fostering trust through responsible regulation, transparent standardization, and comprehensive education. Many of these challenges highlight the necessity for robust monitoring of AI performance while allowing adaptable policies to accommodate the dynamic nature of AI technologies. The authors proposed collaborative efforts across professional organizations, institutions, and individual clinicians to overcome the barriers of AI integration while upholding patient safety and quality of care. Otolaryngologists need to acquire the ability to responsibly select, apply, and oversee AI technologies. Otolaryngologists with AI literacy can proactively engage in national and local initiatives to influence the trajectory of AI implementation within our specialty.

REFERENCES

1. Wiens J, Saria S, Sendak M, et al. Do no harm: a roadmap for responsible machine learning for health care. Nat Med 2019;25(9):1337–40.
2. Gunasekeran DV, Ting DSW, Tan GSW, et al. Artificial intelligence for diabetic retinopathy screening, prediction and management. Curr Opin Ophthalmol 2020; 31(5):357–65.
3. Wells A, Patel S, Lee JB, et al. Artificial intelligence in dermatopathology: Diagnosis, education, and research. J Cutan Pathol 2021;48(8):1061–8.
4. Walradt T, Glissen Brown JR, Alagappan M, et al. Regulatory considerations for artificial intelligence technologies in GI endoscopy. Gastrointest Endosc 2020; 92(4):801–6.
5. He J, Baxter SL, Xu J, et al. The practical implementation of artificial intelligence technologies in medicine. Nat Med 2019;25(1):30–6.
6. Nwosu OI, Crowson MG, Rameau A. Artificial intelligence governance and otolaryngology-head and neck surgery. Laryngoscope 2023;133(11):2868–70.
7. Silkens MEWM, Ross J, Hall M, et al. The time is now: making the case for a UK registry of deployment of radiology artificial intelligence applications. Clin Radiol 2023;78(2):107–14.
8. Reddy S, Allan S, Coghlan S, et al. A governance model for the application of AI in health care. J Am Med Inf Assoc 2020;27(3):491–7.
9. Larson DB, Harvey H, Rubin DL, et al. Regulatory frameworks for development and evaluation of artificial intelligence-based diagnostic imaging algorithms: summary and recommendations. J Am Coll Radiol 2021;18(3 Pt A):413–24.
10. Brady AP, Allen B, Chong J, et al. Developing, purchasing, implementing and monitoring AI tools in radiology: practical considerations. A multi-society statement from the ACR, CAR, ESR, RANZCR & RSNA. Insights Imaging 2024; 15(1):16.
11. U.S. Food and Drug Administration. Proposed regulatory framework for modifications to artificial intelligence/machine learning (AI/ML)-based software as a medical device (SaMD) - discussion paper and request for feedback. 2019. Available at: https://www.fda.gov/files/medical%20devices/published/US-FDA-Artificial-Intelligence-and-Machine-Learning-Discussion-Paper.pdf. [Accessed 15 December 2023].
12. Goodman B, Flaxman S. European Union regulations on algorithmic decision-making and a 'right to explanation'. AI Mag 2017;38(50).
13. U.S. Food and Drug Administration. Artificial intelligence and machine learning in software as a medical device action plan. 2021. Available at: https://www.fda.gov/medical-devices/software-medical-device-samd/artificial-intelligence-and-machine-learning-software-medical-device. [Accessed 10 January 2024].
14. U.S. Food and Drug Administration. Artificial intelligence and machine learning (AI/ML)-Enabled medical devices. Available at: https://www.fda.gov/medical-devices/software-medical-device-samd/artificial-intelligence-and-machine-learning-aiml-enabled-medical-devices. [Accessed 10 January 2024].
15. IMDRF SaMD Working Group. Software as a medical device (SaMD): clinical evaluation. International Medical Device Regulators Forum; 2016. Available at: http://www.imdrf.org/docs/imdrf/final/consultations/imdrf-cons-samd-ce.pdf. [Accessed 10 January 2024].

16. U.S. Food and Drug Administration. Classify your medical device. Available at: https://www.fda.gov/medical-devices/overview-device-regulation/classify-your-medical-device. [Accessed 10 January 2024].

17. Benjamens S, Dhunnoo P, Meskó B. The state of artificial intelligence-based FDA-approved medical devices and algorithms: an online database. NPJ Digit Med 2020;3:118.

18. Muehlematter UJ, Bluethgen C, Vokinger KN. FDA-cleared artificial intelligence and machine learning-based medical devices and their 510(k) predicate networks. Lancet Digit Health 2023;5(9):e618–26.

19. Danese C, Kale AU, Aslam T, et al. The impact of artificial intelligence on retinal disease management: Vision Academy retinal expert consensus. Curr Opin Ophthalmol 2023;34(5):396–402.

20. Chou YB, Kale AU, Lanzetta P, et al. Current status and practical considerations of artificial intelligence use in screening and diagnosing retinal diseases: Vision Academy retinal expert consensus. Curr Opin Ophthalmol 2023;34(5):403–13.

21. U.S. Food and Drug Administration. Class I and Class II Device Exemptions. Available at: https://www.fda.gov/medical-devices/classify-your-medical-device/class-i-and-class-ii-device-exemptions. [Accessed 15 January 2024].

22. Alon N, Stern AD, Torous J. Assessing the Food and Drug Administration's Risk-Based Framework for Software Precertification With Top Health Apps in the United States: Quality Improvement Study. JMIR Mhealth Uhealth 2020;8(10):e20482.

23. U.S. Food and Drug Administration. FDA selects participants for new digital health software precertification pilot program. 2017. Available at: https://www.fda.gov/news-events/press-announcements/fda-selects-participants-new-digital-health-software-precertification-pilot-program. [Accessed 10 January 2024].

24. Warren E, Murray P, Smith T. Lawmakers Request More Information About FDA Pilot Program's Ability to Ensure Device Safety. Available at: https://www.warren.senate.gov/oversight/letters/-senators-warren-murray-and-smith-raise-further-questions-about-the-fdas-oversight-of-digital-health-devices. [Accessed 1 February 2024].

25. Saenz A, Chen E, Marklund H, et al. The MAIDA initiative: establishing a framework for global medical-imaging data sharing. Lancet Digit Health 2024;6(1):e6–8.

26. Allen B, Agarwal S, Coombs L, et al. 2020 ACR data science institute artificial intelligence survey. J Am Coll Radiol 2021;18(8):1153e9.

27. Bidgood WD, Horii SC. Introduction to the ACR-NEMA DICOM standard. Radiographics 1992;12(2):345–55.

28. Data Science Institute. American College of Radiology. Available at: https://www.acrdsi.org/DSI-Services. [Accessed 1 February 2024].

29. Tsai EB, Simpson S, Lungren MP, et al. The RSNA International COVID-19 Open Radiology Database (RICORD). Radiology 2021;299(1):E204–13.

30. Hendel RC, Bozkurt B, Fonarow GC, et al. ACC/AHA 2013 methodology for developing clinical data standards: a report of the American College of Cardiology/American Heart Association Task Force on Clinical Data Standards. Circulation 2014;129(22):2346–57.

31. Reg-ENT American Academy of Otolaryngology—Head and Neck Surgery. About Reg-ent. 2017. Available at: https://www.entnet.org//content/about-Reg-Ent. [Accessed 27 July 2018].

32. Harvey HB, Gowda V. Regulatory Issues and Challenges to Artificial Intelligence Adoption. Radiol Clin North Am 2021;59(6):1075–83.

33. Al-Ruithe M, Benkhelifa E, Hameed K. A systematic literature review of data governance and cloud data governance. Pers Ubiquit Comput 2019;23:839–59.

34. Bur AM, Shew M, New J. Artificial Intelligence for the Otolaryngologist: A State of the Art Review. Otolaryngol Head Neck Surg 2019;160(4):603–11.

35. Walsh G, Stogiannos N, van de Venter R, et al. Responsible AI practice and AI education are central to AI implementation: a rapid review for all medical imaging professionals in Europe. BJR Open 2023;5(1):20230033.

36. Babu CS, Holsinger FC, Zuchowski L, et al. Epistemological challenges of artificial intelligence clinical decision support tools in otolaryngology: the black box problem. Otolaryngol Head Neck Surg 2023;169(6):1697–700.

37. Perchik JD, Smith AD, Elkassem AA, et al. Artificial intelligence literacy: developing a multi-institutional infrastructure for AI education. Acad Radiol 2023; 30(7):1472–80.

38. Charow R, Jeyakumar T, Younus S, et al. Artificial intelligence education programs for health care professionals: scoping review. JMIR Med Educ 2021;7(4):e31043.

39. Wartman S, Combs C. Reimagining medical education in the age of AI. AMA J Ethics 2019;21(2):E146–52.

40. Studts CR. Implementation science: increasing the public health impact of audiology research. Am J Audiol 2022;31(3S):849–63.

41. Solow M, Perry TE. Change management and health care culture. Anesthesiol Clin 2023;41(4):693–705.

42. Karaca O, Çalışkan SA, Demir K. Medical artificial intelligence readiness scale for medical students (MAIRS-MS) - development, validity and reliability study. BMC Med Educ 2021;21(1):112.

43. Santos DP, Giese D, Brodehl S, et al. Medical students' attitude towards artificial intelligence: a multicentre survey. Eur Radiol 2019;29(4):1640–6.

44. Wood MJ, Tenenholtz NA, Geis JR, et al. The need for a machine learning curriculum for radiologists. J Am Coll Radiol 2019;16(5):740–2.

45. Perchik JD, Tridandapani S. AI/ML Education in Radiology: Accessibility is Key. Acad Radiol 2023;30(7):1491–2.

46. Artificial Intelligence for the Practicing Radiologist: Understand AI in Five Lessons. American College of Radiology. Available at: https://pages.acr.org/Informatics-e-learning-hub-ai-for-the-practicing-radiologist.html.

47. RSNAI. Radiology Society of North America. Available at: https://www.rsna.org/rsnai.

48. Masterclass in AI. European Society of Radiology. Available at: https://www.myesr.org/education/masterclass-in-ai/.

The Integration and Impact of Artificial Intelligence in Otolaryngology—Head and Neck Surgery: Navigating the Last Mile

Matthew G. Crowson, MD, MPA, MASc, MBI[a,b,*], Obinna I. Nwosu, MD[a,b]

KEYWORDS

- Otolaryngology • Artificial intelligence • Machine learning • Clinical integration

KEY POINTS

- Data silos in health care: Health care suffers from data silos, notably in otolaryngology, impairing patient data integration and use, challenging imaging data accessibility, and fragmenting patient records across platforms.
- Electronic health records (EHRs) and artificial Intelligence (AI) in otolaryngology: EHRs centralize patient data, crucial for efficient care and AI development. However, they face challenges integrating detailed otolaryngology-specific data and ensuring data quality.
- Challenges and considerations for AI integration: Integrating AI into otolaryngology requires addressing EHR compatibility, maintaining continuous machine learning model validation, ethical patient care considerations, and practical clinical staff training.

INTRODUCTION

Artificial intelligence (AI) is the technological domain where machines emulate human cognitive skills, transforming once-unthinkable ideas into realities. Machine learning (ML), a subset of this field, involves algorithms that evolve through data exposure. In recent years, AI has been at the center of tremendous advances in almost every industry, with health care being no exception.

The surge in recent literature exploring innovative applications of AI in otolaryngology underscores the potential of AI to reshape and advance otolaryngologic care. AI research has demonstrated a potential to increase diagnostic accuracy, novel

[a] Department of Otolaryngology-Head & Neck Surgery, Massachusetts Eye & Ear Hospital, Boston, MA, USA; [b] Department of Otolaryngology-Head & Neck Surgery, Harvard Medical School, Boston, MA, USA
* Corresponding author. 243 Charles Street, Boston, MA 02114.
E-mail address: matthew_crowson@meei.harvard.edu

Otolaryngol Clin N Am 57 (2024) 887–895
https://doi.org/10.1016/j.otc.2024.04.001
0030-6665/24/© 2024 Elsevier Inc. All rights reserved.

therapeutics, and improved techniques for surveillance outcome prediction.[1–4] While there has been a tremendous boom in AI-focused literature in otolaryngology, few studies have deployed these AI tools for clinical use.

Ultimately, the advances promised by AI must be safely integrated into the clinical workspace to realize their complete and intended potential. However, there are several considerations and challenges to consider in navigating this integration smoothly. Herein, the authors discuss key factors impacting the integration of AI into routine otolaryngologic care.

DISCUSSION
Clinical Data Interoperability

In health care, the presence of data silos can hamper the integration and utilization of patient data. These silos appear in various forms, including imaging data, laboratory and pathology data, and unstructured patient narratives.

Imaging data in otolaryngology, essential for diagnostics and treatment planning, often resides in proprietary systems with limited interoperability.[5] This compartmentalization challenges the accessibility and sharing of crucial imaging resources. Similarly, patient records, encompassing medical histories, treatment plans, and follow-up care, are fragmented across different platforms and institutions. Additionally, recording surgical outcomes can inhibit a comprehensive analysis of these data due to the absence of standardized reporting formats and centralized databases.

The impact of these data silos is likely underestimated, affecting patient care, research, and the development of new treatments in otolaryngology. Addressing these challenges necessitates a multifaceted approach:

1. Collaborative frameworks: Developing collaborative frameworks among health care providers, researchers, and technology developers is important given the diversity of data sources required to develop robust models.[6] Such frameworks should encourage data and resource sharing, mitigating the effects of data silos.
2. Data-sharing agreements: Instituting data-sharing agreements between institutions can facilitate secure and efficient data exchange. These agreements must consider legal, ethical, and logistical aspects to ensure data security and efficacy.
3. Standardization initiatives: Standardizing data formats and protocols enhances data interoperability. Adopting universal standards or new approaches like semantic data entry and storage interoperability can simplify data exchange and integration across systems.[7]

High-quality, diverse, and sufficient volumes of data are needed to develop robust AI models. Dismantling data silos in otolaryngology is a key step for advancing AI research. As such, collaborative frameworks, data-sharing agreements, and standardization initiatives are essential to begin overcoming these challenges as we work toward developing AI to foster improved patient care, research, and clinical outcomes.

Electronic Health Records: Utilization in Otolaryngology

Electronic health records (EHRs) are central to modernizing and centralizing patient data in contemporary medicine in the United States. EHRs play a central role in organizing medical information, which is fundamental for efficient patient care and one precursor for amassing patient-level data for AI applications.

Standardizing and centralizing patient data through EHRs are important for consistent patient care. EHRs allow for a unified view of a patient's medical history, treatments, and outcomes, which is essential for effective clinical decision-making. However, the integration of EHRs in otolaryngology presents unique challenges. Capturing detailed information about complex surgical procedures and follow-up care specific to this field requires EHR systems that are both flexible and comprehensive.[8]

Moreover, the role of EHRs extends beyond patient care. They are important for supporting AI application development. AI algorithms require large datasets to develop predictive models, and EHRs are a valuable source of these data.[9] However, the quality and format of the data recorded in EHRs are the lynchpin for training applicable AI models. This necessitates the adoption of best practices in EHR utilization, ensuring data accuracy and consistency.

Despite the potential benefits, several challenges persist. One significant issue is the need for EHR systems to be tailored to capture the nuances of otolaryngology-specific data, such as detailed surgical procedures and follow-up care, which often need to be adequately represented in generic EHR templates.[10] Concerns regarding data privacy, security, and the interoperability of different EHR systems also pose substantial challenges.[11]

While EHRs offer immense potential in standardizing and centralizing patient data, addressing the challenges of integration, data quality, and system specificity is a pressing need. Adopting best practices in EHR utilization and continuously refining these systems will be essential in leveraging their full potential for patient care and AI applications.

Common Data Model: Adaptation for ENT-specific Data

Adapting a common data model (CDM) is a prerequisite for enhancing interoperability and facilitating AI applications in otolaryngology. A CDM provides a standardized way to represent health care data from various sources, enabling seamless integration and analysis. The significance of a CDM in health care, particularly in otolaryngology, lies in its ability to harmonize disparate data types, such as diverse diagnostic testing modalities (eg, audiometry, video-based endoscopic evaluations, genomic testing), which are unique to this specialty. This standardization is needed for effective data exchange and comparison across research teams and health care systems.[12,13]

Tailoring a CDM to accommodate the unique aspects of otolaryngology data involves addressing the specific data elements and structures. For instance, incorporating detailed audiometry test results and voice disorder evaluations into the CDM requires a nuanced understanding of these data types and their clinical implications. This customization ensures that the CDM can effectively manage and represent complex data sets.

However, adopting a CDM for otolaryngology-specific data takes time and effort. One significant hurdle is ensuring that the CDM remains flexible enough to accommodate the evolving nature of otolaryngology data, especially as data arise from diagnostic and treatment modalities. Moreover, aligning the CDM with data privacy and security regulations is essential to protect patient information. Adapting a CDM for otolaryngology-specific data promises improved interoperability, enhanced AI development, and streamlined research. While challenges exist, the ongoing refinement and customization of CDMs are pivotal for leveraging their full potential in advancing otolaryngology.

Health Level Seven International Fast Healthcare Interoperability Resources standards: Application in Otolaryngology

Health Level Seven International (HL7) Fast Healthcare Interoperability Resources (FHIR) standards are a modern framework designed to efficiently exchange and use electronic health data.[14–16] Specifically, HL7 is a set of international standards for exchanging, integrating, sharing, and retrieving electronic health information, aiming to enhance clinical practice and managing, delivering, and evaluating health services. FHIR combines the best features of HL7's previous standards with the latest web standards, including a strong focus on ease of implementation, flexibility, and interoperability.[15] FHIR is built on modular components called "resources," which can be combined to solve clinical and administrative problems practically and agilely.

In otolaryngology, applying HL7 FHIR standards holds promise for integrating diverse health care data. This interoperability is particularly important given the complexity of data in otolaryngology, which spans patient-level data, detailed surgical information, and diverse clinical outcomes. Implementing HL7 FHIR standards facilitates several key improvements; principally, it enables the efficient sharing of detailed clinical data among various health care providers.[17]

However, adopting HL7 FHIR standards presents specific challenges. One significant challenge is adapting these standards to effectively represent the unique data types associated with ear, nose, and throat examinations and treatments. This may involve developing otolaryngology-specific functionality (eg, custom resources or fields) in FHIR or modifying existing ones within the FHIR framework. Additionally, the widespread adoption of HL7 FHIR standards faces hurdles related to the varied technical capabilities and resources of different health care systems. Furthermore, as with any data medium, maintaining data privacy and security in compliance with relevant regulations is a consideration.

Challenges of Integrating Machine Learning Systems into Existing Clinical Workflows in Otolaryngology

Integrating ML systems into the existing clinical workflows in otolaryngology presents distinct challenges. The primary issue is ensuring compatibility with current EHRs. EHRs are central to clinical data management, and ML systems must seamlessly interface with these systems. Another challenge is aligning the outputs of ML algorithms with existing clinical protocols. These algorithms must provide accurate but also interpretable and actionable predictions for human clinicians within existing best clinical practices.

To successfully integrate ML systems into otolaryngology workflows, the following strategies are essential:

1. *Interoperability with EHR systems*: The development of ML systems that can exchange data effectively with EHRs is important. Adhering to interoperability standards like HL7 FHIR can facilitate this integration.
2. *Alignment with clinical protocols*: Ensuring that the ML systems support and enhance human clinical decision-making is essential. This requires a collaborative approach between clinicians and those developing the AI models (eg, data scientists and ML engineers) to ensure that ML outputs are contextually relevant and applicable to existing clinical protocols.

Integrating ML into otolaryngology's clinical workflows involves overcoming challenges related to EHR compatibility and protocol alignment. However, with the right strategies and learnings from successful case studies, ML can be effectively integrated, enhancing both the efficiency and the quality of patient care.

Considerations for Moving Artificial Intelligence Models to Production in Otolaryngology

The transition of AI models to full-scale production requires careful consideration of scalability, data security, regulatory compliance, customization to specialty-specific needs, and collaboration among various stakeholders. Addressing these factors is crucial for AI's successful and sustainable implementation in otolaryngology.

1. Scalability: Scalability is a key consideration in transitioning AI models to production. The models developed during pilot phases must handle an increased volume of data and users without performance degradation. Scalability ensures that the AI system remains efficient and effective as it is expanded to larger patient populations and more complex data sets.
2. Data security: Given the sensitivity of medical data, which often includes high-resolution imaging and detailed patient information, ensuring robust data security measures is paramount. This involves implementing advanced encryption methods and secure data access protocols to protect patient data from unauthorized access and breaches.
3. Regulatory compliance: Compliance with health care regulations such as HIPAA in the United States and GDPR in Europe is necessary. AI models must adhere to best practices for trustworthy AI/ML to protect patient privacy and data. They are incorporating regulatory requirements into designing and implementing AI models to avoid legal and ethical issues.

Moreover, collaboration between clinicians, engineers, data scientists, regulators, and ethicists is vital to ensure AI models' practical applicability and usability. Multidisciplinary collaboration facilitates the development of AI solutions that are not only technically sound but also clinically relevant and user-friendly. Such collaboration ensures that the AI models developed align with clinical needs and can be seamlessly integrated into clinical workflows.

Artificial Intelligence Performance Monitoring: Continuous Testing and Validation

Continuous testing and validation ensure the accuracy and reliability of ML models. The dynamic nature of clinical data and evolving medical practices necessitates a thoughtful approach to maintain the effectiveness of these models.

The ongoing testing and validation of ML models are essential for making informed clinical decisions. Regular testing ensures that the models adapt to the changing landscape of patient data and treatment protocols. Implementing continuous testing involves methods like real-time monitoring and periodic re-evaluation against new data sets. Real-time monitoring assesses the model's performance in clinical settings, offering immediate insights into its effectiveness. Periodic re-evaluation against new data is crucial to ensure the model's relevance and accuracy as new patient data and clinical knowledge become available.

Addressing the challenges of data drift and model degradation over time is another critical aspect of maintaining ML models. Data drift refers to the changes in new data characteristics compared to the training data, potentially reducing model accuracy.[18] Model degradation occurs when the performance of an ML model declines due to shifts in underlying data patterns or clinical practices. Strategies are needed to identify and address data drift and model degradation promptly. These strategies include updating the model with new data, refining algorithms, and retraining the model to adapt to significant changes.[19]

Another aspect of performance monitoring is addressing and mitigating errors and biases in ML models. Inherent biases in training data or algorithmic errors can lead to inaccurate predictions or recommendations, adversely affecting patient care. For instance, an algorithm for detecting skin cancer trained primarily on light skin tones may misdiagnose or overlook conditions in patients with darker skin, potentially leading to delayed treatment and worse outcomes. This illustrates the impact of ensuring that diverse training data are used in health care AI model development. Practitioners and developers must maintain a high suspicion index and continuously scrutinize ML models to identify and correct biases or errors. Scrutiny in this context includes reviewing the data sources, algorithms, and outcomes to ensure that the models provide fair and accurate predictions across diverse patient populations.

Ethical Considerations and Patient Consent

Integrating ML in otolaryngology raises significant ethical considerations, particularly concerning patient care. These considerations revolve around transparency, patient autonomy, and informed consent.

The use of ML in patient care necessitates a high level of transparency. Patients and clinicians must understand how ML models make predictions or recommendations. This transparency is crucial for maintaining trust and ensuring that clinical decisions are made with a clear understanding of the ML model's role. Additionally, patient autonomy must be respected. Decisions influenced by ML should be made with the patient's knowledge and agreement, ensuring their autonomy is preserved in the decision-making process.[20]

Obtaining informed consent is a critical best practice when implementing ML-driven diagnostic or therapeutic approaches. This involves clearly explaining to patients how ML is used in their care, what data are used, and the potential benefits and risks of ML-driven decisions. Informed consent should include a discussion about the accuracy and limitations of ML models, allowing patients to make well-informed decisions about their care.[20] Obtaining informed consent for ML applications should be an ongoing conversation rather than a one-time event. As ML models are updated or their role in patient care evolves, patients should be informed and their consent reaffirmed.

Ethical considerations and patient consent in using ML in otolaryngology are fundamental to ensuring that these advanced technologies are used responsibly and with respect for patient rights. By prioritizing transparency, respecting patient autonomy, and adhering to best practices for informed consent, health care providers can ethically integrate ML into patient care.

Training and Education for Clinical Staff

The successful implementation of ML in otolaryngology depends not only on the technology's sophistication but also on the training and education of clinical staff. Ensuring clinicians and support staff are well equipped to use and understand ML tools is fundamental for effectively applying these technologies in patient care.

Training programs for clinicians and support staff are essential to facilitate the effective use of ML tools in otolaryngology. These programs should focus on enhancing understanding of how ML algorithms function, how they are applied in clinical settings, and how to interpret their outputs. Such training ensures that staff can operate these tools efficiently and integrate ML insights into clinical decision-making processes.

The complexity of ML applications in otolaryngology demands an interdisciplinary approach to training. This means developing modules that cover both the technical aspects of ML (like data analysis and algorithm functionality) and their clinical applications (such as diagnostic procedures and treatment planning). By doing so, clinicians can better understand the capabilities and limitations of ML tools, leading to more informed and effective use in patient care.

Interdisciplinary training should be an ongoing process, adapting to the evolving nature of ML technologies and the changing landscape of medical knowledge. Continuous education ensures that clinical staff remain updated on the latest developments and best practices.

The "AI Ready" Otolaryngology Enterprise: Artificial Intelligence Governance

The "AI Ready" otolaryngology enterprises must establish checkpoints regularly to oversee AI systems used in patient care and research. Governing AI within health care is a multi-stakeholder effort focused on ensuring the development of fair, interpretable, and inclusive AI solutions.

At both national and institutional levels, leaders within otolaryngology must define guidelines for developing, deploying, and monitoring AI systems. These might include rules for ideal reporting of AI methodology in otolaryngology research,[21] recommendations for informed consent regarding the use of AI tools in care,[20] standardized methods for safe data acquisition, and recommended schedules and resources for routine AI system maintenance.

Clinicians will play an integral and critical role in this governance process within the "AI Ready" enterprise. As the first checkpoint in assuring data integrity, providers must carefully guide the collection of organized, meaningful, and task-appropriate data. They must communicate with developers and IT staff to define the clinical context in which AI solutions are employed appropriately and monitor that tools perform their intended task. While perhaps at the center of safe and effective AI utilization, clinicians cannot and should not do this alone. Administration and institutional leadership should be trained to oversee AI systems and involve individuals with appropriate IT expertise in governance processes.

Infrastructure and Resource Allocation

Prioritizing the upgrade of IT infrastructure is essential for the safe and effective implementation of AI in clinical care. This includes enhancing hardware and software capabilities tailored to support AI applications. Otolaryngology stakeholders should consider strategic budgeting, resource allocation, and novel funding sources to support acquiring local and cloud computing and storage resources needed to develop and deploy AI models.

COLLABORATIONS AND PARTNERSHIPS FOR ARTIFICIAL INTELLIGENCE ADVANCEMENT

Collaborations between academic institutions, technology companies, and other health care organizations hold promise for catalyzing AI development. Otolaryngologists should consider internally hiring IT and computer science experts or seek partnerships with these entities to realize their AI development goals. For academic-based otolaryngology practices, collaborations with internal computer science departments are a low-barrier option for partnership. Several universities have created formal collaborations between medical and computer science departments. Examples include the Partnership in AI-Assisted Care At Stanford (https://med.stanford.edu/content/sm/pacresearch.html.html), the Center for Machine Learning and Health at the University of Pittsburgh Medical Center and Carnegie Melon (https://www.cs.cmu.edu/cmlh/), and the Windreich Department of Artificial Intelligence and Human Health at the Icahn School of Medicine (https://icahn.mssm.edu/about/departments/ai-human-health). These types of collaboration are designed to align the specialized knowledge and resources needed to integrate and utilize AI technologies in health care settings effectively.

Measuring Success and Impact

As novel AI approaches are incorporated into clinical practice, we must develop associated processes for evaluating clinical utility. AI solutions intended for patient care should be scrutinized within the established paradigms of clinical outcome metrics, patient-reported outcomes, and patient satisfaction. Alternatively, models intended to increase clinical efficiency, rather than to be directly involved in patient care, should be regularly assessed in their ability to complete their intended task. Benchmarking AI solutions against other industry standards is needed to ensure clinical AI remains robust and current. Formal audit services may be employed, internally and externally, to carry out routine AI maintenance and safeguard against inappropriate use of AI.

SUMMARY

Integrating AI and ML in otolaryngology presents a transformative opportunity for patient care, requiring careful consideration of data management, security, and ethical practices. Successful implementation hinges on interdisciplinary collaboration, continuous innovation, and adherence to regulatory standards, ensuring these technologies enhance clinical outcomes and patient experiences in otolaryngology.

REFERENCES

1. You E, Lin V, Mijovic T, et al. Artificial intelligence applications in otology: a state of the art review. Otolaryngol Neck Surg 2020;163(6):1123–33.
2. Tama BA, Kim DH, Kim G, et al. Recent advances in the application of artificial intelligence in otorhinolaryngology-head and neck surgery. Clin Exp Otorhinolaryngol 2020;13(4):326–39.
3. Bur AM, Shew M, New J. Artificial intelligence for the otolaryngologist: a state of the art review. Otolaryngol–Head Neck 2019;160(4):603–11.
4. Crowson MG, Ranisau J, Eskander A, et al. A contemporary review of machine learning in otolaryngology–head and neck surgery. Laryngoscope 2020;130(1): 45–51.
5. Tahmassebi A, Ehtemami A, Mohebali B, et al. Big data analytics in medical imaging using deep learning. In: Ahmad F, editor. Big data learn anal appl. 2019. p. 13. https://doi.org/10.1117/12.2516014. Published online May 13.
6. Hulsen T. Sharing is caring-data sharing initiatives in healthcare. Int J Environ Res Public Health 2020;17(9):3046.
7. de Mello BH, Rigo SJ, da Costa CA, et al. Semantic interoperability in health records standards: a systematic literature review. Health Technol 2022;12(2): 255–72.
8. Corey KM, Helmkamp J, Simons M, et al. Assessing quality of surgical real-world data from an automated electronic health record pipeline. J Am Coll Surg 2020; 230(3):295–305.e12.
9. Wang M, Sushil M, Miao BY, et al. Bottom-up and top-down paradigms of artificial intelligence research approaches to healthcare data science using growing real-world big data. J Am Med Inf Assoc 2023;30(7):1323–32.
10. Ehrenstein V, Kharrazi H, Lehmann H, et al. Obtaining data from electronic health records. In: Tools and technologies for registry interoperability, registries for evaluating patient outcomes: a user's guide, 3rd edition, addendum 2 [internet]. Agency for Healthcare Research and Quality (US); 2019. Available at: https://www.ncbi.nlm.nih.gov/books/NBK551878/. [Accessed 27 January 2024].
11. Li E, Clarke J, Ashrafian H, et al. The impact of electronic health record interoperability on safety and quality of care in high-income countries: systematic review. J Med Internet Res 2022;24(9):e38144.

12. Johnson AL, Bouvette M, Rangu N, et al. Data-sharing across otolaryngology: comparing journal policies and their adherence to the FAIR principles. Ann Otol Rhinol Laryngol 2024;133(1):105–10.
13. Eckert MA, Husain FT, Jayakody D, et al. An opportunity for constructing the future of data sharing in otolaryngology. JARO J Assoc Res Otolaryngol 2023; 24(4):397–9.
14. Saripalle R, Runyan C, Russell M. Using HL7 FHIR to achieve interoperability in patient health record. J Biomed Inf 2019;94:103188.
15. Ayaz M, Pasha MF, Alzahrani MY, et al. The fast health interoperability resources (fhir) standard: systematic literature review of implementations, applications, challenges and opportunities. JMIR Med Inform 2021;9(7):e21929.
16. Vorisek CN, Lehne M, Klopfenstein SAI, et al. Fast healthcare interoperability resources (FHIR) for Interoperability in Health Research: Systematic Review. JMIR Med Inform 2022;10(7):e35724.
17. Liu TJ, Lee HT, Wu F. Building an electronic medical record system exchanged in FHIR format and its visual presentation. Healthc Basel Switz 2023;11(17):2410.
18. Nelson K, Corbin G, Anania M, et al. Evaluating model drift in machine learning algorithms. IEEE; 2015. p. 1–8. https://ieeexplore.ieee.org/document/7208643.
19. Sahiner B, Chen W, Samala RK, et al. Data drift in medical machine learning: implications and potential remedies. Br J Radiol 2023;96(1150):20220878.
20. Cohen IG. Informed consent and medical artificial intelligence: what to tell the patient? SSRN Electron J 2020. https://doi.org/10.2139/ssrn.3529576.
21. Crowson MG, Rameau A. Standardizing machine learning manuscript reporting in otolaryngology-head & neck surgery. Laryngoscope 2022;132(9):1698–700.

Standardization, Collaboration, and Education in the Implementation of Artificial Intelligence in Otolaryngology
The Key to Scalable Impact

Emily Evangelista, MS[a], Yael Bensoussan, MD, MSc[b],*

KEYWORDS

- Artificial intelligence • Otolaryngology • Collaborative science • Standardization
- Education

KEY POINTS

- Collaboration between academia and industry is essential for scalable and impactful artificial intelligence (AI) implementation in otolaryngology.
- Standardization of AI projects through system reporting and education of practitioners are crucial for responsible AI adoption.
- Academic–industry partnerships can enhance resources and accelerate clinical implementation of AI innovations.
- Multi-institutional collaborations and interdisciplinary teams are vital for overcoming current barriers and advancing AI in otolaryngology.
- Integration of AI into medical education is imperative for continued progress and effective use of AI tools in clinical practice.

INTRODUCTION

"Big data" is a term often used to describe the massively expansive data sets that are necessary for computational artificial intelligence (AI) analysis to reveal patterns, trends, anomalies, and associations.[1] For machine learning (ML) models to be accurate, scalable, and impactful in health care, large amounts of quality data are needed.

[a] Morsani College of Medicine, University of South Florida, Yael Bensoussan and Emily Evangelista, 13330 USF Laurel Drive, Morsani Health, Tampa, FL 33612, USA; [b] Department of Otolaryngology – Head & Neck Surgery, University of South Florida, 13330 USF Laurel Drive, Tampa, FL 33612, USA
* Corresponding author.
E-mail address: yaelbensoussan@usf.edu

Otolaryngol Clin N Am 57 (2024) 897–908
https://doi.org/10.1016/j.otc.2024.04.005
0030-6665/24/Published by Elsevier Inc.

oto.theclinics.com

Big data is generally assessed on 5 qualities[2]:

1. Variability—data within a range of structure, consistency, and contexts.
2. Variety—data in multiple formats (audio, images, and numerical, text) from multiple sources.
3. Velocity—high-speed transmission of data with real-time processing.
4. Veracity—accuracy of data, minimal noise, and uncertainty.
5. Volume—extremely large data sets.

Volume, the last of the "5 Vs," relates overwhelmingly to the statistical replicability, generalizability, and accuracy of AI-generated experimental conclusions.[3,4] Larger datasets help compensate for shortcomings in other characteristics without normalizing or transforming raw data. Smaller sample sizes predispose analysis to flaws that prevent them from being clinically useful, such as overfitting, poor generalizability, biases, or appreciation of rare events.[5]

Publicly available databases that are large enough to be utilized can, in theory, contain data from a variety of sources, not only adding needed volume but also enriching dataset diversity. These sources include commercial, institutional, large-payer, geographic, population-based (statewide, nationwide, and international) registries, state and government administrative databases, and research-based databases.[5]

Otolaryngology is, in part, well suited for AI due to the various instruments utilized for assessment, as medical imagery is a notable natural avenue with big data for AI implementation.[6] AI is already being investigated concerning a wide variety of otolaryngologic diseases. Regarding the communication sciences, applications have been utilized in minimizing the hearing-in-noise problem of cochlear implants and hearing aids, developing AI-driven speech neuroprostheses, analyzing medical imaging, and even classifying and identifying laryngeal lesions using deep learning.[7] Numerous AI techniques are also used for voice-based analysis for early detection, diagnosis and monitoring of disease, optimization of hearing aid performance, and even voice restoration.[6]

Despite the exponential rise in publications and applications of AI in otolaryngology, more collaborative multi-institutional and industry collaborations still need to be improved and needed to produce impactful and scalable results. To build impactful AI models and AI-based solutions and fuel discovery, larger datasets that are standardized need to be developed through multi-institutional collaborations. Moreover, for AI-based solutions to be transferrable to the health care setting and have a broad impact on patient care, industry partners need to be involved as they are experts in market research, business development, and commercially viable solutions.

The purpose of this article is to address interacademic and academic–industry collaborations, standardization of AI projects, system reporting for peer-reviewed publications and AI system performance, and AI education and literacy in the field of otolaryngology and to discuss their potential impact on scalable integration of AI and ML in our field.

CURRENT BARRIERS OF INTEGRATION OF ARTIFICIAL INTELLIGENCE-BASED SOLUTIONS IN OTOLARYNGOLOGY
Siloed Work in Academia

Due to the current academic setting, generating large, diverse databases to train scalable ML models needs collaboration for voluminous data procurement. Of the otolaryngology AI articles reviewed for this article, many reported the robustness of datasets as a limitation to their work.[8–12] Both the small number of available datasets and the limited ability to build voluminous datasets contributed to this claim. Despite this, very few collaborations exist between otolaryngology stakeholders concerning AI advancement and database building.

Another barrier limiting collaboration is that sharing data across multiple institutions or regulatory jurisdictions poses a challenge due to a lack of standardization of sharing practices.[13] A survey of laryngologists performed in 2022 reported disparate regulatory models for inter-institution patient-data sharing in the academic setting.[14]

Moreover, important aspects of data sharing between institutions still lack standardization and are often accompanied by significant administrative burden.

A. Data sharing agreements that require drafting and institutional approval.
B. Clear discernment of data ownership.
C. Informed consents that include data sharing policies.
D. Careful examination of data to minimize risk of reidentification with sharing.

Otolaryngology clinicians are often unfamiliar with these issues, which involve significant administrative research support and are challenging to attend to in busy clinical practices, limiting collaboration between clinical researchers.

Sparse Academic–Industrial Partnerships

A study analyzing the monetary cost of nonreproducible science discerned that as much as 80% of all results of projects undertaken at academic institutions have been reported as nonreproducible in an industry setting.[15,16] This surprising percentage is hypothesized to be a result of multiple challenges. First, academic research is often performed independently of collaboration with industry due to goals and research interests based on different incentives.[15] Moreover, we have historically seen AI-related research being conducted in single-institution or single-geographical location settings, resulting in small databases with poor diversity. Institutional data ownership regulations can also be limiting and prevent use by the broader population of researchers or specify that the institutional data are not available for commercial intent.

SOLUTIONS FOR MORE IMPACTFUL AND SCALABLE ARTIFICIAL INTELLIGENCE IN OTOLARYNGOLOGY
Choosing the Right Team Members for Impactful Implementation of Solutions

Broad implementation of ML models in clinical otolaryngology practice needs the input and collaboration of stakeholders from different backgrounds. **Table 1** describes important stakeholders to consider when building a collaborative team.

Aligning Incentives and Measuring Impact of Collaborations

Each party involved in collaboration has independent priorities within a main shared goal. Therefore, generalized determination of success must include wide-reaching goals that are reflective of the wishes of all partnership members (**Box 1**).

DEFINITION AND SIGNIFICANCE OF DIFFERENT TYPES OF COLLABORATIONS

There are significant shortcomings of each individual sector involved in otolaryngologic research. As such, structured, well-defined, appropriately regulated collaborations between universities and businesses may enhance resources, break down barriers, and lead to accelerated clinical implementation of innovation. These academic–industry partnerships (AIPs) can be defined as mutually beneficial resource-sharing relationships between industry and academia with the shared goal of bringing innovation to the clinical market. **Table 2** demonstrates a few examples of collaborations in otolaryngology.

Table 1
Stakeholders regarding otolaryngology artificial intelligence collaboration

Stakeholders	Description
Clinicians	Otolaryngologists, speech language pathologists, have insight into their patient population, disease physiopathology, strengths and limitations of their institution's capabilities, and clinical relevance and workflow applicability of certain technological ideations.
Clinician-scientists/ researchers	Academic researchers are valuable partners due to their knowledge in methodology design, science implementation.
Bioinformaticians/data scientists	Data science and ML experts will help develop AI solutions that are accurate and reproducible, by partnering with clinicians.
Industry partners	Professionals in biotechnological and pharmaceutical spaces are useful partners to weigh in on financial and outcome expectations, market viability of developed products or solutions, resource and manufacturing abilities, personnel needs, and partnership goals.
Patients and patient advocacy groups	Patient and patient advocacy groups allow for intentional creational processes with the highest utility to end users. They can advocate for real patient needs, safety and privacy concerns, and usability of certain AI technologies.
Regulatory officials	Involving regulatory professionals from the inception of ideas will allow for thoughtful integration with current regulatory requirements and more thoughtful adaptations for new technologies.
Bioethicists	As AI is a new frontier and requires bold innovation, this must be balanced with calculated use of sensitive patient data to facilitate moral and social stewardship over medical AI.

Multi-institutional Collaborations

Multi-institutional collaborations involve teams from multiple universities that may be in different geographic locations. This allows for data diversity in terms of patient population, demographics, and reduces bias due to data homogeneity.

Multidisciplinary Collaborations

Multidisciplinary collaborations can happen within a single institution or in a multi-institutional setting and involve stakeholders from different background including medicine, bioinformatics, and ethics among other.

Box 1
Examples of metrics of success of collaborations

1. Implementation of AI-based solutions into clinical practice.

2. Development of Food and Drug Administration-approved products/solutions.

3. Commercialization of AI-based solutions.

4. Peer-reviewed article publication.

5. Patient outcomes.

6. System efficiency.

Table 2
Examples of collaborative groups in otolaryngology

Name	Description
Bridge2AI - Voice[21]	This consortium aims to integrate the use of voice as biomarker of health in clinical care by generating a substantial multi-institutional, ethically sourced, and diverse voice database linked to multimodal health biomarkers to fuel voice AI research and build predictive models to assist in screening, diagnosis, and treatment of a broad range of diseases.
North American Airway Collaborative (NoAAC)[22]	The NoAAC exists to develop and exchange information concerning the treatment of adult airway disease. It is an international, voluntary, multi-disciplinary group of surgeons, pulmonologists, patient representatives, and a data center who seek to improve continuously the quality, safety, effectiveness, and cost of medical interventions in adult airway disorders.
The Vocal Cord Paralysis Experience (CoPE) Collaborative[23]	The CoPE Collaborative is a multi-institutional collaborative composed of laryngologists from 34 tertiary care institutions across the United States that treat unilateral vocal fold paralysis.

Consortiums

The National Cancer Institute defines a consortium as a group of scientists from multiple institutions who have agreed to participate in cooperative research efforts involving activities such as methods development and validation, pooling of information from more than one study for the purpose of combined analyses, and collaborative projects.[17] Consortiums usually involve multidisciplinary and multi-institutional teams that work together on complex challenges over a significant period of time.

Academic–Industry Partnerships

AIPs are important alliances between academia and industry that help more effectively translate technology to the clinical setting and complete the innovation cycle.[18] AIPs function to lower the barriers to implementation of marketable technology and offer translational research funding.[19]

These partnerships allow the companies involved access to highly qualified researchers and learners, while allowing these researchers access to expensive and time-consuming research and development pipelines.[20] Additionally, AIPs allow for early trainee exposure to innovations and opportunities for continuing education.[20]

IMPORTANCE OF ACADEMIC–INDUSTRY PARTNERSHIPS

As much as 10% of all new medical products/processes to market are secondary to contributions made by academia.[24] Academic projects receiving funding from for-profit companies have traditionally received criticism secondary to potential biases and prior misbehavior by both investigators and companies.[25–27] Though it has been proposed that the nature of the ever-evolving digital era is encouraging greater collaboration between medical practitioners and marketplace stakeholders.[18] Today, government agencies such as the National Institutes of Health (NIH) is encouraging partnerships between the public and private sectors to enhance efficient scientific discovery.[28]

Limitations of Academic Work

There are some obvious benefits to working within an academic setting. By nature, clinical academic patients have more robust access to patients.[7] Additionally, the rigorous and systematic regulatory requirements, such as Insitutional Review Board (IRB) processes, may suggest better patient safety than would be customary in purely industry settings. As academic teams are customarily composed of physicians and other health care practitioners that have recited oaths promising to uphold the principles of beneficence and nonmaleficence, these institutions typically hold more stringent ethical perspectives. Additionally, such multidisciplinary teams are more readily available in academia, adding to diversity of perspective and skillset.

However, with the privilege of greater patient access, comes high levels of administrative burden. This burden exists due to the aforementioned rigorous review process and high-integrity ethical considerations.[29] Many institutions also have differing opinions on data ownership and data sharing agreements between partners, with no legal or regulatory consensus.[30] These disparities in views can lead to bulky processes related to access and collaboration, slowing the process and adding to resource consumption.

Administrative Delays in Extramural Funding

Academic research can be unfunded, funded by intramural or extramural funding. Intramural funding pertains to institutional grants and are often of smaller financial amounts. Extramural funding includes government funding coming from various government agencies and grant mechanisms, foundation funding, and industry funding. Government-funded agencies have different grant mechanisms that are often very competitive. The 2022 report from the NIH's research project grants applications showed a 20.7% rate of funded projects compared to applications.[31] Moreover, the deadline for award funding from submission can take 8 to 20 months, representing a significant barrier to the completed work.[31] Industry funding usually arrives much quicker, with less administrative barrier.

Limitations of Industry/Pharma Work

While industry has the capital to fund clinical research without the resource constraints present in academia, the goals and expectations for outcomes may differ from what is historically acceptable in the academic realm. The motivation for research may be centered around financial return to investors rather than patient impact.

Additionally, due to medicine's history of biased research, industry players often must rely on partnerships with trusted institutions and medical professionals to gain access to the breadth of patients necessary for robust research trials.

STANDARDIZING ARTIFICIAL INTELLIGENCE PROJECTS THROUGH SYSTEM REPORTING

Explainability is one of the most heavily debated aspects of AI in health care, opening a labyrinth of medical, ethical, legal, and technological questions. Deep learning tools are often considered "black box" systems. The "black box" or explainability problem relates to the inability to explicitly state how internal mechanisms of AI tools determine a given solution.[32] The explainability problem thus creates a dilemma for reproducibility and reliability of results. How, without precise and reproducible methods, are physicians and scientists to trust these systems? Reporting results for ML publications should include details about the training datasets including detailed demographics, methodology of data collection and data preparation, and explicit models

Table 3
Artificial intelligence performance reporting guidelines

Reporting Guidelines	Study Type (Stage)	AI Intervention	Algorithm Version and Modifications[a]	Intended Use of AI	Input Training Data[b]	Human Factors/ Interaction	Output and AI Contribution	AI Evaluation/ Validation	Performance Errors[c]	Limits of AI	Ethics/ Fairness	Generalizability	Safety Profile/ Risks	Data Availability	Explainability
								Recommended AI-specific Parameters							
CONSORT-AI[34,35]	RCT (phase 3)	Y	Y	Y	Y	Y	Y	—	Y	Y	—	Y	Y	—	—
SPIRIT-AI[34]	RCT	Y	Y	Y	Y	Y	Y	—	Y	Y	—	Y	Y	—	—
STARD-AI[36]	Diagnostic accuracy	Y	Y	Y	Y	Y	—	Y	Y	—	Y	—	—	—	Y
CLAIM[37]	Imaging AI	Y	Y	Y	Y	—	—	Y	Y	Y	—	Y	—	—	Y
MI-CLAIM[38]	Diagnostic accuracy	Y	Y	Y	Y	—	—	Y	Y	—	Y	—	Y	Y	—
MINIMAR[39]	Diagnostic accuracy	Y	Y	Y	Y	Y	Y	—	Y	—	Y	—	—	Y	—
DECIDE-AI[40]	Early clinical evaluation	Y	Y	Y	Y	Y	Y	Y	—	—	Y	—	—	—	—
TRIPOD-AI[41]	Prediction study	Development in progress													

a Setting of integration, input/output handling, human–AI interaction, provision of analysis of error cases.
b Where it was collected, how it was selected, processed, handled, how missingness was accounted for, the output, eligibility criteria at the level of the participant, and input data.
c Result of any performance errors, how they were identified, if no error analysis performed.

trained to ensure reproducibility of the results, accuracy of the models, and avoidance of bias.

Furthermore, a main barrier to successful AI/ML implementation that has been reported include the need for standardized methodological performance reporting.[33] Reporting guidelines are structured tools developed using explicit methodology that specify the minimum information required by researchers when reporting a study.[34] Reporting guidelines are important as they can address potential bias sources, allow for transparency and reproducibility and this verifiability of AI-driven results. A number of experts have created parallel recommendations for reporting.[34] The guidelines reported in the literature are demonstrated in **Table 3**.

ARTIFICIAL INTELLIGENCE EDUCATION AND LITERACY

As AI remains at the forefront of academia, industry, and media headlines, its potential to revolutionize patient care needs to be improved by misconceptions and a lack of knowledge of what AI is and how it is to be applied to otolaryngology.[42] Otolaryngology trainees and professionals are important stakeholders who need to be educated in novel technologies to shape the way they are utilized for the greatest clinical benefit.

In a 2023 survey of otolaryngology practitioners, only 8% of respondents reported having AI training in residency, though 72% had familiarity with general AI concepts; no respondents had personal experience with AI in clinical settings.[43]

When assessed with the otolaryngology residency in-service examination, ChatGPT (a generative AT chatBot) demonstrated a correct answer rate of 53%.[44] Demonstrating that while AI has great promise in otolaryngology, it must be thoroughly questioned by medical professionals before acceptance of results. Critical appraisal of the validity of AI tools requires a level of technical literacy in order to foster responsible AI adoption that is methodologically sound. This level of understanding is also necessary for discernment of appropriate generalizability and application of AI outputs. It is difficult to discern whether a certain instrument will be accurate for your use case without comprehension of its mechanisms.

Many subspecialties are implementing specialty-specific entrustable professional activities (EPAs).[45] An avenue for exploration of enhancement of AI education could be the facilitation of AI-specific, otolaryngology-specific EPAs.

Additionally, the landscape of surgical training is rapidly evolving to integrate AI into education and simulation.[46] For example, *Theator* is a video-based surgical feedback tool that uses computer vision AI technology to analyze videos of the surgical performances of trainees. It can annotate critical moments and key steps during procedures and compares performance against established benchmarks, allowing for objectivity and personalization similar to what an athlete experiences during a film review.

SUMMARY

Soon, it is exceedingly likely that AI will revolutionize the intricacies of the practice of otolaryngology. To ensure that AI lives up to its hype, AI engineers, physicians, and regulatory and legislative officials must collaborate to standardize the knowledge base surrounding the uses and limitations of otolaryngologic AI tools.

Otolaryngologists are instrumental to the assurance of meaningful clinical integration of AI technologies that will safely and effectively improve patient care. As such, specialists should work collaboratively with a variety of stakeholders in different sectors to maximize resources and propel AI integration into otolaryngology. Though it is imperative to adapt to the growing breadth of AI applications in the field, physicians must be critical in their appraisal and adoption of such technologies, as to protect the trust in the medical innovation process.

High-quality, high-volume data collection is essential for the development of accurate AI algorithms. As such, efforts to build such databases and algorithms should be distributed over the collective otolaryngology community. Not only would this allow for swift progress but also infuse diversity of perspective, expand applicable patient populations, and increase data richness.

AI has been thought to chip away at the patient–physician relationship, to threaten the status of physicians in certain specialties.[47] Though as Dr Aaron Moberly of Vanderbilt's department of head and neck surgery so plainly stated, "AI's role is not to replace physicians, but to augment our abilities."[47] In order to do so, otolaryngologists should seek opportunities to collaborate with clinical teams, statisticians, engineers, and patients to guide them toward significant answers for important clinical questions.

CLINICS CARE POINTS

- Critically evaluate any AI tool you plan to use.
- Collaborate with a team of diverse professionals to enhance success.
- Integration into medical and continuing education is imperative to continued progress and savvy use of AI.

DISCLOSURE

Y. Bensoussan is funded by the National Institutes of Health, United States through the Common Fund for the project "Voice as a biomarker of Health." Award number: 3OT2OD032720-01S1. E. Evangelista has no disclosures.

REFERENCES

1. Baro E, Degoul S, Beuscart R, et al. Toward a literature-driven definition of big data in healthcare. BioMed Res Int 2015;2015:1–9.
2. Benke K, Benke G. Artificial intelligence and big data in public health. Int J Environ Res Publ Health 2018;15(12):2796.
3. Isbmda Aveiro P, Author IC. On sample size and classification accuracy: a performance comparison. Biological and Medical Data Analysis 2005;3745: 193–201.
4. Rahman MS, Sultana M. Performance of firth-and logf-type penalized methods in risk prediction for small or sparse binary data. BMC Med Res Methodol 2017; 17(1). https://doi.org/10.1186/s12874-017-0313-9.
5. Kunze KN, Williams RJ, Ranawat AS, et al. Artificial intelligence (AI) and large data registries: Understanding the advantages and limitations of contemporary data sets for use in AI research. Knee Surg Sports Traumatol Arthrosc 2024; 32(1):13–8.
6. Tama BA, Kim DH, Kim G, et al. Recent advances in the application of artificial intelligence in otorhinolaryngology-head and neck surgery. Clinical and Experimental Otorhinolaryngology 2020;13(4):326–39.
7. Wilson BS, Tucci DL, Moses DA, et al. Harnessing the power of artificial intelligence in otolaryngology and the communication sciences. Journal of the Association for Research in Otolaryngology 2022;23(3):319–49.

8. Wolff J, Pauling J, Keck A, et al. Success factors of artificial intelligence implementation in healthcare. Frontiers in Digital Health 2021;3. https://doi.org/10.3389/fdgth.2021.594971.

9. Yao P, Usman M, Chen YH, et al. Applications of artificial intelligence to office laryngoscopy: a scoping review. Laryngoscope 2022;132(10):1993–2016.

10. Ren J, Jing X, Wang J, et al. Automatic recognition of laryngoscopic images using a deep-learning technique. Laryngoscope 2020;130(11). https://doi.org/10.1002/lary.28539.

11. Crowson MG, Dixon P, Mahmood R, et al. Predicting postoperative cochlear implant performance using supervised machine learning. Otol Neurotol 2020;41(8):e1013–23.

12. Goldstein CA, Berry RB, Kent DT, et al. Artificial intelligence in sleep medicine: background and implications for clinicians. J Clin Sleep Med 2020;16(4):609–18.

13. Fang C, Dziedzic A, Zhang L, et al. Decentralised, collaborative, and privacy-preserving machine learning for multi-hospital data. EBioMedicine 2024;101:105006.

14. Evangelista E, Kale R, Mccutcheon D, et al. Current practices in voice data collection and limitations to voice <scp>AI</scp> research: a national survey. Laryngoscope 2023. https://doi.org/10.1002/lary.31052.

15. Levin LA, Behar-Cohen F. The academic-industrial complexity: failure to launch. Trends Pharmacol Sci 2017;38(12):1052–60.

16. Freedman S, Mullane K. The academic–industrial complex: navigating the translational and cultural divide. Drug Discov Today 2017;22(7):976–93.

17. NCI. Consortia to advance collaboration in epidemiologic and cancer research, 2023, NIH National Cancer Institute, Center for biomedical informatics and information technology.

18. Ankrah S, Omar ALT. Universities–industry collaboration: A systematic review. Scand J Manag 2015;31(3):387–408.

19. Pantanowitz L, Bui MM, Chauhan C, et al. Rules of engagement: promoting academic-industry partnership in the era of digital pathology and artificial intelligence. Academic Pathology 2022;9(1):100026.

20. Rybnicek R, Königsgruber R. What makes industry–university collaboration succeed? A systematic review of the literature. J Bus Econ 2019;89(2):221–50.

21. Bridge2AI-Voice. Bidge2AI-Voice. Available at: www.b2ai-voice.org.

22. Gelbard A, Kinnard C. North American Airway Collaborative (NOAAC). Available at: https://noaac.net/.

23. Collaborative C. Vocal Cord Paralysis Experiment. 2024.

24. Rudi B, Isabel M. Analysing knowledge transfer channels between universities and industry: To what degree do sectors also matter? Res Pol 2008;37(10):1837–53.

25. Campbell EG. Doctors and drug companies — scrutinizing influential relationships. N Engl J Med 2007;357(18):1796–7.

26. Relman AS. The new medical-industrial complex. N Engl J Med 1980;303(17):963–70.

27. Bero L. When big companies fund academic research, the truth often comes last. The Conversation US; 2019. Available at: https://nexus.od.nih.gov/all/2023/03/01/fy-2022-by-the-numbers-extramural-grant-investments-in-research/#:~:text=Like%20RPGs%2C%20the%20R01%2Dequivalent,to%2021.6%25%20in%20FY%202022.

28. Tierney WM, Meslin EM, Kroenke K. Industry support of medical research: important opportunity or treacherous pitfall? J Gen Intern Med 2016;31(2):228–33.

29. Rao SK, Kimball AB, Lehrhoff SR, et al. The impact of administrative burden on academic physicians: results of a hospital-wide physician survey. Acad Med 2017;92(2):237–43.

30. Mirchev M, Mircheva I, Kerekovska A. The academic viewpoint on patient data ownership in the context of big data: scoping review. review. J Med Internet Res 2020;22(8):e22214.

31. Lauer M. FY 2022 by the numbers: extramural grant investments in research, . Extramural NEXUS. National Institute of Health, Office of extramural research; 2023.

32. Babu CS, Holsinger FC, Zuchowski L, et al. Epistemological challenges of artificial intelligence clinical decision support tools in otolaryngology: the black box problem. Otolaryngology-Head Neck Surg (Tokyo) 2023;169(6):1697–700.

33. Mäkitie AA, Alabi RO, Ng SP, et al. Artificial intelligence in head and neck cancer: a systematic review of systematic reviews. Adv Ther 2023;40(8):3360–80.

34. Ibrahim H, Liu X, Denniston AK. Reporting guidelines for artificial intelligence in healthcare research. Clin Exp Ophthalmol 2021;49(5):470–6.

35. Liu X, Cruz Rivera S, Moher D, et al. Reporting guidelines for clinical trial reports for interventions involving artificial intelligence: the CONSORT-AI extension. Nat Med 2020;26(9):1364–74.

36. Sounderajah V, Ashrafian H, Golub RM, et al. Developing a reporting guideline for artificial intelligence-centred diagnostic test accuracy studies: the STARD-AI protocol. BMJ Open 2021;11(6):e047709.

37. Mongan J, Moy L, Kahn CE. Checklist for artificial intelligence in medical imaging (CLAIM): a guide for authors and reviewers. Radiology: Artif Intell 2020;2(2):e200029.

38. Norgeot B, Quer G, Beaulieu-Jones BK, et al. Minimum information about clinical artificial intelligence modeling: the MI-CLAIM checklist. Nat Med 2020;26(9):1320–4.

39. Hernandez-Boussard T, Bozkurt S, Ioannidis JPA, et al. MINIMAR (MINimum information for medical AI reporting): developing reporting standards for artificial intelligence in health care. J Am Med Inf Assoc 2020;27(12):2011–5.

40. Vasey B, Nagendran M, Campbell B, et al. Reporting guideline for the early-stage clinical evaluation of decision support systems driven by artificial intelligence: DECIDE-AI. Nat Med 2022;28(5):924–33.

41. Collins GS, Dhiman P, Andaur Navarro CL, et al. Protocol for development of a reporting guideline (TRIPOD-AI) and risk of bias tool (PROBAST-AI) for diagnostic and prognostic prediction model studies based on artificial intelligence. BMJ Open 2021;11(7):e048008.

42. Bur AM, Shew M, New J. Artificial intelligence for the otolaryngologist: a state of the art review. Otolaryngology-Head Neck Surg (Tokyo) 2019;160(4):603–11.

43. Asokan A, Massey CJ, Tietbohl C, et al. Physician views of artificial intelligence in otolaryngology and rhinology: a mixed methods study. Laryngoscope Investigative Otolaryngology 2023;8(6):1468–75.

44. Mahajan AP, Shabet CL, Smith J, et al. Assessment of artificial intelligence performance on the otolaryngology residency in-service exam. OTO Open 2023;7(4):e98.

45. Hanna K, Gupta S, Hurst R, et al. Specialty-specific entrustable professional activities: a bridge to internship. Cureus 2023. https://doi.org/10.7759/cureus.35547.

46. Varas J, Coronel BV, Villagrán I, et al. Innovations in surgical training: exploring the role of artificial intelligence and large language models (LLM). Rev Col Bras Cir 2023;50. https://doi.org/10.1590/0100-6991e-20233605-en.
47. Fink J. Artificial intelligence helps otolaryngologists give excellent patient care. ENT Today; 2023. Available at: https://www.enttoday.org/article/artificial-intelligence-helps-otolaryngologists-give-excellent-patient-care/. [Accessed 18 January 2023].

Transforming Otolaryngology—Head and Neck Surgery
The Pivotal Role of Artificial Intelligence in Clinical Workflows

Ross W. Green, MD[a],*, Harvey Castro, MD, MBA[b,1]

KEYWORDS

- Artificial intelligence • Machine learning • Clinical workflows • Outpatient AI
- Inpatient AI • Surgical AI

KEY POINTS

- Artificial intelligence has applications in otolaryngology—head and neck surgery to optimize clinical workflows in the following areas:
  - Outpatient/clinic
  - Inpatient
  - Surgical (inpatient and ambulatory)

INTRODUCTION

Artificial intelligence (AI) is increasingly becoming a cornerstone in the evolution of health care practices. In otolaryngology—head and neck surgery (OHNS), a specialty that deals with complex and varied disorders, AI promises to bring about a transformative shift in clinical workflows. A whirlwind of AI firms targeting otolaryngologists will continue to sprout up claiming to provide a new value proposition, new utilizations of data to create value, and/or a shift in current "general business reasoning"[1] aimed at improving clinical workflows. One such example is Medical Intelligence Ops, a startup led by one of the authors as Chief Executive Officer, which focuses on customizing AI solutions for hospitals using large language models (LLMs) that can be used for clinical workflows improvement.[2] The otolaryngologist interested in the AI space should be familiar with the Gartner hype cycle (**Fig. 1**) to understand the ebbs and flows of startup ideas when assessing what is best for their clinical workflows.

The current hyped AI innovation phase we are experiencing offers some potential advances for patient care. As Crowson and colleagues[3] (2019) mentioned in their review of

a Opollo Technologies, Buffalo, NY, USA; b Medical Intelligence Ops, Dallas, TX, USA
1 Present address: 2109 Morgan Drive, Flower Mound, TX 75028.
* Corresponding author. 61 Eastern Parkway, Apartment 2D, Brooklyn, NY 11238.
E-mail address: Ross@opollo.ai

Otolaryngol Clin N Am 57 (2024) 909–918
https://doi.org/10.1016/j.otc.2024.04.003
0030-6665/24/© 2024 Elsevier Inc. All rights reserved.
oto.theclinics.com

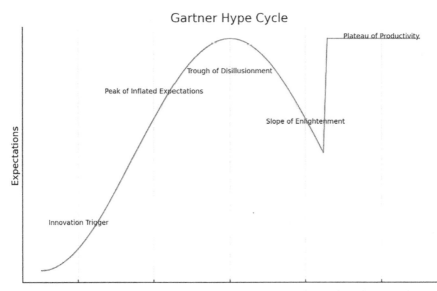

Fig. 1. Gartner hype cycle. Innovation trigger: introduction of AI in health care, where expectations begin to build, typically starting with innovative experiments. Peak of inflated expectations: over-enthusiasm and unrealistic projections for AI applications in medical diagnosis, treatment plans, and outcome predictions. Trough of disillusionment: realization of the challenges in AI, such as data privacy concerns, integration with existing systems, and the need for large data sets. Slope of enlightenment: incremental improvements in AI algorithms, better understanding of its capabilities and limitations, leading to more practical applications. Plateau of productivity: AI becomes mainstream in health care, with established best practices and widespread understanding of its value.

machine learning in OHNS, "investigators have realized significant success in validated models with model sensitivities and specificities approaching 100%," thereby offering the potential for advances in the quality of patient care. To be sure, *potential* is a key word pertaining to AI in clinical workflows as few models currently are validated on external data sets[4] and most algorithms end up never realizing clinical use.[5] With the amount of medical data doubling every 73 days,[6] there is an opportunity to use these data for training and improving AI models for clinical workflow purposes. As such, one research company estimated that AI will boost medical outcomes by as much as 40% while optimistically arguing that AI will reduce treatment costs by 50%.[7] Whether otolaryngologists "like AI" or not within clinical workflows, it is here to stay and grow, and it is expected that the AI health care market will attain a value of $1.3 billion by 2025.[7]

This article aims to shed light on the multifaceted applications of AI in otolaryngologic workflows, emphasizing its impact on outpatient settings, hospital environments, and operating rooms. Integrating AI in these settings can potentially enhance patient care, streamline operational efficiencies, reduce physician burnout, and positively impact the environment.

DISCUSSION
Artificial Intelligence in Outpatient Settings

Outpatient care is one of the mainstays of OHNS, where most patient interactions and preliminary diagnoses occur. Integrating AI in this setting can significantly enhance the efficiency and effectiveness of care provided in the pivotal outpatient setting. For example, one study suggested that for each 10-min increase in wait time, patients were 43.4% less likely to report satisfaction with their visit.[8] Patient satisfaction has increasingly played a paramount role in evaluating the quality of patient care in the outpatient setting, while also being a key factor in reimbursements.[9] Therefore, the otolaryngologist should consider AI as one tool to provide patients with a more efficient and effective visit.

Automated processes

i. Automated coding and note-taking: AI algorithms can revolutionize administrative tasks in OHNS clinics. By automating the coding of diagnoses and procedures, AI can reduce physicians' time on paperwork, allowing for more patient-focused care. Similarly, LLM-driven note-taking solutions can transcribe and organize patient interactions, ensuring accurate and comprehensive medical records.[10] The popular electronic health records (EHR) company EPIC, for instance, has an AI-driven note summarization solution it is now offering.[11]
ii. Streamlined health record management: AI can also be pivotal in managing electronic health records. AI systems can efficiently organize and retrieve patient information through advanced data analytics, aiding in better treatment planning and follow-up care. These systems can analyze patient history, radiology images,[12] and laboratory results, providing otolaryngologists with a comprehensive overview of the patient's health status.

Enhanced diagnostic and treatment planning

i. AI-assisted diagnostic tools: Accurate diagnosis is crucial for effective treatment in OHNS. AI-powered diagnostic tools can assist in identifying conditions such as hearing loss, vocal cord disorders, and sinus issues more accurately and swiftly. Using machine learning algorithms, these tools can analyze patterns in clinical data, helping clinicians make more informed decisions. Sections by other authors will cover in more detail the specific uses of AI in these subspecialties.
ii. Personalized treatment recommendations/triage: AI's ability to process vast amounts of data can also aid in creating customized treatment plans. AI systems can suggest customized treatment approaches by considering a patient's unique medical history, genetic information, and current health status.[13] This enhances the effectiveness of treatments and minimizes the risk of side effects. As an example, triaging using AI was effectively used during the coronavirus disease 2019 pandemic in which an AI model used conversational agents programmed within a phone "visit" to stratify patients based on the acuity of their symptoms,[14] thereby reducing the risk of patients exposing other patients to the virus[15] while also treating the sicker patients first.

Patient engagement and follow-up

i. AI-driven communication tools: Patient engagement is key to the quality of outpatient care. AI can facilitate this through intelligent communication tools such as chatbots and automated reminders.[16] These tools can provide patients with timely information about their conditions, medication schedules, and follow-up appointments, enhancing their engagement in their care.
ii. Remote monitoring and telehealth applications: AI also extends its benefits to remote monitoring and telehealth, which is especially crucial in managing chronic ear, nose, and throat (ENT) conditions. Wearable devices equipped with AI can monitor patient symptoms and digital biomarkers and alert clinicians about any

concerning changes.[17] Moreover, AI-enhanced telehealth platforms can offer virtual consultations, making health care more accessible.

Artificial Intelligence in Hospital Settings

The integration of AI in hospital settings is redefining patient care in OHNS. With its ability to process and analyze vast amounts of data, AI enhances patient monitoring, decision-making processes, and resource management.

Patient monitoring and care

i. Real-time data analysis for patient monitoring: AI systems can continuously monitor patient vitals and detect and diagnose anomalies that might indicate complications or the need for intervention. For example, AI algorithms can analyze data from monitoring devices in real-time, alerting health care providers to changes in a patient's condition, such as fluctuations in oxygen levels or heart rate, which are critical in postoperative care in OHNS. In this light, studies have shown that AI can improve patient safety outcomes in the inpatient setting.[18]
ii. AI in critical care and emergency response: In emergencies, AI tools can assist in quickly analyzing patient data to diagnose conditions like severe allergic reactions or respiratory distress. This rapid analysis aids clinicians in making swift, life-saving decisions.[19]

Decision support systems

i. Integration with hospital information systems: AI can integrate with electronic health records (EHRs) and other hospital information systems, providing clinicians with comprehensive patient insights. This integration helps identify potential health risks, suggest preventive measures, and aid in formulating treatment strategies. It is worth noting that "interoperability" with EHR systems and between different EHR systems remains challenging[20] and involves laws/governmental intervention; though there has been some improvement with regard to interoperability over the recent years (as one example, the federal government's requirements around the use of the United States Core Data for Interoperability[21] and the role of Fast Healthcare Interoperability Resources[22]), this still remains a challenge within the AI space and for otolaryngologists. In fact, EPIC is, "Leveraging Nuance's Dragon Ambient eXperience (DAX) technology…[to] further enhanc[e] a seamless workflow experience for users" via "seamless" integration with EHRs.[23]
ii. Evidence-based treatment suggestions: Leveraging the vast medical literature and clinical data, AI systems can provide otolaryngologists with evidence-based treatment recommendations. These suggestions are based on the latest research findings and data-driven insights, ensuring patients receive the most effective and current treatments. As such, some cardiologists are already doing this using large data sources to provide personalized inpatient medical diagnoses and treatments.[24] EPIC has recently come out with a solution for treatment suggestions, "…using Azure OpenAI Service… via SlicerDicer to fill gaps in clinical evidence using real-world data and to study rare diseases and more."[11]

Management

i. AI in hospital administration and logistics: AI can optimize hospital operations by forecasting patient admissions,[25] managing staff schedules,[26] and ensuring the availability of necessary equipment.[27] This efficiency is crucial in OHNS departments where timely access to specialized equipment and expertise are often needed.

ii. Predictive analytics for resource allocation: AI-driven predictive analytics can anticipate future trends in patient influx, common ENT conditions during certain times of the year,[28] and resource requirements. This foresight enables better preparedness and resource allocation, ensuring that the OHNS department is well-equipped to handle patient volume and needs.

Artificial Intelligence in Operating Rooms

AI's role in operating rooms, particularly in OHNS, is among the most exciting developments. AI is set to revolutionize surgical procedures from preoperative planning to postoperative care.

Preoperative planning

i. AI-driven surgical simulations and planning: AI can aid surgeons in preoperative planning by providing simulations and predictive analyses of surgical procedures. For instance, AI algorithms can analyze imaging data to map out the surgical area, predict potential complications, and suggest the most effective surgical approach.
ii. Customization of surgical procedures: AI enables the customization of surgical procedures to each patient's unique anatomy and condition. This is particularly beneficial in complex otolaryngologic surgeries where precision and personalization are key to successful outcomes.
iii. Increased revenue generation and reduced costs through better surgical duration forecasts: Surgeries are an important revenue stream for health care facilities including ambulatory surgical centers.[29] Accurate and precise surgery duration forecasts are essential for maximizing surgical suite efficiency—one study suggests running operating rooms (ORs) cost $36-$37 per minute.[30] Existing duration forecasting methods such as moving averages and surgeon estimates have been shown by peer-reviewed journal articles to be both inaccurate and imprecise.[31] AI has the potential to predict the duration of surgery and to book additional cases if the ORs will run shorter than the original "block" was scheduled for, or to close down ORs early if the surgical cases for the day will end earlier than the forecasted duration. One such solution is Opollo offered by Opollo Technologies, of which one of the authors is a principal owner. Opollo is an AI algorithm that has been designed to use both surgeon-factor data and patient-factor data to provide more accurate and precise duration forecasts. In one test data set with *only* patient factors (with no surgeon data being available), Opollo more than doubled the percentage of surgery durations accurately forecasted within 10 minutes of the actual duration, as compared to the method the facility was using prior to consulting with Opollo Technologies (71.8% versus 31.8%, respectively). With these efficiencies, the facility would have achieved almost $1 million in cost savings and potentially $6.4 million in additional revenue growth with the use of an AI model such as Opollo.[32]

Intraoperative assistance

i. AI in surgical navigation and precision: During surgeries, AI can provide real-time guidance[33] by enhancing the precision of surgical interventions. This is especially important in delicate ENT procedures, where millimeter-level accuracy is required.
ii. Real-time data analysis during surgeries: AI systems can analyze data during surgeries by monitoring vital signs and providing alerts on critical changes. This real-time analysis supports the surgical team in making informed decisions during the procedure.[34]

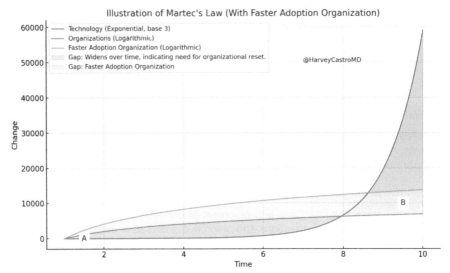

Fig. 2. Martec's Law. Technology change (exponential): AI technology advances rapidly, out-pacing the ability of health care organizations to keep up. Organizational change (logarithmic): health care organizations adapt more slowly due to bureaucracy, resistance to change, and regulatory compliance. Gap illustrates the challenge health care organizations face in adopting AI technologies at a pace that matches technological advancements. Faster adoption organization: some health care organizations adopt AI more quickly, leveraging it for operational efficiency and improved patient care.

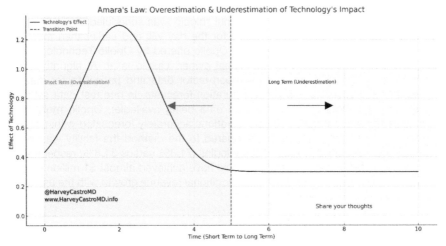

Fig. 3. Amara's Law. Short-term overestimation: initial overestimation of AI's impact on health care, expecting rapid changes in clinical practice and patient outcomes. Transition point: acknowledgment of the hurdles, such as regulatory issues, required training for health care professionals, and ethical considerations. Long-term underestimation: underappreciation of the profound, transformative effects AI will have on health care over decades, including personalized medicine and predictive analytics.

Postoperative care and analysis

i. AI in recovery monitoring and management: Postoperative care is crucial in OHNS procedures. AI can monitor patients' recovery progress, predict potential complications, and suggest interventions to enhance recovery and reduce the likelihood of readmissions.[35]

ii. Analyzing surgical outcomes for quality improvement: AI can also play a significant role in analyzing surgical outcomes. By evaluating data on patient recovery, complications, and overall results, AI can provide insights into areas of improvement, leading to enhanced surgical techniques and patient care protocols.[36]

SUMMARY

Otolaryngologists are key stakeholders in the creation and clinical implementation of AI technologies that can improve the care of patients. Integrating AI in an otolaryngologic practice represents a paradigm shift in health care delivery, promising to enhance clinical workflows, patient care, and overall operational efficiency. Change, to be sure, does not happen overnight as exemplified by Martec's Law (**Fig. 2**) and an otolaryngologist who wants to be part of the AI revolution and the evolution inherently associated with machine learning should be aware of the general environmental factors that influence health care-related AI advances. Amara's Law (**Fig. 3**) nicely demonstrates how an otolaryngologist should appreciate the lifecycle of expectations as it pertains to AI innovations as a means to temper enthusiasm for a novel AI startup or solution, while also appreciating the potential long-term upsides of the technology. As explored in this article, AI's applications in otolaryngologic workflows are diverse and impactful, ranging from outpatient care to hospital settings to operating rooms.

AI has the potential to revolutionize patient interactions and preliminary diagnoses in outpatient settings through automated coding, efficient record management, and enhanced diagnostic and treatment planning. In inpatient environments, AI's ability to process and analyze vast amounts of data significantly improves patient monitoring and critical care response. The operating room, a critical arena in OHNS, witnesses AI's transformative impact in preoperative planning, intraoperative assistance, and postoperative care. However, not every aspect of an otolaryngologist's practice needs to be "AI-driven"; thoughtful consideration should be made by otolaryngologists to understand what solutions, if any, will benefit their specific clinical workflows as it pertains to the patient population(s) they treat, their practice's dynamics, etc.

In conclusion, AI stands at the forefront of revolutionizing OHNS practice workflows, offering unprecedented opportunities to enhance health care delivery. Its ability to reduce physician burnout, positively impact the environment, and improve patient experiences highlights its transformative role. As we embrace this new era of technology in health care, the collaboration between AI and human expertise will be instrumental in shaping a future where enhanced patient care and operational excellence are the norms in ENT.

CLINICS CARE POINTS

- In otolaryngology—head and neck surgery (OHNS), AI promises to bring about a transformative shift in clinical workflows. Whether otolaryngologists "like AI" or not within clinical workflows, it is here, and it is expected that the AI health care market will attain a value of $1.3 billion by 2025.
  - However, the excitement around what AI can do for patient care and clinical workflows needs to be tempered and thoughtful considerations need to be made by

> otolaryngologists to decide on the correct workflow AI solutions for their patient population, their practice, etc.

- AI revolutionizes patient interactions and preliminary diagnoses in outpatient settings through automated coding, efficient record management, and enhanced diagnostic and treatment planning.
- In inpatient environments, AI's ability to process and analyze vast amounts of data significantly improves patient monitoring and critical care response.
- The operating room, a critical arena in OHNS, witnesses AI's transformative impact in preoperative planning, intraoperative assistance, and postoperative care.
  - Startups like Opollo Technologies, a company where one of the lead authors is an advisor, offer solutions to more accurately predict OR scheduling times as a means to boost revenue (i.e., by increasing the number of cases a facility can accommodate in a given day) while offering the potential for reducing costs (i.e., by shutting down ORs early if cases will not run the entire day).

DISCLOSURES

R.W. Green is the Chief Medical Officer at Opollo Technologies. H. Castro is the CEO of Medical Intelligence Ops.

REFERENCES

1. Widayanti R, Meria L. Business Modeling Innovation Using Artificial Intelligence Technology. International Transactions on Education Technology (ITEE) 2023; 1(2):95–105.
2. Medical intelligence Ops, Available at: http://mi-ops.ai. Accessed May 2, 2024.
3. Crowson MG, Ranisau J, Eskander A, et al. A contemporary review of machine learning in otolaryngology–head and neck surgery. Laryngoscope 2019;130(1): 45–51.
4. Panch T, Mattie H, Celi LA. The "inconvenient truth" about AI in healthcare. Npj Digital Medicine 2019;2(1):77.
5. Wilkinson J, Arnold KF, Murray EJ, et al. Time to reality check the promises of machine learning-powered precision medicine. The Lancet Digital Health 2020; 2(12):e677–80.
6. Densen P. Challenges and opportunities facing medical education. Trans Am Clin Climatol Assoc 2011;122:48–58.
7. Artificial Intelligence In Healthcare Market Size Report, 2019-2025. (n.d.). Available at: Www.grandviewresearch.com https://www.grandviewresearch.com/industry-analysis/artificial-intelligence-ai-healthcare-market.
8. Redding TS, Keefe KR, Stephens AR, et al. Evaluating Factors That Influence Patient Satisfaction in Otolaryngology Clinics. Ann Otol Rhinol Laryngol 2022; 132(1):19–26.
9. Jacobs DB, Schreiber M, Seshamani M, et al. Aligning Quality Measures across CMS — The Universal Foundation. N Engl J Med 2023;388:776–9.
10. Wang J, Yang J, Zhang H, et al. PhenoPad: Building AI enabled note-taking interfaces for patient encounters. NPJ DigitalMedicine 2022;5(1):12.
11. Diaz N. Epic, Microsoft add new AI capabilities to EHR software. 2023. Available at: Www.beckershospitalreview.com; https://www.beckershospitalreview.com/ehrs/epic-microsoft-add-new-ai-capabilities-to-ehr-software.html.

12. Wu Q, Wang X, Liang G, et al. Advances in Image-Based Artificial Intelligence in Otorhinolaryngology-Head and Neck Surgery: A Systematic Review. Otolaryngol Head Neck Surg 2023;169(5):1132–42.

13. Johnson KB, Wei W, Weeraratne D, et al. Precision Medicine, AI, and the Future of Personalized Health Care. Clinical and Translational Science 2020;14(1):86–93.

14. Kuziemsky C, Maeder AJ, John O, et al. Role of Artificial Intelligence within the Telehealth Domain. Yearbook of Medical Informatics 2019;28(01):035–40.

15. Wosik J, Fudim M, Cameron B, et al. Telehealth transformation: COVID-19 and the rise of virtual care. J Am Med Inf Assoc 2020;27(6):957–62.

16. Lalwani T, Bhalotia S, Pal A, et al. Implementation of a Chatbot System using AI and NLP. Papers.ssrn.com. 2018. Available at: https://papers.ssrn.com/sol3/papers.cfm?abstract_id=3531782.

17. Tran V-T, Riveros C, Ravaud P. Patients' views of wearable devices and AI in healthcare: findings from the ComPaRe e-cohort. Npj Digital Medicine 2019;2(1):53.

18. Choudhury A, Asan O. Role of Artificial Intelligence in Patient Safety Outcomes: Systematic Literature Review. JMIR Medical Informatics 2020;8(7):e18599.

19. Gutierrez G. Artificial Intelligence in the Intensive Care Unit. In: Vincent JL, editor. Annual update in intensive care and emergency medicine. Cham: Springer; 2020. p. 667–81.

20. M. S, Chacko AM. 2 - Interoperability issues in EHR systems: Research directions. ScienceDirect. 2021. https://www.sciencedirect.com/science/article/abs/pii/B9780128193143000021. 2020, 13-28.

21. United States Core Data for Interoperability (USCDI) [Review of United States Core Data for Interoperability (USCDI)]. HealthIT.gov. Retrieved from December 29, 2023. Available at: https://www.healthit.gov/isa/united-states-core-data-interoperability-uscdi.

22. Braunstein ML. Health Informatics on FHIR: How HL7's API is Transforming Healthcare. In Computers in health care. 2022. Available at: https://doi.org/10.1007/978-3-030-91563-6.

23. Umapathy VR, Rajinikanth BS, Raj RDS, et al. Perspective of Artificial Intelligence in Disease Diagnosis: A Review of Current and Future Endeavours in the Medical Field. Cureus 2023;15(9):e45684.

24. Dilsizian SE, Siegel EL. Artificial Intelligence in Medicine and Cardiac Imaging: Harnessing Big Data and Advanced Computing to Provide Personalized Medical Diagnosis and Treatment. Curr Cardiol Rep 2013;16(1):441.

25. Zhou L, Zhao P, Wu D, et al. Time series model for forecasting the number of new admission inpatients. BMC Med Inf Decis Making 2018;18(1):39.

26. Leung F, Lau Y-C, Law M, et al. Artificial intelligence and end user tools to develop a nurse duty roster scheduling system. Int J Nurs Sci 2022;9(3):373–7.

27. Munavalli JR, Boersma HJ, Rao S, et al. Real-Time Capacity Management and Patient Flow Optimization in Hospitals Using AI Methods. 55–69, 2020. Available at: https://doi.org/10.1007/978-3-030-45240-7_3.

28. Indhumathi K, Sathesh Kumar K. Prediction of Seasonal Ailments Using Big Data. 485–491. 2023. Available at: https://doi.org/10.1002/9781119879831.ch27.

29. Li F, Gupta D, Potthoff S. Improving operating room schedules. Health Care Manag Sci 2016;19(3):261–78.

30. Childers CP, Maggard-Gibbons M. Understanding Costs of Care in the Operating Room. JAMA Surgery 2018;153(4):e176233.

31. Laskin DM, Abubaker AO, Strauss RA. Accuracy of predicting the duration of a surgical operation. J Oral Maxillofac Surg 2013;71(2):446–7.

32. Young R., Opollo technologies whitepaper, In: Green R. and Turner P., *[Review of Opollo technologies whitepaper]*, 2023, Opollo Technologies, Available at: https://www.opollo.ai/white_paper.pdf. Buffalo, NY.

33. Siemionow K, Katchko K, Lewicki P, et al. Augmented reality and artificial intelligence-assisted surgical navigation: Technique and cadaveric feasibility study. J Craniovertebral Junction Spine 2020;11(2):81–5.

34. Birkhoff DC, van Dalen ASHM, Schijven MP. A Review on the Current Applications of Artificial Intelligence in the Operating Room. Surg Innovat 2021;28(5):611–9.

35. Hashimoto DA, Witkowski E, Gao L, et al. Artificial Intelligence in Anesthesiology. Anesthesiology 2020;132:379–94.

36. Salati M, Migliorelli L, Moccia S, et al. A Machine Learning Approach for Postoperative Outcome Prediction: Surgical Data Science Application in a Thoracic Surgery Setting. World J Surg 2021;45(5):1585–94.

UNITED STATES POSTAL SERVICE ®

Statement of Ownership, Management, and Circulation
(All Periodicals Publications Except Requester Publications)

1. Publication Title
OTOLARYNGOLOGIC CLINICS OF NORTH AMERICA

2. Publication Number
466 – 550

3. Filing Date
9/18/2024

4. Issue Frequency
FEB, APR, JUN, AUG, OCT, DEC

5. Number of Issues Published Annually
6

6. Annual Subscription Price
$478.00

7. Complete Mailing Address of Known Office of Publication *(Not printer) (Street, city, county, state, and ZIP+4®)*
ELSEVIER INC.
230 Park Avenue, Suite 800
New York, NY 10169

Contact Person
Malathi Samayan

Telephone *(include area code)*
91-44-4299-4507

8. Complete Mailing Address of Headquarters or General Business Office of Publisher *(Not printer)*
ELSEVIER INC.
230 Park Avenue, Suite 800
New York, NY 10169

9. Full Names and Complete Mailing Addresses of Publisher, Editor, and Managing Editor *(Do not leave blank)*

Publisher *(Name and complete mailing address)*
Dolores Meloni, ELSEVIER INC.
1600 JOHN F KENNEDY BLVD. SUITE 1600
PHILADELPHIA, PA 19103-2899

Editor *(Name and complete mailing address)*
Stacy Eastman, ELSEVIER INC.
1600 JOHN F KENNEDY BLVD. SUITE 1600
PHILADELPHIA, PA 19103-2899

Managing Editor *(Name and complete mailing address)*
PATRICK MANLEY, ELSEVIER INC.
1600 JOHN F KENNEDY BLVD. SUITE 1600
PHILADELPHIA, PA 19103-2899

10. Owner *(Do not leave blank. If the publication is owned by a corporation, give the name and address of the corporation immediately followed by the names and addresses of all stockholders owning or holding 1 percent or more of the total amount of stock. If not owned by a corporation, give the names and addresses of the individual owners. If owned by a partnership or other unincorporated firm, give its name and address as well as those of each individual owner. If the publication is published by a nonprofit organization, give its name and address.)*

Full Name	Complete Mailing Address
WHOLLY OWNED SUBSIDIARY OF REED/ELSEVIER, US HOLDINGS	1600 JOHN F KENNEDY BLVD. SUITE 1600 PHILADELPHIA, PA 19103-2899

11. Known Bondholders, Mortgagees, and Other Security Holders Owning or Holding 1 Percent or More of Total Amount of Bonds, Mortgages, or Other Securities. If none, check box → ☐ None

Full Name	Complete Mailing Address
N/A	

12. Tax Status *(For completion by nonprofit organizations authorized to mail at nonprofit rates) (Check one)*
The purpose, function, and nonprofit status of this organization and the exempt status for federal income tax purposes:
☒ Has Not Changed During Preceding 12 Months
☐ Has Changed During Preceding 12 Months *(Publisher must submit explanation of change with this statement)*

PS Form **3526**, July 2014 *[Page 1 of 4 (see instructions page 4)]* PSN: 7530-01-000-9931 PRIVACY NOTICE: See our privacy policy on www.usps.com.

---

13. Publication Title
OTOLARYNGOLOGIC CLINICS OF NORTH AMERICA

14. Issue Date for Circulation Data Below
AUGUST 2024

15. Extent and Nature of Circulation

		Average No. Copies Each Issue During Preceding 12 Months	No. Copies of Single Issue Published Nearest to Filing Date
a. Total Number of Copies *(Net press run)*		166	166
b. Paid Circulation *(By Mail and Outside the Mail)*	(1) Mailed Outside-County Paid Subscriptions Stated on PS Form 3541 *(include paid distribution above nominal rate, advertiser's proof copies, and exchange copies)*	89	89
	(2) Mailed In-County Paid Subscriptions Stated on PS Form 3541 *(include paid distribution above nominal rate, advertiser's proof copies, and exchange copies)*	0	0
	(3) Paid Distribution Outside the Mails Including Sales Through Dealers and Carriers, Street Vendors, Counter Sales, and Other Paid Distribution Outside USPS®	52	54
	(4) Paid Distribution by Other Classes of Mail Through the USPS *(e.g. First-Class Mail®)*	22	20
c. Total Paid Distribution *(Sum of 15b (1), (2), (3), and (4))*		163	163
d. Free or Nominal Rate Distribution *(By Mail and Outside the Mail)*	(1) Free or Nominal Rate Outside-County Copies included on PS Form 3541	2	2
	(2) Free or Nominal Rate In-County Copies Included on PS Form 3541	0	0
	(3) Free or Nominal Rate Copies Mailed at Other Classes Through the USPS *(e.g. First-Class Mail)*	0	0
	(4) Free or Nominal Rate Distribution Outside the Mail *(Carriers or other means)*	1	1
e. Total Free or Nominal Rate Distribution *(Sum of 15d (1), (2), (3) and (4))*		3	3
f. Total Distribution *(Sum of 15c and 15e)*		166	166
g. Copies not Distributed *(See Instructions to Publishers #4 (page #3))*		0	0
h. Total *(Sum of 15f and g)*		166	166
i. Percent Paid *(15c divided by 15f times 100)*		98.29%	98.19%

* If you are claiming electronic copies, go to line 16 on page 3. If you are not claiming electronic copies, skip to line 17 on page 3.

16. Electronic Copy Circulation

PS Form **3526**, July 2014 *(Page 2 of 4)*

	Average No. Copies Each Issue During Preceding 12 Months	No. Copies of Single Issue Published Nearest to Filing Date
a. Paid Electronic Copies →		
b. Total Paid Print Copies (Line 15c) + Paid Electronic Copies (Line 16a) →		
c. Total Print Distribution (Line 15f) + Paid Electronic Copies (Line 16a) →		
d. Percent Paid (Both Print & Electronic Copies) (16b divided by 16c × 100) →		

☒ I certify that 50% of all my distributed copies (electronic and print) are paid above a nominal price.

17. Publication of Statement of Ownership

☒ If the publication is a general publication, publication of this statement is required. Will be printed
in the **October 2024** issue of this publication.

☐ Publication not required.

18. Signature and Title of Editor, Publisher, Business Manager, or Owner

Malathi Samayan Date 9/18/2024

Malathi Samayan – Distribution Controller

I certify that all information furnished on this form is true and complete. I understand that anyone who furnishes false or misleading information on this form or who omits material or information requested on the form may be subject to criminal sanctions (including fines and imprisonment) and/or civil sanctions (including civil penalties).

PS Form **3526**, July 2014 *(Page 3 of 4)* PRIVACY NOTICE: See our privacy policy on www.usps.com

Moving?

Make sure your subscription moves with you!

To notify us of your new address, find your **Clinics Account Number** (located on your mailing label above your name), and contact customer service at:

Email: journalscustomerservice-usa@elsevier.com

800-654-2452 (subscribers in the U.S. & Canada)
314-447-8871 (subscribers outside of the U.S. & Canada)

Fax number: 314-447-8029

Elsevier Health Sciences Division
Subscription Customer Service
3251 Riverport Lane
Maryland Heights, MO 63043

*To ensure uninterrupted delivery of your subscription, please notify us at least 4 weeks in advance of move.

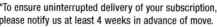
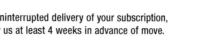

Printed and bound by CPI Group (UK) Ltd, Croydon, CR0 4YY

08/05/2025

01864752-0004